Reproductive Aging

Editors

NANETTE SANTORO
HOWARD M. KRAVITZ

OBSTETRICS AND GYNECOLOGY CLINICS OF NORTH AMERICA

www.obgyn.theclinics.com

Consulting Editor
WILLIAM F. RAYBURN

December 2018 • Volume 45 • Number 4

ELSEVIER

1600 John F. Kennedy Boulevard • Suite 1800 • Philadelphia, Pennsylvania, 19103-2899

http://www.theclinics.com

OBSTETRICS AND GYNECOLOGY CLINICS OF NORTH AMERICA Volume 45, Number 4
December 2018 ISSN 0889-8545, ISBN-13: 978-0-323-64326-9

Editor: Kerry Holland
Developmental Editor: Kristen Helm

Obstetrics and Gynecology Clinics (ISSN 0889-8545) is published quarterly by Elsevier Inc., 360 Park Avenue South, New York, NY 10010-1710. Months of issue are March, June, September, and December. Periodicals postage paid at New York, NY, and additional mailing offices. Subscription price per year is $313.00 (US individuals), $652.00 (US institutions), $100.00 (US students), $393.00 (Canadian individuals), $823.00 (Canadian institutions), $225.00 (Canadian students), $459.00 (international individuals), $823.00 (international institutions), and $225.00 (international students). To receive student/resident rate, orders must be accompanied by name of affiliated institution, date of term, and the signature of program/residency coordinator on institution letterhead. Orders will be billed at individual rate until proof of status is received. Foreign air speed delivery is included in all *Clinics* subscription prices. All prices are subject to change without notice. POSTMASTER: Send address changes to *Obstetrics and Gynecology Clinics*, Elsevier Health Sciences Division, Subscription Customer Service, 3251 Riverport Lane, Maryland Heights, MO 63043. **Customer Service: Telephone: 1-800-654-2452 (U.S. and Canada); 314-447-8871 (outside U.S. and Canada). Fax: 314-447-8029. E-mail: journalscustomerservice-usa@elsevier.com (for print support); journalsonlinesupport-usa@elsevier. com (for online support).**

Reprints. For copies of 100 or more of articles in this publication, please contact the Commercial Reprints Department, Elsevier Inc., 360 Park Avenue South, New York, New York 10010-1710. Tel.: 212-633-3874; Fax: 212-633-3820; E-mail: reprints@elsevier.com.

Obstetrics and Gynecology Clinics of North America is also published in Spanish by McGraw-Hill Interamericana Editores S.A., P.O. Box 5-237, 06500, Mexico; in Portuguese by Reichmann and Affonso Editores, Rio de Janeiro, Brazil; and in Greek by Paschalidis Medical Publications, Athens, Greece.

Obstetrics and Gynecology Clinics of North America is covered in *MEDLINE/PubMed (Index Medicus), Excerpta Medica, Current Concepts/Clinical Medicine, Science Citation Index, BIOSIS, CINAHL, and ISI/BIOMED.*

Contributors

CONSULTING EDITOR

WILLIAM F. RAYBURN, MD, MBA
Associate Dean, Continuing Medical Education and Professional Development,
Distinguished Professor and Emeritus Chair, Obstetrics and Gynecology, University
of New Mexico School of Medicine, Albuquerque, New Mexico

EDITORS

NANETTE SANTORO, MD
Professor and E. Stewart Taylor Chair, Department of Obstetrics and Gynecology,
University of Colorado School of Medicine, Aurora, Colorado

HOWARD M. KRAVITZ, DO, MPH
Emeritus Professor, Departments of Psychiatry and Preventive Medicine, Rush Medical
College, Rush University Medical Center, Chicago, Illinois

AUTHORS

AMANDA ALLSHOUSE, MS
Instructor, Department of Biostatistics, Colorado School of Public Health, Aurora,
Colorado

NANCY E. AVIS, PhD
Professor, Department of Social Sciences and Health Policy, Wake Forest School of
Medicine, Winston-Salem, North Carolina

JOYCE T. BROMBERGER, PhD
Professor of Epidemiology and Psychiatry, Departments of Epidemiology and Psychiatry,
University of Pittsburgh, Pittsburgh, Pennsylvania

SHERRI-ANN M. BURNETT-BOWIE, MD, MPH
Assistant Professor of Medicine, Endocrinology Division, Massachusetts General
Hospital, Harvard Medical School, Boston, Massachusetts

MARCELLE I. CEDARS, MD
Department of Obstetrics, Gynecology and Reproductive Sciences, University of
California, San Francisco, San Francisco, California

CAROLYN J. CRANDALL, MD, MS
Professor of Medicine, Division of General Internal Medicine and Health Services
Research, David Geffen School of Medicine at UCLA, Los Angeles, California

SYBIL L. CRAWFORD, PhD
Professor, Graduate School of Nursing, University of Massachusetts Medical School,
Worcester, Massachusetts

CAROL A. DERBY, PhD
Research Professor, Saul R. Korey Departments of Neurology, and Epidemiology
and Population Health, Albert Einstein College of Medicine, Bronx, New York

SHEILA A. DUGAN, MD
Departments of Physical Medicine and Rehabilitation, and Preventive Medicine,
Rush University Medical Center, Chicago, Illinois

SAMAR R. EL KHOUDARY, PhD, MPH
Associate Professor, Department of Epidemiology, Graduate School of Public Health,
Epidemiology Data Center, University of Pittsburgh, Pittsburgh, Pennsylvania

CYNTHIA NEILL EPPERSON, MD
Departments of Psychiatry, Obstetrics and Gynecology, Perelman School of Medicine,
University of Pennsylvania, Penn PROMOTES Research on Sex and Gender
in Health, University of Pennsylvania, Philadelphia, Pennsylvania

ELLEN W. FREEMAN, PhD
Research Professor, Departments of Obstetrics and Gynecology, and Psychiatry,
University of Pennsylvania School of Medicine, Philadelphia, Pennsylvania

KELLEY PETTEE GABRIEL, MS, PhD
Department of Epidemiology, Human Genetics, and Environmental Sciences, University
of Texas Health Science Center at Houston, School of Public Health, Austin Campus,
Michael and Susan Dell Center for Healthy Living, Department of Women's Health,
The University of Texas at Austin, Dell Medical School, Austin, Texas

CAREY E. GLEASON, PhD, MS
Associate Professor (CHS), Division of Geriatrics, Department of Medicine, University of
Wisconsin School of Medicine and Public Health, Madison Geriatric Research Education
and Clinical Center (GRECC) (11G), William S. Middleton Memorial Veterans Hospital,
Madison, Wisconsin

CLARISA R. GRACIA, MD
Professor, Department of Obstetrics and Gynecology, Division of Reproductive
Endocrinology and Infertility, University of Pennsylvania School of Medicine,
Philadelphia, Pennsylvania

ROBIN GREEN, PsyD
Assistant Professor, The Saul R. Korey Department of Neurology, Albert Einstein College
of Medicine, Bronx, New York

SIOBÁN D. HARLOW, PhD
Professor, Department of Epidemiology, School of Public Health, Professor, Department
of Obstetrics and Gynecology, Medical School of the University of Michigan, Ann Arbor,
Michigan

RACHEL HESS, MD, MS
Professor of Medicine and Population Health Sciences, Departments of Population Health
Sciences and Internal Medicine, University of Utah, Salt Lake City, Utah

HADINE JOFFE, MD, MSc
Executive Director, Connors Center for Women's Health, Vice Chair for Research,
Department of Psychiatry, Brigham and Women's Hospital, Dana Farber Cancer Institute,
Harvard Medical School, Boston, Massachusetts

ARUN S. KARLAMANGLA, PhD, MD
Professor of Medicine, Division of Geriatrics, David Geffen School of Medicine at UCLA,
Los Angeles, California

CARRIE KARVONEN-GUTIERREZ, MPH, PhD
Department of Epidemiology, University of Michigan, School of Public Health, Ann Arbor, Michigan

RASA KAZLAUSKAITE, MD, MSc, FACE
Associate Professor, Department of Medicine, Division of Endocrinology and Metabolism, Director, Diabetes Technology Program, Rush University Medical Center, Chicago, Illinois

HOWARD M. KRAVITZ, DO, MPH
Emeritus Professor, Departments of Psychiatry and Preventive Medicine, Rush Medical College, Rush University Medical Center, Chicago, Illinois

BRITTNEY S. LANGE-MAIA, MPH, PhD
Department of Preventive Medicine, Rush University Medical Center, Center for Community Health Equity, Chicago, Illinois

CAROLINE M. MITCHELL, MD
Assistant Professor, Department of Obstetrics, Gynecology and Reproductive Biology, Vincent Center for Reproductive Biology, Massachusetts General Hospital, Boston, Massachusetts

KELLY N. MORGAN, PsyD
Neuropsychology Postdoctoral Fellow, Division of Neuropsychology, The Institute of Living/Hartford Hospital, Hartford, Connecticut

GENEVIEVE S. NEAL-PERRY, MD, PhD
Professor of Obstetrics and Gynecology and Reproductive Endocrinology and Infertility, Department of Obstetrics and Gynecology, University of Washington, Seattle, Washington

JELENA PAVLOVIC, MD, PhD
Assistant Professor, Department of Neurology, Albert Einstein College of Medicine, Bronx, New York

MOLLY M. QUINN, MD
Department of Obstetrics, Gynecology and Reproductive Sciences, University of California, San Francisco, San Francisco, California

NANETTE SANTORO, MD
Professor and E. Stewart Taylor Chair, Department of Obstetrics and Gynecology, University of Colorado School of Medicine, Aurora, Colorado

HOLLY N. THOMAS, MD, MS
Assistant Professor of Medicine and Clinical and Translational Research, Center for Women's Health Research and Innovation, Department of Medicine, University of Pittsburgh, Pittsburgh, Pennsylvania

REBECCA C. THURSTON, PhD
Professor, Departments of Psychiatry and Epidemiology, School of Medicine, Graduate School of Public Health, University of Pittsburgh, Pittsburgh, Pennsylvania

L. ELAINE WAETJEN, MD
Professor, Department of Obstetrics and Gynecology, University of California, Davis, Sacramento, California

Contents

Foreword: A More Complete Picture of Reproductive Aging and the Menopause Transition   xiii

William F. Rayburn

Preface: The Disruptive Changes of Midlife: A Biopsychosocial Adventure   xv

Nanette Santoro and Howard M. Kravitz

Declining Fertility with Reproductive Aging: How to Protect Your Patient's Fertility by Knowing the Milestones   575

Molly M. Quinn and Marcelle I. Cedars

> Protection of fertility shares many of the same concepts as optimization of general health, such as smoking cessation, maintenance of a healthy body weight, and moderation of alcohol intake. Increasing attention has been placed on minimizing exposures to known reproductive toxicants. There are few conclusive data to support specific diet patterns or supplements for fertility. Ovarian reserve testing has been explored as potential diagnostic tests for assessment of reproductive aging with some controversy. Finally, the development of vitrification in the assisted reproduction laboratory has increased the success and, therefore, access to fertility preservation by way of oocyte or embryo cryopreservation.

Onset of the Menopause Transition: The Earliest Signs and Symptoms   585

Clarisa R. Gracia and Ellen W. Freeman

> Although more than 80% of women experience some degree of psychological or physical symptoms around menopause, both women and clinicians have misconceptions about how hormonal changes relate to menopausal symptoms and psychological conditions. Recently, several large-scale, longitudinal studies have been conducted to better characterize symptoms and changes that occur around menopause. This article offers current evidence for symptoms that occur in the early menopause transition, including vasomotor symptoms, mood changes, sleep problems, and changes in sexual functioning.

Menstrual Cycle Changes as Women Approach the Final Menses: What Matters?   599

Siobán D. Harlow

> Increased variability in menstrual cycle length marks the onset of the menopausal transition, with the likelihood of long cycles increasing as women approach menopause. This article describes the STRAW+10 bleeding criteria for recognizing onset of the early and late menopausal transition, as well as the specific bleeding changes a woman may experience during this life stage, including how women's bleeding experiences differ. The high probability of episodes of excessive and prolonged bleeding as women approach their final menstrual period is documented, as is the continuing probability of ovulation as women reach their final menstrual period.

Menstrual Cycle Hormone Changes Associated with Reproductive Aging and How They May Relate to Symptoms   613

Amanda Allshouse, Jelena Pavlovic, and Nanette Santoro

> Key cycle changes occur as women transition from reproductive life to menopause, and they can be roughly linked to menopausal staging. It is important to understand the types of studies that inform the current knowledge. Patterns of symptoms within menstrual cycles (sleep, headache) generally favor worsening in association with the perimenstrual phase of the cycle, and patterns of chronic symptoms, such as hot flashes and adverse mood, appear to be worse when hormones are more variable.

Vasomotor Symptoms Across the Menopause Transition: Differences Among Women   629

Nancy E. Avis, Sybil L. Crawford, and Robin Green

> Vasomotor symptoms (VMS) are the primary menopausal symptoms, occurring in up 80% of women and peaking around the final menstrual period. The average duration is 10 years, longer in women with an earlier onset. Compared with non-Hispanic white women, black and Hispanic women are more likely and Asian women are less likely to report VMS. Risk factors include greater body composition (in the early stage of menopausal transition), smoking, anxiety, depression, sensitivity to symptoms, premenstrual syndrome, lower education, and medical treatments, such as hysterectomy, oophorectomy, and breast cancer-related therapies. VMS patterns over time and within higher-risk subgroups are heterogeneous across women.

Cardiovascular Implications of the Menopause Transition: Endogenous Sex Hormones and Vasomotor Symptoms   641

Samar R. El Khoudary and Rebecca C. Thurston

> The menopause transition (MT) is a critical period of women's lives marked by several physiologic changes and menopause-related symptoms that have implications for health. Risk for cardiovascular disease, the leading cause of death in women, increases after menopause, suggesting a contribution of the MT to its development. This article focuses on the relationship between 2 main features of the MT and women's cardiovascular health: (1) dynamic alterations of sex hormones, particularly endogenous estradiol and follicle-stimulating hormone, and (2) vasomotor symptoms, the cardinal symptom of the menopause. Limitations and future directions are discussed.

Depression During and After the Perimenopause: Impact of Hormones, Genetics, and Environmental Determinants of Disease   663

Joyce T. Bromberger and Cynthia Neill Epperson

> Vulnerability to depression is increased across the menopause transition and in the early years after the final menstrual period. Clinicians should systematically screen women in this age group; if depressive symptoms or disorder are present, treatment of depression should be initiated. Potential treatments include antidepressants for moderate to severe symptoms, psychotherapy to target psychological and interpersonal factors,

and hormone therapy for women with first-onset major depressive disorder or elevated depressive symptoms and at low risk for adverse effects. Behavioral interventions can improve physical activity and sleep patterns.

Sleep, Health, and Metabolism in Midlife Women and Menopause: Food for Thought   679

Howard M. Kravitz, Rasa Kazlauskaite, and Hadine Joffe

Sleep and metabolism are essential components of health. Metabolic health depends largely on individual's lifestyle. Disturbances in sleep health, such as changes in sleep patterns that are associated with menopause/reproductive aging and chronologic aging, may have metabolic health consequences. Sleep restriction and age-related changes in sleep and circadian rhythms may influence changes in appetite and reproductive hormones, energy expenditure, and body adiposity. In this article, the authors describe how menopause-related sleep disturbance may affect eating behavior patterns, immunometabolism, immunometabolic dysfunction, and associations between sleep and metabolic outcomes.

Bone Health During the Menopause Transition and Beyond   695

Arun S. Karlamangla, Sherri-Ann M. Burnett-Bowie, and Carolyn J. Crandall

The menopause transition is a critical period for bone health, with rapid losses in bone mass and strength occurring in a 3-year window bracketing the date of the final menstrual period. Declines in bone mass are accompanied by deleterious changes in bone macrostructure and microarchitecture, which may be captured by changes in composite strength indices and indices of trabecular thickness and connectivity. The onset of the rapid bone loss phase is preceded by changes in sex steroid hormones and increases in markers of bone resorption, measurements of which may be clinically useful in predicting the onset of the rapid loss phase and in identifying the women who will lose the most bone strength over the menopause transition.

Female Sexual Function at Midlife and Beyond   709

Holly N. Thomas, Genevieve S. Neal-Perry, and Rachel Hess

Sexual function is an important component of quality of life for women. Midlife poses several challenges to optimal sexual function and intimacy for women. In addition to anatomic factors related to estrogen deficiency, such as genitourinary syndrome of menopause, vulvovaginal atrophy, and pelvic organ prolaps, psychosocial factors, including prior sexual trauma, play an important role in sexual function in women. Several treatments have emerged for female sexual dysfunction; long-term studies and head-to-head comparisons are lacking.

Physical Activity and Physical Function: Moving and Aging   723

Sheila A. Dugan, Kelley Pettee Gabriel, Brittney S. Lange-Maia, and Carrie Karvonen-Gutierrez

Evidence supports that the physical disablement process starts earlier than previously thought, in midlife when women still have many years to live. Physical activity participation and interventions have been successful in preventing disability in older adults and may be promising for maintaining function at younger ages. Changing the conversation to more relevant topics in midlife, like positive changes in body composition, sleep, and improved mood, may move the dial on participation, as midlife women do not meet guidelines for physical activity. Exploring the role of reproductive aging beyond chronologic aging may provide gender-specific insights on both disablement and participation.

Genitourinary Changes with Aging   737

Caroline M. Mitchell and L. Elaine Waetjen

Both chronologic aging and menopause affect the physical, physiologic, and microbiological characteristics of the genitourinary tract. The genitourinary syndrome of menopause, characterized by vulvovaginal and lower urinary tract signs and symptoms, is prevalent and has a significant negative impact on women's lives. In this article, the authors detail the genitourinary tract changes associated with menopause and/or aging. They also review the 2014 North American Menopause Society's definition of the genitourinary syndrome of menopause and present the epidemiology and impact of genitourinary aging in midlife and older women, namely, vulvovaginal, urinary, and sexual symptoms.

Cognitive Changes with Reproductive Aging, Perimenopause, and Menopause   751

Kelly N. Morgan, Carol A. Derby, and Carey E. Gleason

This article reviews the role of endogenous estrogen in neural and cognitive processing, followed by an examination of longitudinal cognitive data captured in various stages of the menopausal transition. The remaining text reviews the contradictory results from major hormone therapy trials to date, evidence for the "timing hypothesis," and closes with recommendations for future research and for practicing clinicians.

OBSTETRICS AND GYNECOLOGY CLINICS

FORTHCOMING ISSUES

March 2019
Gynecologic Cancer Care: Innovative Progress
Carolyn Y. Muller, *Editor*

June 2019
Patient Safety in Obstetrics and Gynecology
Paul A. Gluck, *Editor*

September 2019
Well Woman Health and Prevention
Jeanne Conry, *Editor*

RECENT ISSUES

September 2018
Perinatal Mental Health
Constance Guille and
Roger B . Newman, *Editors*

June 2018
Medical Disorders in Pregnancy
Erika Peterson and Judith U. Hibbard,
Editors

March 2018
Reproductive Genetics
Lorraine Dugoff, *Editor*

Foreword

A More Complete Picture of Reproductive Aging and the Menopause Transition

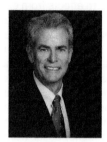

William F. Rayburn, MD, MBA
Consulting Editor

This issue of the *Obstetrics and Gynecology Clinics of North America*, co-edited by Nanette Santoro, MD and Howard M. Kravitz, DO, MPH, deals with reproductive aging. A prior issue devoted to the perimenopause, which was published in September 2011 and was also edited by Dr Santoro, highlighted the findings of several worldwide, longitudinal cohort studies of midlife women. The present issue provides a more complete picture of reproductive aging and the menopause transition beginning with declining fertility with reproductive aging and menstrual cycle changes as women approach their final menses. A staging system was developed that is now considered to be the gold standard for characterizing reproductive aging.

Natural menopause is defined as the permanent cessation of menstrual periods after 12 months of amenorrhea without any other cause. It occurs at a median age of 51.4 years and is a reflection of complete, or near complete, ovarian follicular depletion. Menopausal transition typically occurs four years before the final menstrual period. Virtually all women experience some menstrual irregularity and gradual hormonal fluctuations before menopause. This issue outlines menstrual cycle hormone changes associated with reproductive aging and how they may relate to symptoms.

This issue describes how those longitudinal cohort studies evaluated the phases of change in hormones, reproductive milestones, and outcomes to better understand the age of onset and pace of the menopause transition. Women who present at midlife for evaluation of possible menopausal transition are interested in hormone replacement therapy, while others simply want to know what is expected. In addition, the physician or provider caring for these women should provide or encourage patient education materials written in plain language for those desiring either a general overview or more sophisticated and detailed information.

Obstet Gynecol Clin N Am 45 (2018) xiii–xiv
https://doi.org/10.1016/j.ogc.2018.08.002
0889-8545/18/© 2018 Published by Elsevier Inc.

obgyn.theclinics.com

The initial evaluation should assess the woman's menstrual cycle history using a menstrual calendar, and a detailed history of any menopausal symptoms (hot flashes, sleep disturbances, depression, mood symptoms, vaginal dryness, skin aging and wrinkling, dyspareunia, and sexual dysfunction). Up to 80% develop vasomotor symptoms (or hot flashes) despite only about two-thirds seeking medical treatment. Searching for a high serum follicle-stimulating hormone (FSH) is not routinely required to make the diagnosis. Women aged 45 or less would benefit from excluding causes of oligo/amenorrhea, including a serum FSH, human chorionic gonadotropin, prolactin, and thyroid-stimulating hormone.

Separate articles deal with valuable information about long-term effects from estrogen deficiency, including cardiovascular implications, osteoporosis and bone health, and cognitive changes. The risk of cardiovascular disease increases after menopause. Any relation to estrogen deficiency may be mediated by changes in cardiovascular risk factors, such as lipid profiles that begin to change. Loss of bone mineral density appears to be highest during the one year before the final menses and two years thereafter. Estrogen deficiency after menopause may contribute to the development of osteoarthritis, but data are limited. There is limited epidemiologic support that estrogen preserves overall cognitive changes in nondemented women, yet replacement therapy has no known global cognitive benefits in older postmenopausal women. Impaired balance in postmenopausal women may be a central effect of estrogen deficiency and could lead to more falls that place a greater risk of forearm fractures.

This issue provides useful, evidence-based information for the practitioner. I wish to thank the editors and experienced authors in providing counseling and medical therapeutic guidelines for most patients later in their reproductive aging. The commitment of the many women who shared their experiences as part of these longitudinal studies deserves our acknowledgment and sincere appreciation to future generations.

William F. Rayburn, MD, MBA
Department of Obstetrics and Gynecology
Continuing Medical Education and Professional Development
University of New Mexico School of Medicine
MSC10 5580
1 University of New Mexico
Albuquerque, NM 87131-0001, USA

E-mail address:
wrayburn@salud.unm.edu

Preface

The Disruptive Changes of Midlife: A Biopsychosocial Adventure

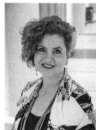

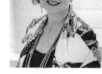

Nanette Santoro, MD   Howard M. Kravitz, DO, MPH
Editors

In addition to the psychosocial challenges of evolving family relationships, midcareer job stressors, and the recrudescence of childhood and sexual trauma, unpredictable changes in reproductive hormones may result in further destabilization of tissue function and end-organ manifestations.

Our knowledge of how reproductive aging and menopause affects women has grown tremendously in recent decades. Menopause transects aging, and somatic aging is an essential confounding factor that must be addressed in studies of the menopausal transition. The journey began with a series of cross-sectional studies that attempted to group women by age as a proxy for menopause, an approach now known to be inadequate. The critical need for serial study of the same woman over time to fully capture the impact of menopausal milestones on health was appreciated and embraced by a number of worldwide, longitudinal cohort studies, some of which collected data for over 20 years. These include but are not limited to the Study of Women's Health Across the Nation, the Penn Ovarian Aging Study, the Melbourne Women's Midlife Health Project, the Seattle Midlife Women's Health Study, and the Rotterdam Study. There remain few large-scale clinical trials that have specifically focused on the menopause transition, but some that have addressed the hypothesis that there is a window of opportunity to intervene with hormone therapy to reduce later-life disease include the Kronos Early Estrogen Prevention Study,[1] the Early versus Late Postmenopausal Treatment with Estradiol[2] trials, and the Women's Health Initiative.[3] The advent of the Staging of Reproductive Aging Workshop (STRAW)[4] classification system and its update, STRAW+10,[5] which has now become well validated, helped define the signposts along the way to menopause and

Obstet Gynecol Clin N Am 45 (2018) xv–xvii
https://doi.org/10.1016/j.ogc.2018.08.001
0889-8545/18/© 2018 Published by Elsevier Inc.

thereafter. A prior issue of the *Obstetrics and Gynecology Clinics of North America* devoted to the menopausal transition (Perimenopause; September 2011) highlighted the findings of these longitudinal studies, most of which did not have a complete capture of the final menstrual period in the entire sample. Now, 7 years later, we can provide a more complete picture of how the menopausal transition in its entirety is related to women's health, because we are able to center findings on the final menstrual period and can thereby begin to separate the process of aging from the process of menopause. As you will see, the relative contributions of both processes differ for most outcomes.

Our work is not done, however. The next phase of these cohort studies seeks to evaluate the trajectories of change in hormones, reproductive milestones, and outcomes, and to develop within-woman predictive models that take into account the age of onset and pace of the transition, and relevant genetic factors that influence health outcomes. You will see the beginnings of this work in some of the articles. Already, these data are being mobilized to inform clinical trials, leading to the ultimate goal of evidence-based improvements in clinical practice.

The research described herein is painstaking and requires a great commitment from the women who have shared their lives with us for so many years. Their contribution to future generations is incalculable, and we thank them from the bottom of our hearts. Finally, we wish to dedicate this issue of the *Obstetrics and Gynecology Clinics of North America* to two extraordinary visionaries, Kim Sutton-Tyrrell and Sherry Sherman, who captained the Study of Women's Health for a number of years and who were taken from us far too soon.

Nanette Santoro, MD
University of Colorado School of Medicine
12631 East 17th Avenue
Mail Stop B-198
Aurora, CO 80045, USA

Howard M. Kravitz, DO, MPH
Psychiatry and Preventive Medicine
Rush Medical College
Rush University Medical Center
2150 West Harrison Street
Room 278
Chicago, IL 60612, USA

E-mail addresses:
Nanette.Santoro@ucdenver.edu (N. Santoro)
hkravitz@rush.edu (H.M. Kravitz)

REFERENCES

1. Harman SM, Black DM, Naftolin F, et al. Arterial imaging outcomes and cardiovascular risk factors in recently menopausal women: a randomized trial. Ann Intern Med 2014;161:249–60.

2. Hodis HN, Mack WJ, Henderson VW, et al. Vascular effects of early versus late postmenopausal treatment with estradiol. N Engl J Med 2016;374:1221–31.

3. Rossouw JE, Anderson GL, Prentice RL, et al. Risks and benefits of estrogen plus progestin in healthy postmenopausal women: principal results from the Women's Health Initiative randomized controlled trial. JAMA 2002;288:321–33.

4. Soules MR, Sherman S, Parrott E, et al. Executive summary: stages of reproductive aging workshop (STRAW). Fertil Steril 2001;76:874–8.
5. Harlow SD, Gass M, Hall JE, et al. Executive summary of the Stages of Reproductive Aging Workshop + 10: addressing the unfinished agenda of staging reproductive aging. J Clin Endocrinol Metab 2012;97:1159–68.

Declining Fertility with Reproductive Aging

How to Protect Your Patient's Fertility by Knowing the Milestones

Molly M. Quinn, MD, Marcelle I. Cedars, MD*

KEYWORDS

- Fertility • Reproductive aging • Lifestyle • Ovarian reserve testing
- Fertility preservation

KEY POINTS

- Smoking cessation, maintenance of a healthy body weight, and moderation of alcohol intake are important for optimization of fertility and general health.
- There are few data to support a specific diet or supplement regimen for fertility.
- Ovarian reserve testing with ultrasound assessment of antral follicle count or serum antimüllerian hormone assays have limited value for planning reproductive timelines.
- Fertility preservation by oocyte or embryo cryopreservation is an option for some women planning to delay childbearing, although cost-effectiveness has not yet been demonstrated.

INTRODUCTION

Although infertility manifests in the reproductive years (Stages of Reproductive Aging Workshop [STRAW] stages −4 to −3a), it has been increasingly associated with reduction in long-term health and increased risk of disease postmenopause (STRAW stages +1a to +2). Therefore, it is not surprising that optimization, or protection, of fertility involves many of the same concepts as optimization of general health, such as smoking cessation, maintenance of a healthy body weight, and moderation of alcohol intake. Additionally, increasing attention has been placed on minimizing exposures to known reproductive toxicants. A significant body of literature has explored the role of diet patterns and supplements in the promotion of fertility, with few conclusive data. Ovarian reserve testing, including assessment of antral follicle count (AFC) by transvaginal ultrasound and serum assays for antimüllerian hormone (AMH) have

Disclosures: Funding support: 1R01AG053332-01A1 (NIA).
Department of Obstetrics, Gynecology and Reproductive Sciences, University of California, San Francisco, 550 16th Street, 7th Floor, San Francisco, CA 94158-2519, USA
* Corresponding author.
E-mail address: marcelle.cedars@ucsf.edu

been explored as potential diagnostic tests for assessment of reproductive aging with some controversy. Finally, the development of vitrification in the assisted reproduction laboratory has increased the success and, therefore, access to fertility preservation by way of oocyte or embryo cryopreservation.

OPTIMIZING HEALTH

Cigarette smoking is well known to increase the risk for cardiovascular disease, cancer, and overall morbidity and mortality. The general population may be unaware, however, of the association between smoking and both infertility and earlier age at menopause. In a large, prospective, population-based study of factors associated with fertility, the number of cigarettes smoked per day was, in addition to advancing age, the most consistent finding associated with decreased fertility.[1] A meta-analysis of 12 studies demonstrated an odds ratio of 1.6 (95% CI, 1.34–1.91) for risk of infertility in female smokers versus nonsmokers.[2] Mechanisms for this finding include an increase in pelvic inflammatory disease[3] and, therefore, tubal factor infertility in addition to more rapid reproductive aging.[4,5] Exposure to tobacco smoke may reduce ovarian reserve via increased follicular apoptosis and oxidative stress.[6] Finally, cigarette smoking has been associated with an increased risk of spontaneous abortion.[7] Knowledge of the association between smoking and adverse reproductive outcomes may serve as a powerful motivator for young women to stop smoking and, therefore, offers providers an opportunity to engage young patients in preventative health care.

Being underweight or overweight has been associated with increased time to conception.[8] Although anovulation is the primary culprit for a reduction in fecundity for both extremes of body mass index (BMI), obesity has also been associated with increased rates of miscarriage, congenital anomalies, and intrauterine fetal demise. Rodent data suggest that diet-induced obesity causes follicle apoptosis, oxidative stress in cumulus-oocyte complexes, and meiotic defects in oocytes in addition to impaired fertilization, abnormal embryogenesis, and impaired fetal growth.[9,10] A reduction in pregnancy rates among surrogates with a BMI greater than or equal to 35 compared with those with a BMI less than 35 has supported the hypothesis that the endometrial environment is also altered in obesity.[11] Weight loss in obese women has been associated with improved rates of spontaneous ovulation and conception.[12] In a prospective cohort study of physical activity and time to pregnancy, moderate physical activity was associated with an increase in fecundability regardless of BMI whereas vigorous physical activity was associated with a reduction in fecundability among women with BMI less than 25 kg/m^2. The investigators concluded that physical activity of any type might improve fertility among overweight and obese women whereas for lean women, substitution of vigorous activity with moderate activity might improve fertility.[13] Nevertheless, in a recent randomized controlled trial of a lifestyle intervention for obese women, participation in the intervention prior to compared with immediate infertility treatment did not result in a higher rate of healthy singleton live birth within 2 years.[14] This suggests that acute weight loss may not improve pregnancy outcomes; therefore, maintenance of normal weight from an earlier age is likely superior.

Studies of the effect of moderate alcohol consumption on female fertility are inconclusive. A prospective study of 7393 women in Sweden suggested that consumption of 2 alcoholic drinks per day was associated with increased risk of infertility (relative risk 1.59; 95% CI, 1.09–2.31) whereas the risk was decreased for those who consumed less than 1 drink per day (relative risk 0.64; 95% CI, 0.46–0.90).[15] Another large prospective cohort study demonstrated no effect of consumption of less than 14 servings of alcohol per week on fertility.[16] Thus, although heavy alcohol consumption is not recommended when attempting conception, there is limited evidence guiding a threshold of moderate consumption that may be permissible.

MINIMIZING EXPOSURES

There are increasing data relating environmental exposures, such as natural gas, endocrine-disrupting chemicals, and outdoor air pollution, to reproductive outcomes. A variety of organic pollutants, including many polychlorinated biphenyls, pesticides, and phthalates, have been associated with early menopause using data from the US National Health and Nutrition Examination Survey.[17] Furthermore, in a recent study, higher consumption of high-pesticide residue fruits and vegetables was associated with lower probability of pregnancy and live birth after infertility treatment.[18] Pesticide exposure within the range of usual human exposure is thus hypothesized to be associated with adverse reproductive outcomes. Additionally, it has been shown that high mercury levels from excess seafood consumption are associated with infertility.[19] As a result, it is recommended that consumption of seafood high in mercury be limited in the population, particularly in those desiring conception. Exposure to pesticides may be reduced through the consumption of organic products. Additional data are needed to further elucidate the mechanisms behind the impact of environmental exposures on reproductive outcomes and to compel policy change that will reduce such exposures at the population level.

FERTILITY DIETS AND SUPPLEMENTS

There is little evidence that variations in diet or the addition of vitamins and/or supplements affords substantial improvements in fertility. Healthier diets have been associated with reduced rates of infertility, yet healthy diets have been defined differently across studies and no randomized trials have been performed to date.[20] Limited evidence suggests that intake of red meat and trans fats may be associated with increased infertility.[21] Intake of polyunsaturated fatty acids, however, in particular long-chain omega-3 fatty acids, seems associated with increased female fertility.[20]

Although antioxidants have been posited to improve semen analysis parameters in men with infertility, a 2013 Cochrane review concluded that there was a lack of evidence for antioxidant supplementation in women for improvement in pregnancy and/or live birth rates.[22] A reduction in serum levels of CoQ10, an antioxidant component of the electron transport chain, however, has been associated with aging, and aged mice supplemented with CoQ10 demonstrated significantly improved mitochondrial function, spindle formation, and chromosome alignment.[23] Nevertheless, a clinical study of older women undergoing in vitro fertilization (IVF) randomized to CoQ10, 600 mg, for 2 months revealed no significant effect on aneuploidy in oocytes.[24] Thus, although many women undergoing treatment of infertility supplement with CoQ10, this practice is not currently evidence based and impact on spontaneous conception is unknown.

Supplementation with dehydroepiandrosterone (DHEA), an androgen precursor produced primarily in the adrenal glands, at a dose of 25 mg 3 times daily up to 4 months prior to IVF, was suggested to improve response to ovarian stimulation in observational reports of patients with diminished ovarian reserve undergoing IVF.[25] An initial small, randomized controlled trial of DHEA in a similar cohort of patients resulted in an improved live birth rate for those who received DHEA relative to controls.[26] The largest study to date, however, investigated 12 weeks of DHEA supplementation in 104 poor responders compared with 104 women without pretreatment and found no significant difference in pregnancy outcomes between groups.[27] Finally, randomized controlled trials of DHEA supplementation in poor[28] and normal[29] ovarian responders found no significant difference in AFC or response to stimulation after 12 weeks of DHEA prior to IVF treatment relative to placebo. In summary, there are few data to support the use of DHEA in patients undergoing fertility treatment.

Finally, a daily dose of folic acid, 400 µg, is recommended for women attempting to conceive to reduce risk of neural tube defects, yet a higher intake of preconception supplemental folate (up to 800 µg) may increase a woman's chances of conception and live birth.[20] Nevertheless, these data are limited to observational studies and require further investigation in the setting of a randomized controlled trial.

OVARIAN RESERVE TESTING

Female fertility is known to decrease over time (**Fig. 1**),[30] but the rate of follicular depletion is uncertain for any given individual. Biomarkers of ovarian reserve have been increasingly used not only to predict treatment response in those undergoing assisted reproduction but also to estimate ovarian reserve and time to menopause in populations not actively attempting to conceive. Although follicle-stimulating hormone and inhibin B have been used in the past to diagnose reproductive aging, it has been recognized that neither is a good marker of ovarian reserve or even predictive of time to menopause for women in the menopausal transition.

AFC describes the number of follicles measuring 2 mm to 10 mm in diameter on a transvaginal ultrasound. The number of antral follicles is believed to correlate with the size of the remaining follicular pool and the number of oocytes that may be retrieved after ovarian stimulation for IVF. The AFC exhibits a gradual acceleration of follicular loss with age (**Fig. 2**) and is the most accurate noninvasive measure of reproductive aging.[31] In experienced centers, AFC has good intercycle and interobserver reliability.

Straw -4	-3b	-3a

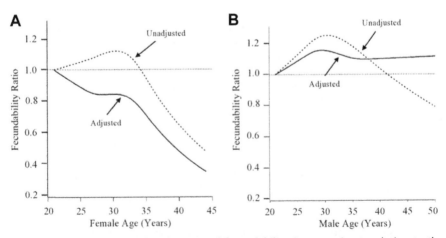

Fig. 1. Association between female age and fecundability, in approximate relation to the corresponding stages of reproductive aging. (*Adapted from* Wesselink AK, Rothman KJ, Hatch EE, et al. Age and fecundability in a North American preconception cohort study. Am J Obstet Gynecol 2017;217(6):667.e5; with permission.)

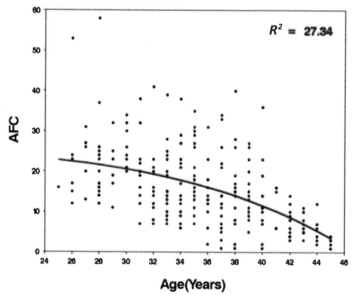

$R^2 = 27.34$

Fig. 2. AFC by age in a cross-sectional community-based population. (*Reprinted by* permission from the American Society for Reproductive Medicine. *From* Rosen MP, Johnstone E, McCulloch CE, et al. A characterization of the relationship of ovarian reserve markers with age. Fertility and Sterility 2012;97(1):238–43.)

Although a low AFC is associated with poor response to ovarian stimulation for IVF, it has been shown poorly predictive of failure to conceive.[32,33]

AMH is a member of the transforming growth factor β superfamily of cytokines and is a product of granulosa cells from preantral and small antral follicles. Concentrations are gonadotropin independent; therefore, values remain relatively consistent across the menstrual cycle. AMH is highly correlated with AFC[34,35] and low AMH levels have been shown predictive of menopause.[36] Concerns exist, however, about the performance of AMH assays after variations in collection and storage practices.[37] Further limiting the utility of the AMH assay is that multiple disparate AMH assays are commercially available with considerable interassay and intra-assay variability in addition to poor comparability.[38]

A recent publication indicated that among women aged 30 to 44 without a history of infertility trying to conceive for 3 months or less, a low AMH was not associated with a reduction in natural fertility.[39] Additional data demonstrated that neither AMH, AFC, nor follicle-stimulating hormone levels predicted time to pregnancy in a cohort of healthy women planning pregnancy.[40] Thus, although AMH may reflect the quantity of oocytes remaining, it does not reliably predict oocyte quality or individual fecundability.

In a population of women with a low prevalence of diminished ovarian reserve or poor fecundability (eg, those who are young and have not tried to conceive), the positive predictive value of any screening test—such as AFC or AMH—is low. Therefore, a low AMH or AFC in a young patient who has not tried to conceive has a high probability of being a false positive and, therefore, misleading and is not recommended for the purpose of creation of timelines for family building.

FERTILITY PRESERVATION

Declining fertility rates are seen among women beginning at age 35. Women in their late 30s experience a 50% reduction in fertility compared with women in their late

20s.[41] Nevertheless, in the United States childbearing is increasingly delayed. From 2000 to 2014, the proportion of first births to women aged 30 to 34 rose 28% and first births to women aged 35 or over rose 23%.[42] Over this same time period, there have been substantial improvements in mature oocyte cryopreservation technology with the application of vitrification, allowing for improved cryopreserved oocyte survival. Furthermore, recent data have indicated that fertilization and pregnancy rates are similar when fresh oocytes or vitrified/warmed oocytes are used as part of IVF/intracytoplasmic sperm injection.[43] Data tend to arise, however, from young, highly selected populations and may not apply to older women or to patients undergoing treatment at less experienced centers.

Oocyte cryopreservation, therefore, may allow women to have an opportunity to have biologic children at advanced ages, yet there are few data on the efficacy of this treatment of elective indications. A decision-analytic model suggested oocyte cryopreservation at the age of 37 years seemed to have the largest benefit over no action and was the most cost effective.[44] Another publication suggested that at least 8 to 10 metaphase II oocytes were necessary to achieve reasonable success in women 36 years of age or younger, but data are limited in older age groups.[45]

Additional data are needed to further understand not only the efficacy but also the cost-effectiveness of elective oocyte cryopreservation. Furthermore, there remains concern that the widespread use of this technology may give women a false hope, because there are no thresholds of number of cryopreserved oocytes that guarantee a woman a live birth in the future. Therefore, elective oocyte cryopreservation cannot be universally recommended, but individualized and detailed counseling of risks and benefits may guide some patients to pursue this technology to reduce the impact of reproductive aging.

SUMMARY

Providers may counsel women desiring to optimize future fertility that smoking cessation, maintenance of a healthy body weight, and avoidance of known reproductive toxicants will improve their overall health and may have a beneficial effect on fertility. There are few data, however, to support specific diet or lifestyle interventions to delay reproductive aging. Markers of ovarian reserve have not proved useful in pregnancy planning. Fertility preservation by oocyte or embryo cryopreservation may be an option for some women looking to delay childbearing, although its cost-effectiveness has not yet been demonstrated.

REFERENCES

1. Howe G, Westhoff C, Vessey M, et al. Effects of age, cigarette smoking, and other factors on fertility: findings in a large prospective study. Br Med J 1985; 290(6483):1697–700.
2. Augood C, Duckitt K, Templeton AA. Smoking and female infertility: a systematic review and meta-analysis. Hum Reprod 1998;13(6):1532–9.
3. Marchbanks PA, Lee NC, Peterson HB. Cigarette smoking as a risk factor for pelvic inflammatory disease. Am J Obstet Gynecol 1990;162(3):639–44.
4. Jick H, Porter J. Relation between smoking and age of natural menopause. Report from the Boston Collaborative Drug Surveillance Program, Boston University Medical Center. Lancet 1977;1(8026):1354–5.
5. Whitcomb BW, Purdue-Smithe AC, Szegda KL, et al. Cigarette smoking and risk of early natural menopause. Am J Epidemiol 2018;187(4):696–704.

6. Vabre P, Gatimel N, Moreau J, et al. Environmental pollutants, a possible etiology for premature ovarian insufficiency: a narrative review of animal and human data. Environ Health 2017;16:37.

7. Ness RB, Griffo JA, Hirschinger N, et al. Cocaine and tobacco use and the risk of spontaneous abortion. N Engl J Med 1999;340:330–9.

8. Kawwass JF, Kulkarni AD, Hipp HS, et al. Extremities of body mass index and their association with pregnancy outcomes in women undergoing in vitro fertilization in the United States. Fertil Steril 2016;106(7):1742–50.

9. Wu LL, Dunning KR, Yang X, et al. High-fat diet causes lipotoxicity responses in cumulus-oocyte complexes and decreased fertilization rates. Endocrinology 2010;151:5438–45.

10. Jungheim ES, Schoeller EL, Marquard KL, et al. Diet-induced obesity model: abnormal oocytes and persistent growth abnormalities in the offspring. Endocrinology 2010;151:4039–46.

11. Deugarte D, Deugarte C, Sahakian V. Surrogate obesity negatively impacts pregnancy rates in third-party reproduction. Fertil Steril 2010;93:1008–10.

12. Clark AM, Thornley B, Tomlinson L, et al. Weight loss in obese infertile women results in improvement in reproductive outcome for all forms of fertility treatment. Hum Reprod 1998;13:1502–5.

13. Wise LA, Rothman KJ, Mikkelsen EM, et al. A prospective cohort study of physical activity and time to pregnancy. Fertil Steril 2012;97(5):1136–42.

14. Mutsaerts MA, van Oeras AM, Groen H, et al. Randomized trial of a lifestyle program in obese infertile women. N Engl J Med 2016;374:1942–53.

15. Eggert J, Theobald H, Engfeldt P. Effects of alcohol consumption on female fertility during an 18-year period. Fertil Steril 2004;81(2):379–83.

16. Mikkelsen EM, Riis AH, Wise LA, et al. Alcohol consumption and fecundability: prospective Danish cohort study. BMJ 2016;354:i4262.

17. Grindler NM, Allsworth JE, Macones GA, et al. Persistent organic pollutants and early menopause in U.S. women. PLoS One 2015;10(1):e0116057.

18. Chiu Y, Williams PL, Gillman MW, et al. Association between pesticide residue intake from consumption of fruits and vegetables and pregnancy outcomes among women undergoing infertility treatment with assisted reproductive technology. JAMA Intern Med 2018;178(1):17–26.

19. Choy CM, Lam CW, Cheung LT, et al. Infertility, blood mercury concentrations and dietary seafood consumption: a case-control study. BJOG 2002;109:1121–5.

20. Gaskins AJ, Chavarro JE. Diet and fertility: a review. Am J Obstet Gynecol 2018; 218(4):379–89.

21. Chavarro JE, Rich-Edwards JW, Rosner BA, et al. Protein intake and ovulatory infertility. Am J Obstet Gynecol 2008;198:210.e1-7.

22. Showell MG, Brown J, Clarke J, et al. Antioxidants for female subfertility. Cochrane Database Syst Rev 2013;(7):CD007807.

23. Ben-Meir A, Burstein E, Borrego-Alvarez A, et al. Coenzyme q10 restores oocytes mitochondrial function and fertility during reproductive aging. Aging Cell 2015; 14(5):887–95.

24. Bentov Y, Hannam T, Jurisicova A, et al. Coenzyme Q10 supplementation and oocyte aneuploidy in women undergoing IVF-ICSI. Clin Med Insights Reprod Health 2014;8:31–6.

25. Barad D, Gleicher N. Effect of dehydroepiandrosterone on oocyte and embryo yields, embryo grade and cell number in IVF. Hum Reprod 2006;21: 2845–949.

26. Wiser A, Gonen O, Ghetler Y, et al. Addition of dehydroepiandrosterone (DHEA) for poor-responder patients before and during IVF treatment improves the pregnancy rate: a randomized prospective study. Hum Reprod 2010;25(10): 2496–500.

27. Kara M, Aydin T, Aran T, et al. Does dehydroepiandrosterone supplementation really affect IVF-ICSI outcome in women with poor ovarian reserve? Eur J Obstet Gynecol Reprod Biol 2014;173:63–5.

28. Yeung TW, Chai J, Li RH, et al. A randomized, controlled, pilot trial on the effect of dehydroepiandrosterone on ovarian response markers, ovarian response, and in vitro fertilization outcomes in poor responders. Fertil Steril 2014;102(1):108–15.

29. Yeung T, Chai J, Li R, et al. A double-blind randomized controlled trial on the effect of dehydroepiandrosterone on ovarian reserve markers, ovarian response and number of oocytes in anticipated normal ovarian responders. BJOG 2016; 123(7):1097–105.

30. Wesselink AK, Rothman KJ, Hatch EE, et al. Age and fecundability in a North American preconception cohort study. Am J Obstet Gynecol 2017;217:667.e1-8.

31. Rosen MP, Johnstone E, McCulloch CE, et al. A characterization of ovarian reserve markers with age. Fertil Steril 2012;97:238–43.

32. Hendriks DJ, Mol BW, Bancsi LF, et al. Antral follicle count in the prediction of poor ovarian response and pregnancy after in vitro fertilization: a meta-analysis and comparison with basal follicle-stimulating hormone level. Fertil Steril 2005; 83:291–301.

33. Broekmans FJ, Kwee J, Hendriks DJ, et al. A systematic review of tests predicting ovarian reserve and IVF outcome. Hum Reprod Update 2006;12:685–718.

34. Fanchin R, Schonauer LM, Righini C, et al. Serum anti-Mullerian hormone is more strongly related to ovarian follicular status than serum inhibin B, estradiol, FSH and LH on day 3. Hum Reprod 2003;18:323–7.

35. Van Rooij IA, Broekmans FJ, Te Velde ER, et al. Serum AMH levels: a novel measure of ovarian reserve. Hum Reprod 2002;17:3065–71.

36. Freeman EW, Sammel MD, Lin H, et al. Anti-mullerian hormone as a predictor of time to menopause in late reproductive age women. J Clin Endocrinol Metab 2012;97(5):1673–80.

37. Broer SL, Broekmans FJM, Laven JSE, et al. Anti-mullerian hormone: ovarian reserve testing and its potential clinical implications. Hum Reprod Update 2014;20(5):688–701.

38. Su HI, Sammel MD, Homer MV, et al. Comparability of AMH levels among commercially available immunoassays. Fertil Steril 2014;101(6):1766–72.

39. Steiner AZ, Pritchard D, Stanczyk FZ, et al. Association between biomarkers of ovarian reserve and infertility among older women of reproductive age. JAMA 2017;318(14):1367–76.

40. Depmann M, Broer SL, Eijkemans MJC, et al. Anti-mullerian hormone does not predict time to pregnancy: results of a prospective cohort study. Gynecol Endocrinol 2017;33(8):644–8.

41. Dunson D, Baird D, Colombo B. Increased infertility with age in men and women. Obstet Gynecol 2004;103(1):51–6.

42. Mathews TJ, Hamilton BE. Mean age of mothers is on the rise: United States, 2000-2014. NCHS Data Brief No 232. 2016. Available at: http://www.cdc.gov/nchs/data/databriefs/db232.pdf. Accessed November 26, 2017.

43. Practice Committee of the American Society for Reproductive Medicine. Mature oocyte cryopreservation: a guideline. Fertil Steril 2013;99:37–43.

44. Messen TB, Mersereau JE, Kane JB, et al. Optimal timing for elective egg freezing. Fertil Steril 2015;103(6):1551 6.
45. Cobo A, Garcia-Velasco JA, Coello A, et al. Oocyte vitrification as an efficient option for elective fertility preservation. Fertil Steril 2016;105(3):755–64.

Onset of the Menopause Transition

The Earliest Signs and Symptoms

Clarisa R. Gracia, MD[a,b,*], Ellen W. Freeman, PhD[a,c]

KEYWORDS

- Menopause • Menopause transition • Menopausal symptoms
- Vasomotor symptoms • Depression • Anxiety • Poor sleep • Libido

KEY POINTS

- The transition to menopause is often marked by physiologic and psychosocial changes in varying degrees of severity and disruption for midlife women.
- Menopausal symptoms, particularly hot flushes and depressed mood, can begin early in the menopause transition, well before menstrual irregularities occur, and can continue well beyond the final menstrual period.
- These and other acute symptoms of menopause are primarily multifactorial in nature, with biological changes interacting with other psychological, cultural, and socioeconomic characteristics of women.
- It is critical to determine whether symptoms are primarily associated with the menopause transition, and are thus likely to be time-limited, or whether the symptoms are a continuum of medical or psychiatric illnesses.

INTRODUCTION

Four of 5 women experience psychological or physical symptoms around menopause, with varying degrees of severity and disruption in their lives.[1] Clinicians and women normally identify the transition to menopause by the onset of irregular menstrual cycles or the experience of vasomotor symptoms that commonly occur at this time. However, in addition to vasomotor symptoms that are readily recognized, other common menopausal symptoms, such as mood changes, sleep difficulties, and changes

The authors state that there are no funding sources or conflicts of interest in relation to this article.

[a] Department of Obstetrics/Gynecology, University of Pennsylvania School of Medicine, 3400 Spruce Street, Philadelphia, PA 19104, USA; [b] Division of Reproductive Endocrinology and Infertility, University of Pennsylvania School of Medicine, 3400 Spruce Street, Philadelphia, PA 19104, USA; [c] Department of Psychiatry, University of Pennsylvania School of Medicine, 3400 Spruce Street, Philadelphia, PA 19104, USA
* Corresponding author. Penn Fertility Care, 3701 Market Street, Suite 800, Philadelphia, PA 19104.
E-mail address: cgracia@uphs.upenn.edu

Obstet Gynecol Clin N Am 45 (2018) 585–597
https://doi.org/10.1016/j.ogc.2018.07.002
0889-8545/18/© 2018 Elsevier Inc. All rights reserved.

obgyn.theclinics.com

in sexual functioning, may increase early in the menopause transition.[2–4] This transition period, termed perimenopause, is highly variable but can extend for 5 to 10 years before menopause (marked by the final menstrual period [FMP], which is identified by the absence of menstrual bleeding for at least 12 months).

Information on the normal process of reproductive aging and its acute consequences has been limited by many factors. Research has been dominated by cross-sectional study designs, small clinical samples, suboptimal assessment, and lack of adjustment for confounding factors. However, in recent years, several large population-based, longitudinal cohort studies have been conducted that more fully characterize changes during this transition period. This article focuses on current evidence, primarily from large, population-based studies, for symptoms that increase during the menopausal transition. Specifically, we address vasomotor symptoms, mood changes, sleep problems, and changes in sexual functioning.

VASOMOTOR SYMPTOMS
Characteristic Symptoms

The sudden sensation of extreme heat in the upper body, particularly the face, neck, and chest is referred to as a "hot flush." Flushing, chills, clamminess, sweating, anxiety, and occasionally palpitations can occur lasting 1 to 5 minutes.[5,6] These episodes vary in frequency and duration and include night sweats. Some studies show that up to 87% of women reporting hot flushes experience daily symptoms, with one-third experiencing more than 10 per day. Sleep disruption has been demonstrated with physiologic measures of hot flushes.[7]

Prevalence and Duration

Vasomotor symptoms are the most common symptom of menopause experienced by up to 80% of women.[8,9] In the United States, the prevalence of vasomotor symptoms among naturally menopausal women is approximately 40% in the early menopause transition, with the peak prevalence of 60% to 80% in the first 2 years after the FMP.[10]

On average, hot flushes commence before the FMP and continue for several years *after* the FMP. More than one-third of women who experience moderate/severe hot flushes will continue to have them for more than 10 years *after* the FMP.[11,12]

Pathophysiology

The pathophysiology of the hot flush is not clearly understood. A current hypothesis is that the thermoregulatory mechanisms change during the transition so that the thermoregulatory zone is narrowed and becomes more sensitive to subtle changes in core body temperature. Small increases in temperature lead to what we know as a hot flush (vasodilatation, sweating, and decreased skin resistance). Freedman[5,13] postulates that noradrenergic stimulation in conjunction with estrogen may trigger thermoregulatory changes resulting in hot flushes.

Although there is little doubt that estrogen is important in the pathophysiology of hot flushes, changes in estrogen alone do not account for vasomotor symptoms. Instead, the mechanism of action appears to be centrally mediated. Some evidence indicates that hot flushes are temporally related to luteinizing hormone (LH) pulses, but other findings showed that LH is not the direct cause. In another study, cortisol dysregulation was related to more frequent, severe, and bothersome hot flushes, which supports a potential role of the hypothalamic pituitary adrenal axis in the etiology of the symptoms.[14]

The relationship of genetic variation and hot flushes was recently evaluated using data from the Women's Health Initiative and found that genetic variation in tachykinin receptor 3 (TACR3) might contribute to the risk of hot flushes.[15] The hypothalamic neuron neurokinin B (NKB) and its receptor NK3R (which is encoded by TACR3) may also be involved in the pathophysiology of hot flushes.[16,17]

Risk Factors

Epidemiologic studies have identified numerous risk factors for vasomotor symptoms, including racial/ethnicity and body weight (body mass index [BMI]). In the Study of Women's Health Across the Nation (SWAN), African American women reported significantly more vasomotor symptoms, white women reported more psychosomatic symptoms, and Asian women reported the fewest symptoms compared with other groups in a cross-sectional survey of 14,906 multiethnic women aged 40 to 55 years in the United States.[18] In the Penn Ovarian Again Study (POAS), African American women reported more physiologic symptoms (hot flushes, dizziness, clumsiness, urine leaks, and vaginal dryness) compared with white women even when adjusting for age, BMI, and demographic factors.[4,12] Such racial and cross-cultural variability in the prevalence of self-reported hot flushes is substantiated by other studies.[19–21] Although physiologic or dietary differences may account for variable symptomatology, it is also possible that ethnic variations are largely due to differences in cross-cultural perceptions and reporting[2,22,23] (see the article by Nancy E. Avis and colleagues' article, "Vasomotor Symptoms Across the Menopause Transition: Differences Among Women," elsewhere in this issue for more details).

POAS, SWAN, and other studies have reported that obese women have more frequent vasomotor symptoms than nonobese women independent of race, age, and smoking.[4,24–27]

Smoking is a strong risk factor for hot flushes. Smokers in SWAN had a more than 60% greater likelihood of reporting vasomotor symptoms overall and moderate to severe hot flushes compared with nonsmokers.[28,29]

Physical activity has not significantly reduced vasomotor symptoms in a number of studies.[24,30–32] Moreover, highly active women (ages 35–40 years) were significantly *more likely* to report moderate to severe hot flushes than minimally active women, which may be explained by a rise in core body temperature.[33,34]

Many other behavioral, social, and demographic factors have been associated with hot flushes. Negative or depressed mood, a history of depression, higher anxiety levels, and greater perceived stress are associated with increased hot flushes in SWAN and POAS.[2,12,24]

Depressed Mood

Identifying the risk of depression is clinically important because of the significant disability that accompanies depression and conditions related to depression, including cardiovascular disease, metabolic syndrome, and osteoporosis.[27,35–37] Although the National Institutes of Health State-of-Science Report of 2005 concluded that evidence for an association of depression and menopausal status was poor or mixed, more recent population-based, longitudinal cohort studies have challenged this conclusion.[8]

Increase in Depressive Symptoms Related to Menopausal Status

Several population-based studies show that the likelihood of depressed mood is 30% to 3 times greater in the menopause transition compared with the premenopausal stage, even after adjustment for important variables, such as history of depression, hot flushes, and poor sleep.[38–44] Women with a history of depression are nearly 5 times more likely to have a depression in the menopause transition.[38,43,45,46]

Investigation of the longitudinal pattern of depressive symptoms around natural menopause shows that the FMP is pivotal in the overall pattern of decreasing depressive symptoms in midlife women, with higher risk *before* and lower risk *after* the FMP.[12] Importantly, women who had no history of depression before the menopause transition had a low risk of depressive symptoms 2 or more years after the FMP, which suggests the transient nature of menopausal depression for some women.

Associations between perimenopausal depressed mood and changes in the hormonal milieu have been observed.[38,43] An association between follicle-stimulating hormone and depressive symptoms has been demonstrated and suggests that the changing hormonal milieu may contribute to a transient dysphoric mood. However, studies suggest that psychosocial and lifestyle factors, together with health experience may have more effect on mood than endocrine changes.[45,47] Indeed, there are many health and demographic factors that are associated with depression in the perimenopause, including health problems, marital problems, "empty nest" issues, financial difficulty, lack of physical exercise, and environmental stresses.[27,38]

Depressive Symptoms Related to Vasomotor Symptoms

Vasomotor symptoms are strongly correlated with depressive symptoms. It has long been postulated that the depressive symptoms are secondary to hot flushes,[18] but the temporal associations and causal pathways between these symptoms in perimenopausal women are not clear.[34,48] In the Massachusetts Women's Health Study, the association between perimenopause and increased depression was explained by increased reporting of vasomotor symptoms.[49] In contrast, by studying symptoms over 10 years, the POAS study demonstrated that although both hot flushes and depressive symptoms occurred early in the menopause transition, depressive symptoms were more likely to *precede* hot flushes in women without previous symptoms.[48]

Depression is episodic and multifactorial, associated with numerous health and psychosocial factors, which makes it difficult to determine causality. However, it is clinically important to identify and treat depression regardless of cause.

Anxiety

Anxiety manifests in many ways, ranging from symptoms to fully diagnosed disorders that include generalized anxiety disorder, panic disorder, phobias, and posttraumatic stress disorder. Anxiety syndromes or high anxiety symptoms have been shown to diminish quality of life.[50–52]

In the POAS cohort of midlife women, the likelihood of anxiety was similar to that of depression in the menopause transition, and together with irritability and mood swings, anxiety peaked early in the transition.[53] Reports from SWAN similarly indicated that "psychological distress" (combination of irritability, depression, and tension) was greatest in early perimenopausal women and was highest among whites compared with other ethnicities.[42] A follow-up study confirmed these associations even when the analysis was adjusted for vasomotor and sleep symptoms, factors thought to mediate the relationship between emotional symptoms and menopause.[41] Additional studies have suggested that women with low anxiety levels premenopausally are more likely to report high anxiety levels in the transition, whereas those with high anxiety before menopause continue to experience these symptoms throughout the transition.[54,55]

There are many reports of anxiety as a risk factor for hot flushes and many conflicting findings, which are in part due to the varied manifestations of anxiety disorders and to the similarity of the somatic symptoms of anxiety and the somatic complaints of hot flushes.[12,54,56–61] A recent POAS study showed that somatic anxiety, but not affective anxiety, was a strong predictor of menopausal hot flushes.[62] Therefore, somatic anxiety may be a potential target for treatments of menopausal hot flushes.

Poor Sleep

The prevalence of sleep problems in women increases dramatically during middle age. Among women between the ages of 45 and 49, 23.6% report sleep difficulties, and by the early 50s, 39.7% complain of such trouble.[63] Reported problems include trouble falling asleep, disturbed sleep, and frequent awakenings. Midlife sleep difficulties are often attributed to symptoms of menopause. Poor sleep is clearly associated with hot flushes, but evidence indicating that biological decline in ovarian function has direct effects on sleep is limited and controversial.[64,65]

Sleep and Menopausal Status

Many studies have reported an association between self-reported sleep problems and menopausal status, with more sleep problems reported in the menopause transition.[66,67] Findings from SWAN indicate that perimenopausal and postmenopausal women are more likely to report "difficulty sleeping over the past 2 weeks" compared with premenopausal women,[68] and that symptoms are more prevalent in late perimenopause.[69] Although the POAS study also reported a high prevalence of moderate/severe poor sleep in midlife, only a small subgroup had worse sleep in relation to the FMP.[70] Premenopausal poor sleep is an important predictor of poor sleep during the transition.[71]

Although hot flushes appear to contribute to poor sleep during the menopause transition, physiologic studies have not found a direct link.[7,68,72–74] In addition, a variety of other factors during menopause may contribute to poor sleep, including poor health, chronic illness or pain, anxiety, depression, and medications.

Objective Sleep Measures

Objective measures of sleep during the menopause have recently been conducted using polysomnography. Shaver and Zenk[75,76] assessed 17 sleep-quality parameters with polysomnography in 3 groups of women of different menopausal status and could not demonstrate a significant difference in sleep quality. In the Wisconsin Sleep Cohort Study, which is an ongoing population-based longitudinal study of sleep disorders, a cross-sectional study examined 589 women who underwent extensive interview and overnight polysomnography. Based on self-report questionnaires, both perimenopausal and postmenopausal women were twice as likely to report that they were never or not usually satisfied with sleep compared with premenopausal women.[64] Although perimenopausal women were more likely to complain of difficulty initiating sleep, polysomnographic measures of sleep quality did not differ by menopausal stage. In fact, postmenopausal women had the best sleep architecture, with less stage 1 sleep and more stage 3 to 4 sleep compared with premenopausal women. In addition, even though women with sleep-related hot flushes were more likely to report dissatisfaction with sleep, no differences in objective sleep quality were noted.[64] This study challenges the hypothesis that menopause diminishes sleep quality and suggests that other factors likely explain the sleep difficulties. Therefore, sleep problems during the transition should not be attributed to hormonal changes alone, and should prompt further investigation of other sleep-related conditions.

Sleep-Disordered Breathing

A report from the Wisconsin Sleep Cohort Study demonstrated that the menopausal transition is associated with an increased likelihood of sleep-disordered breathing.[77] Postmenopausal women were 3.5 times more likely to have 15 or more apnea and hypopnea events per hour compared with premenopausal women. Although disordered breathing was associated with worse sleep architecture in all women, postmenopausal women overall had better sleep architecture than premenopausal women. Evidence suggests that this disordered breathing is not related to vasomotor symptoms or estradiol levels.

The subjective nature of sleep quality makes it difficult to assess. Unfortunately, current objective measures of sleep quality from polysomnography do not necessarily reflect subjective sleep quality. Although it is clear that the prevalence of poor sleep clearly increases in the transition to menopause, only a small proportion of this problem can be attributed to menopausal status. Many other health, lifestyle, and relationship factors are associated with poor sleep, and these require careful evaluation for women who seek treatment.

Sexual Functioning

Female sexual dysfunction is extremely prevalent in the United States, affecting more than 40% of women ages 18 to 59.[78] There is substantial evidence that sexual dysfunction increases through the menopausal transition.[79,80] Estimates of sexual dysfunction during the transition are as high as 88%.[81]

There is relatively little research on the sexual problems of women in relation to reproductive aging. This may in part be due to the complexity of female sexuality, which is influenced by a variety of emotional, social, and physiologic factors.[79–83] It may also be due to the complexities of the menopausal transition, when other significant psychosocial and physiologic changes occur and concomitant illnesses arise.[83] Studies differ dramatically with respect to patient population, research design, the assessment of female sexuality and other potential determinants of sexual function, making it difficult to come to clear conclusions regarding sexuality during the menopausal transition.

Characteristics

Several investigators have attempted to characterize the types of sexual problems affecting women during the transition. In a longitudinal study of 438 middle-aged Australian women using a validated questionnaire of sexual function, a significant overall decline in sexual functioning during the menopause transition was observed.[79] This decline was particularly dramatic from early to late perimenopause. This and other studies suggest that sexual responsivity, libido, sexual frequency, and positive feelings for the partner decrease while vaginal dyspareunia increase over the transition.[79,84]

The SWAN study showed that sexual function did not change until 20 months before the FMP, after which sexual function scores decreased annually and continued to decline more than 1 year after the FMP but at a slower rate.[85] Vaginal dryness, depressive symptoms, or anxiety did not explain the decline in sexual function. The decline was smaller in African American than in white women.

Pathophysiology

Until recently, the decline in sexual function has largely been attributed to physical changes that occur in the genitourinary system after menopause. For instance, there is evidence that after menopause, the physiologic sexual response is altered by decreased skin flushing, muscle tension, Bartholin gland secretion, vaginal lubrication, clitoral reactivity, vaginal expansion and congestion, and uterine contractions with orgasm.[86] Community-based studies of self-reported sexual function in postmenopausal women appear consistent with the physiologic findings. For example, menopausal women reported decreased desire, vaginal dryness, decreased clitoral sensitivity, orgasmic intensity, and orgasmic frequency.[87] However, physiologic studies of sexual responsiveness during the menopausal transition are lacking, and further studies are needed to confirm or refute these self-reported findings.

Hormone links

Although some of the physiologic changes that occur with sexual functioning are related to the decline in estrogen that follows menopause, sexual changes that occur early in the transition cannot be attributed to estrogen-related genitourinary atrophy. Indeed, circulating estrogen levels do not fall to their low postmenopausal levels until after the FMP.[88] Nonetheless, a longitudinal study of 438 middle-aged women indicated that decreasing scores for self-reported sexual functioning correlated with decreasing estradiol levels.[81] In contrast, in the Massachusetts Women's Health Study, estradiol levels were related only to pain, not other aspects of sexual functioning.[89] In the POAS, estradiol levels were similar between women with and without a self-reported decline in libido in the early menopausal transition.[82]

Androgens

The relationship between androgens and sexuality during the menopausal transition remains elusive. Coincident with decreasing sexual interest, circulating androgens decline during the late reproductive years with levels of circulating androgens at age 45 approximately one-half that of women in their 20s.[90] It has been presumed that the age-related decline in androgens contributes to the decline in sexual function well before menopause because androgen insufficiency has been associated with decreased sexual functioning in many domains.[83] However, studies have not consistently been able to demonstrate that sexual dysfunction is related to decreased androgen levels in women during the menopausal transition.[81,91] In POAS, preliminary data suggest that the variability in total testosterone levels is associated with decreased libido during the late reproductive years.[82] Of 326 women, 87 (27%) reported a decreased libido, whereas 239 (73%) did not. Although hormone levels were similar between groups, women with the greatest fluctuation in total testosterone over the study were more likely to report decreased libido (odds ratio 4.0 [95% confidence interval 1.6–10.0]). Possibly the variability in testosterone, rather than absolute level, relates to sexual problems in women during this period, but further investigation is needed.

Although evidence suggests that testosterone supplementation to supraphysiologic levels may improve sexual satisfaction in menopausal women,[92–95] the benefits and risks of testosterone supplementation are not clear, and further research is needed.

Other factors affecting sexual functioning

Epidemiologic studies have highlighted numerous factors affecting women's sexuality during the menopausal transition, including health, marital status, mental health, and smoking[89]; depression and children living at home[82]; feelings for partner, and the partner's sexual problems[47]; and social variables, such as paid work, interpersonal stress, daily hassles, and educational level.[47]

In summary, many women suffer from a decline in sexual function during the menopausal transition. Numerous factors appear to be involved in the sexual changes that occur during this time. Hormone changes may contribute to sexual problems, but stronger contributors are likely to be relationship issues, mental health, sociocultural influences, and medical illnesses. Current studies are limited by lack of validated measures of sexual functioning, small sample sizes, and insufficiently sensitive hormone assays. The International Consensus Development Conference on Female Sexual Dysfunctions classified sexual dysfunction into 4 major categories: desire disorders, arousal disorders, orgasmic disorders, and sexual pain disorders.[96] Validated measures of sexual functioning that correspond with this new classification system exist and should be used to investigate specific areas of dysfunction to identify potential areas for therapeutic interventions.

SUMMARY

The transition to menopause marks a time of profound change in a woman's life. Hormonal, physiologic, and psychosocial factors are in flux. Acute symptoms of hot flushes, sleep disruption, psychological symptoms, and decreased sexual functioning may accompany these biological and psychosocial changes. Contrary to common beliefs, these symptoms can begin early in the menopausal transition during the late reproductive years, well before menstrual irregularities occur. Importantly, studies show that these acute symptoms are multifactorial in nature, with biological changes interacting with other psychological, cultural, and socioeconomic characteristics of women. Indeed, inasmuch as women's experience of menopause varies widely, it is obvious that the severity of menopausal symptoms cannot be attributed solely to the changing reproductive hormonal milieu that defines the transition to menopause.

It is important for clinicians to understand the complexity of acute menopausal symptoms. It is not sufficient to attribute these complaints to menopause, or to dismiss them as not related to menopause, but rather to provide treatment options for relief of the symptoms and recognize when further investigation is warranted. Most importantly, one must determine whether these symptoms are primarily associated with the menopausal transition, and are thus likely to be time-limited, or whether the symptoms are a continuum of medical or psychiatric illnesses. In addition, this is an ideal time to reevaluate a woman's psychosocial history to determine whether she has an adequate support system to deal with life stressors. The clinician should have a wide understanding of changes that occur during the transition to maximize women's health and well-being.

Finally, continued epidemiologic and basic research is needed to better understand the symptoms and changes of the menopause transition. Longitudinal studies with sample sizes sufficient for statistical validity, appropriate hormone measurement, and validated instruments to assess menopausal symptoms and potential confounders are essential to disentangle the complex relationships between hormones and symptoms and other factors that mediate these relationships.

REFERENCES

1. McKinlay SM, Jefferys M. The menopausal syndrome. Br J Prev Soc Med 1974; 28:108–15.
2. Freeman EW, Sammel MD, Lin H, et al. Symptoms associated with menopausal transition and reproductive hormones in midlife women. Obstet Gynecol 2007; 110(2 Pt 1):230–40.
3. Blumel JE, Chedraui P, Baron F, et al. Menopausal symptoms appear before the menopause and persist 5 years beyond: a detailed analysis of a multinational study. Climacteric 2012;15:542–51.

4. Freeman EW, Sammel MD, Grisso JA, et al. Hot flashes in the late reproductive years: risk factors for Africa American and Caucasian women. J Womens Health Gend Based Med 2001;10(1):67–76.
5. Freedman RR. Physiology of hot flashes. Am J Hum Biol 2001;13:453–64.
6. Kronenberg F. Hot flashes: epidemiology and physiology. Ann N Y Acad Sci 1990; 592:52–86.
7. Erlik Y, Tatryn IV, Meldrum DR, et al. Association of waking episodes with menopausal hot flushes. JAMA 1981;245:1741–4.
8. National Institutes of Health. National Institutes of Health State of the Science Panel 2005, Conference Statement. Management of menopause related symptoms. Ann Intern Med 2005;142:1003–13.
9. Williams RE, Kalilani L, DeBenedetti DB, et al. Frequency and severity of vasomotor symptoms among peri- and postmenopausal women in the United States. Climacteric 2008;11:32–43.
10. Freeman EW, Sammel MD, Lin H, et al. Duration of menopausal hot flushes and associated risk factors. Obstet Gynecol 2011;117(5):1095–104.
11. Avis NE, Crawford SL, Greendale G, et al. Duration of menopausal vasomotor symptoms over the menopause transition. JAMA Intern Med 2015;175(4):531–9.
12. Freeman EW, Sammel MD, Sanders RJ. Risk of long term hot flashes after natural menopause: evidence from the Penn Ovarian Aging Study. Menopause 2014; 21(9):924–32.
13. Freedman RR. Core body temperature variation in symptomatic and asymptomatic postmenopausal women: brief report. Menopause 2002;9:399–401.
14. Gibson CJ, Thurston RC, Matthews KA. Cortisol dysregulation is associated with daily diary-reported hot flashes among midlife women. Clin Endocrinol 2016; 85(4):645–51.
15. Crandall CJ, Manson JE, Hohensee C, et al. Association of genetic variation in the tachykinin receptor 3 locus with hot flashes and night sweats in the Women's Health Initiative Study. Menopause 2017;24(3):252–61.
16. Rance NE, Dacks PA, Mittelman-Smith MA, et al. Modulation of body temperature and LH secretion by hypothalamic KNDy (kisspeptin, neurokinin B and dynorphin) neurons: a novel hypothesis on the mechanism of hot flushes. Front Neuroendocrinol 2013;34:211–27.
17. Prague JK, Roberts RE, Comninos AN, et al. Neurokinin 3 receptor antagonism as a novel treatment for menopausal hot flushes: a phase 2, randomised, double-blind, placebo-controlled trial. Lancet 2017;389:1809–17.
18. Avis NE, Stellato R, Crawford S, et al. Is there a menopausal syndrome? Menopausal status and symptoms across racial/ethnic groups. Soc Sci Med 2001; 52:345–56.
19. Dennerstein L, Smith AM, Morse C, et al. Menopausal symptoms in Australian women. Med J Aust 1993;159:232–6.
20. Beyene Y. Cultural significance and physiological manifestations of menopause: a bicultural analysis. Cult Med Psychiatry 1986;10:47–71.
21. Tang GW. The climacteric of Chinese factory workers. Maturitas 1994;19:177–82.
22. Green R, Santoro N. Menopausal symptoms and ethnicity: the study of women's health across the nation. Womens Health 2009;5(2):127–33.
23. Richard-Davis G, Wellons M. Racial and ethnic differences in the physiology and clinical symptoms of menopause. Semin Reprod Med 2013;31:380–6.
24. Gold EB, Colvin A, Avis N, et al. Longitudinal analysis of the association between vasomotor symptoms and race/ethnicity across the menopausal transition: study of women's health across the nation. Am J Public Health 2006;96:1226–35.

25. Gracia CR, Sammel MD, Freeman EW, et al. Defining menopause status: creation of a new definition to identify the early changes of the menopausal transition. Menopause 2005;12(2):128–35.

26. Su HI, Sammel MD, Freeman EW, et al. Body size affects measures of ovarian reserve in late reproductive age women. Menopause 2008;15(5):857–61.

27. Freeman EW, Sammel MD, Lin H, et al. Obesity and reproductive hormone levels in the transition to menopause. Menopause 2010;17(4):718–26.

28. Gold EB, Bromberger J, Crawford S, et al. Factors associated with age at natural menopause in a multiethnic sample of midlife women. Am J Epidemiol 2001; 153(9):865–74.

29. Butts SF, Freeman EW, Sammel MD, et al. Joint effects of smoking and gene variants involved in sex steroid metabolism on hot flashes in late reproductive-age women. J Clin Endocrinol Metab 2012;97(6):1032–42.

30. Nelson DB, Sammel MD, Freeman EW, et al. Effect of physical activity on menopausal symptoms among urban women. Med Sci Sports Exerc 2008;40(1):50–8.

31. Greendale GA, Gold EB. Lifestyle factors: are they related to vasomotor symptoms and do they modify the effectiveness or side effects of hormone therapy? Am J Med 2005;118(suppl):148–54.

32. Thurston RC, Joffe H, Soares CN, et al. Physical activity and risk of vasomotor symptoms in women with and without a history of depression: results from the Harvard Study of Moods and Cycles. Menopause 2006;13(4):553–60.

33. Whitcomb BW, Whiteman MK, Langenberg P, et al. Physical activity and risk of hot flashes among women in midlife. J Womens Health 2007;16(1):124–33.

34. Thurston RC, Joffe H. Vasomotor symptoms and menopause: findings from the Study of Women's Health Across the Nation. Obstet Gynecol Clin North Am 2011;38(3):489–501.

35. Lopez AD, Murray AC. The global burden of disease, 1990-2020. Nat Med 1998; 4:1241–3.

36. Bromberger JT, diScalea TL. Longitudinal associations between depression and functioning in midlife women. Maturitas 2009;64:145–59.

37. Wariso BA, Guerrieri GM, Thompson K, et al. Depression during the menopause transition: impact on quality of life, social adjustment, and disability. Arch Womens Ment Health 2017;20(2):273–82.

38. Freeman EW, Sammel MD, Lin H, et al. Associations of hormones and menopausal status with depressed mood in women with no history of depression. Arch Gen Psychiatry 2006;63(4):375–82.

39. Cohen LS, Soares CN, Vitonis AF, et al. Risk for new onset of depression during the menopausal transition: the Harvard study of moods and cycles. Arch Gen Psychiatry 2006;63:385–90.

40. Bromberger JT, Matthews KA, Schott LL, et al. Depressive symptoms during the menopausal transition: the Study of Women's Health Across the Nation (SWAN). J Affect Disord 2007;103:267–72.

41. Bromberger JT, Assmann SF, Avis NE, et al. Persistent mood symptoms in a multiethnic community cohort of pre- and perimenopausal women. Am J Epidemiol 2003;158:347–56.

42. Bromberger JT, Meyer PT, Kravitz HM, et al. Psychological distress and natural menopausal: a multiethnic study. Am J Public Health 2001;91:1435–42.

43. Freeman EW, Sammel MD, Liu L, et al. Hormones and menopausal status as predictors of depression in women in transition to menopause. Arch Gen Psychiatry 2004;61(1):62–70.

44. Woods NF, Smith-DiJulio K, Percival DB, et al. Depressed mood during the menopausal transition and early postmenopause: observations from the Seattle Midlife Women's Health Study. Menopause 2008;15:223–32.
45. Harlow BL, Wise LA, Otto MW, et al. Depression and its influence on reproductive endocrine and menstrual cycle markers associated with perimenopause: the Harvard Study of Moods and Cycles. Arch Gen Psychiatry 2003;60:29–36.
46. Schmidt PJ, Haq N, Rubinow DR. A longitudinal evaluation of the relationship between reproductive status and mood in perimenopausal women. Am J Psychiatry 2004;161:2238–44.
47. Dennerstein L, Lehert P, Burger H, et al. Mood and the menopausal transition. J Nerv Ment Dis 1999;187:685–91.
48. Freeman EW, Sammel MD, Lin H. Temporal associations of hot flashes and depression in the transition to menopause. Menopause 2009;16(4):728–34.
49. Avis NE, Brambilla E, McKinlay SM, et al. A longitudinal analysis of the association between menopause and depression. Ann Epidemiol 1994;4:214–20.
50. Greenblum CA, Rowe MA, Neff DF, et al. Midlife women: symptoms associated with menopausal transition and early postmenopause and quality of life. Menopause 2013;20:22–7.
51. Whitely J, DiBonaventura MD, Wagner J-S, et al. The impact of menopausal symptoms on quality of life, productivity and economic outcomes. J Womens Health 2013;22:983–90.
52. Uguz F, Sahingoz M, Gezgine K, et al. Quality of life in postmenopausal women: the impact of depressive and anxiety disorders. Int J Psychiatry Med 2011;41:281–92.
53. Freeman EW, Sammel MD, Lin H, et al. Symptoms in the menopausal transition: hormone and behavioral correlates. Obstet Gynecol 2008;111(1):127–36.
54. Bromberger JR, Kravitz HM, Chang Y, et al. Does risk for anxiety increase during the menopausal transition? Menopause 2013;20:488–95.
55. Flores-Ramos M, Silvestri-Tomassoni R, Guerrero-Lopez JB, et al. Evaluation of trait and state anxiety levels in a group of peri- and postmenopausal women. Women Health 2017;58(3):305–19.
56. Freeman EW, Sammel MD, Lin H, et al. The role of anxiety and hormonal changes in menopausal hot flashes. Menopause 2005;12(3):258–66.
57. Woods NF, Mitchell ES, Landis C. Anxiety, hormonal changes and vasomotor symptoms during the menopause transition. Menopause 2005;12:242–5.
58. Lermer MA, Morra A, Moineddin T, et al. Somatic and affective anxiety symptoms and menopausal hot flashes. Menopause 2011;18:129–32.
59. Hanisch LJ, Hantsoo L, Freeman EW, et al. Hot flashes and panic attacks: a comparison of symptomatology, neurobiology, treatment, and a role for cognition. Psychol Bull 2008;134(2):247–69.
60. Maki PM. Menopause and anxiety: immediate and long-term effects. Menopause 2008;15:1033–5.
61. Bryant C, Judd FK, Hickey M. Anxiety during the menopause transition: a systematic review. J Affect Disord 2012;139:141–8.
62. Freeman EW, Sammel MD. Anxiety as a risk factor from menopausal hot flashes: evidence from the Penn Ovarian Aging Cohort. Menopause 2016;23(9):942–9.
63. Cirignotta F, Mondini S, Zucconi M, et al. Insomnia: an epidemiological survey. Clin Neuropharmacol 1985;8:S49–54.
64. Young T, Rabago D, Zgierska A, et al. Objective and subjective sleep quality in premenopausal, perimenopausal and postmenopausal women in the Wisconsin sleep cohort study. Sleep 2003;26:667–72.

65. Sharkey KM, Bearpark HM, Acebo C, et al. Effects of menopausal status on sleep in midlife women. Behav Sleep Med 2003;1:69–80.

66. Kuh DL, Wadsworth M, Hardy R. Women's health in midlife: the influence of the menopause, social factors and health in earlier life. Br J Obstet Gynaecol 1997;104:923–33.

67. Owen JF, Matthews KA. Sleep disturbance in healthy middle-aged women. Maturitas 1998;30:41–50.

68. Kravitz HM, Ganz PA, Bromberger J, et al. Sleep difficulty in women at midlife: a community survey of sleep and the menopausal transition. Menopause 2003;10: 19–28.

69. Ciano C, King TS, Wright RR, et al. Longitudinal study of insomnia symptoms among women during perimenopause. J Obstet Gynecol Neonatal Nurs 2017; 46(6):804–13.

70. Freeman EW, Sammel MD, Gross SA, et al. Poor sleep in relation to natural menopause: a population-based 14-year follow-up of midlife women. Menopause 2015;22(7):719–26.

71. Oyayon MM. Severe hot flashes are associated with chronic insomnia. Arch Intern Med 2006;166:1262–8.

72. Ensrud KE, Stone KL, Blackwell TL, et al. Frequency and severity of hot flashes and sleep disturbance in postmenopausal women with hot flashes. Menopause 2009;16:286–92.

73. Hollander LE, Freeman EW, Sammel MD, et al. Sleep quality, estradiol levels, and behavioral factors in late reproductive age women. Obstet Gynecol 2001;98(3): 391–7.

74. Xu H, Thurston RC, Matthews KA, et al. Are hot flashes associated with sleep disturbance during midlife? Results from the STRIDE cohort study. Maturitas 2012;71:34–8.

75. Shaver JLF, Zenk SN. Sleep disturbance in menopause. J Womens Health Gend Based Med 2000;9:109–18.

76. Young T, Finn L, Austin D, et al. Menopausal status and sleep-disordered breathing in the Wisconsin sleep cohort study. Am J Respir Crit Care Med 2003;167: 1181–5.

77. Polo-Kantola P, Rauhala E, Saaresranta T, et al. Climacteric vasomotor symptoms do not predict nocturnal breathing abnormalities in postmenopausal women. Maturitas 2001;39:29–37.

78. Laumann EO, Paik A, Rosen RC. Sexual dysfunction in the United States: prevalence and predictors. JAMA 1999;281:537–44.

79. Dennerstein L, Dudly E, Burger H. Are changes in sexual functioning during midlife due to aging or menopause? Fertil Steril 2001;76:456–60.

80. Osborn M, Hawton K, Gath D. Sexual dysfunction among middle-aged women in the community. BMJ 1988;296:959–62.

81. Dennerstein L, Randolph J, Taffe J, et al. Hormones, mood, sexuality, and the menopausal transition. Fertil Steril 2002;77:S42–8.

82. Gracia CR, Sammel MD, Freeman EW, et al. Predictors of decreased libido in women during the late reproductive years. Menopause 2004;11(2):144–50.

83. Palacios S, Robar AC, Menendez C. Sexuality in the climacteric years. Maturitas 2002;43:S69–77.

84. Rosen RC, Taylor JF, Leiblum SR, et al. Prevalence of sexual dysfunction in women: results of a survey study of 329 women in an outpatient gynecological clinic. J Sex Marital Ther 1993;19:171–88.

85. Avis NE, Colvin A, Karlamangla AS, et al. Change in sexual functioning over the menopausal transition: results from the Study of Women's Health Across the Nation. Menopause 2016;24(4):379–90.
86. Masters WH, Johnson VE. Human sexual response. Boston: Little, Brown; 1966.
87. Sarrel PM. Sexuality and menopause. Obstet Gynecol 1990;75:26s.
88. Burger H, Dudley E, Hopper J, et al. Prospectively measured levels of serum FSH, estradiol, and the dimeric inhibins during the menopausal transition in a population-based cohort of women. J Clin Endocrinol Metab 1999;84:4025–30.
89. Avis NE, Stellato R, Crawford S, et al. Is there an association between menopause status and sexual functioning? Menopause 2000;7:297–309.
90. Zumoff B, Strain GW, Miller LK, et al. Twenty-four hour mean plasma testosterone concentration declines with age in normal premenopausal women. J Clin Endocrinol Metab 1995;80:1429–30.
91. Guay AT, Jacobson J. Decreased free testosterone and dehydroepiandrosterone-sulfate levels in women with decreased libido. J Sex Marital Ther 2002;28:129–42.
92. Davis SR, McCloud PI, Strauss BSG, et al. Testosterone enhances estradiol effects on postmenopausal bone density and sexuality. Maturitas 1995;21:227–36.
93. Sarrel PM, Dobay B, Wiita B. Sexual behavior and neuroendocrine response in estrogen and estrogen-androgen replacement in postmenopausal women dissatisfied with estrogen-only therapy. J Reprod Med 1998;43:847–56.
94. Shifren JL, Braunstein GD, Simon JA, et al. Transdermal testosterone treatment in women with impaired sexual function after oophorectomy. N Engl J Med 2000; 343:682–8.
95. Korkidakis AK, Reid RL. Testosterone in women: measurement and therapeutic use. J Obstet Gynaecol Can 2017;39(3):124–30.
96. Basson R, Berman J, Burnett A, et al. Report of the international consensus development conference on female sexual dysfunction: definitions and classifications. J Urol 2000;163:888–9.

Menstrual Cycle Changes as Women Approach the Final Menses: What Matters?

Siobán D. Harlow, PhD

KEYWORDS

- Menstruation • Menopause • Abnormal uterine bleeding • Menopausal transition

KEY POINTS

- The STRAW+10 bleeding criterion for onset of the early menopausal transition is increased variability (persistent, 7-days or more difference in length of consecutive cycles) and for onset of the late menopausal transition is occurrence of amenorrhea of 60 days or more.
- Twelve percent to 25% of women experience minimal or no change in their menstrual cycle length before their final menstrual period (FMP).
- Women with earlier onset of the menopausal transition have longer transitions. When the transition is not sudden, it may last from approximately 4 to 10 years, with longer duration associated with earlier age at onset.
- Excessive flow and prolonged menstrual bleeding is a hallmark of the menopausal transition. Most women experience repeated bleeding episodes lasting 10 or more days, whereas one-third have heavy menstrual bleeding lasting 3 or more days, with blood loss frequently exceeding 80 mL.
- Anovulation is common in the menopausal transition, but hormonally normal, ovulatory cycles occur up until the FMP.

Since the pioneering publications of Vollman[1] and Treloar and colleagues[2] in the 1950s and 1960s, it has been well-established that marked changes occur in the length and variability of menstrual cycles as women enter the menopausal transition (MT). Classically, increased variability in cycle length marks the onset of the MT, with the likelihood of long cycles increasing as women approach their final menstrual period (FMP), or menopause. Menopause is defined, retrospectively, after 12 months of amenorrhea in women aged 40 and older, although another menstrual bleed may occur in up to 10% of women, especially in women who are younger when they reach this milestone.[3] The challenge for women and their health care providers has been to

Disclosure Statement: The author no conflicts of interest.
Department of Epidemiology, School of Public Health of the University of Michigan, 1415 Washington Heights, Ann Arbor, MI 48109-2029, USA
E-mail address: harlow@umich.edu

Obstet Gynecol Clin N Am 45 (2018) 599–611
https://doi.org/10.1016/j.ogc.2018.07.003
0889-8545/18/© 2018 Elsevier Inc. All rights reserved.

understand what change in menstrual patterns specifically signals that a woman has entered the MT and what signals that she is nearing the FMP.

Over the past 2 decades, longitudinal cohort studies have followed midlife women as they transitioned from reproductive life through to and beyond the menopause, providing a more precise understanding of the specific bleeding changes that mark the onset of the MT and a nuanced understanding of the changes in menstrual bleeding that women may expect at this life stage. These studies, in which midlife women maintained menstrual calendars for various lengths of time, include the multisite, multiethnic Study of Women's Health Across the Nation (SWAN),[4] the Massachusetts Women's Health Study (MWHS),[5] The Melbourne Women's Midlife Health Project (MWMHP),[6] The Seattle Midlife Women's Health Study (SMWHS),[7] and the Penn reproductive aging Study (POAS),[8] among others. Similar to the observations by Treloar and colleagues[2] and Vollman,[1] the MWHS reported that short menstrual cycles were more frequent in early perimenopause whereas cycles longer than 90 days became frequent late in the transition.[5] The MWMHP documented that increasingly longer menstrual cycles were a signal of the approach of the FMP, most notably in the last 20 menstrual cycles before the FMP.[9]

STAGING REPRODUCTIVE AGING: WHAT ARE THE SPECIFIC CHANGES IN MENSTRUAL BLEEDING THAT MARK ONSET OF EARLY AND LATE MENOPAUSAL TRANSITION?

Treloar's landmark paper that defined the concept of an MT[10] was based on visual examination of women's menstrual histories over the 12 years leading to the FMP. He described the phenomenon of increased variability followed by the onset of very long cycles and estimated the average age at entry into the transition to be 45.5 years. In the 1990s, several of the previously mentioned cohort studies proposed different approaches to staging reproductive aging and proposed markers for recognizing the onset of increased variability and of increasingly long cycles. In recognition of the need for consensus regarding stages of reproductive aging and for valid, reliable, and clinically useful criteria to characterize the onset of each stage, the Stages of Reproductive Aging Workshop (STRAW)[11] made initial recommendations for a 7-stage model of reproductive life based on a consensus discussion of the available evidence in 2001. Subsequently, the ReSTAGE Collaboration empirically assessed the validity and reliability of STRAW's menstrual criteria using Treloar's data[10] and data from 3 of the contemporary cohort studies of midlife women: SWAN, the MWMHP, and the SMWHS.[12] The ReSTAGE findings clarified STRAW's recommendations and lead to the 2011 empirically based STRAW+10 recommendations.[13–16]

The STRAW+10 model divides reproductive life into 7 stages: the reproductive years (3 stages), the transition years (2 stages: early and late), and the postmenopausal years (2 stages). Given limitations in the availability of valid, reliable, and widely available assays, STRAW focused on menstrual markers and qualitative changes in follicle-stimulating hormone (FSH) (with quantitative values now defined for the late transition), and to a lesser extent inhibin-B and anti-Mullerian hormone (AMH):

- Entry into the early transition is characterized by increased levels of FSH and increased variability in menstrual cycle length, defined as a persistent, 7-days or more difference in the length of consecutive cycles.
- Entry into the late transition is characterized by the continued elevation of FSH and the occurrence of amenorrhea of 60 days or more.

The bleeding changes that mark onset of the early MT are subtle, yet often apparent to women before they are assessable clinically. No validated standardized questionnaire yet exists that accurately captures these bleeding changes. Longitudinal cohort studies relied on self-reported change or irregularity in menstrual function, with no clear definition of what constituted "change" or "irregularity."The STRAW+10 criterion for ascertaining the change in variability marking entry into the early MT follows from the SMWHS[17] and ReSTAGE,[18] with persistence operationalized as a recurrence within 10 cycles of the first variable-length cycle. After age 40, the median time from occurrence of a persistent 7-day or more difference in consecutive cycle lengths to FMP is 5 to 8 years. SWAN[19] and the Michigan Bone Health and Metabolism Study (MBHMS)[20] found that the initial rise in FSH occurs on average approximately 7 years before the FMP, consistent with the timing of onset of the early transition by this criterion. Other studies[17,21–23] provide further evidence that STRAW's proposed bleeding criteria are valid based on concurrent changes in hormone profiles. Ongoing research suggests that declines in inhibin-B and AMH are also useful qualitative correlates of the onset of the early transition, with more definitive hormonal criteria potentially possible once standardized assays and longitudinal population data on patterns of change in these hormones are available.[24–26]

Menstrual changes associated with the late MT are easier to identify. Although a criterion of amenorrhea of 90 days[27] was in common usage at the time of STRAW, a reanalysis of Treloar's data[28] and data from both SMWHS[17] and MWMHP[9] suggested that a shorter interval of amenorrhea was equally predictive of the approach of the FMP and less likely to misclassify menopausal women as being in late transition. ReSTAGE empirically demonstrated that the optimal bleeding marker of the late transition is an episode of amenorrhea of 60 days or longer.[29] In approximately one-third of women, the first cycle of ≥60 days is in fact ≥90 days. After age 40, the median time from occurrence of ≥60 days of amenorrhea to the FMP is approximately 2.5 to 3.0 years. This criterion also correlates with further elevations in FSH.[30] Clinically, requiring a repeated episode of amenorrhea ≥60 days in women younger than 45 may help ensure women are in fact in late menopause as opposed to experiencing amenorrhea secondary to transient stress.[31] Given the availability of international standards for FSH assays, STRAW+10 provided quantitative criteria for FSH, levels greater than 25 IU/L in a random blood draw, being characteristic of late transition. Notably, in SWAN and MWMHP, an episode of amenorrhea ≥60 days was a better predictor of proximity to the FMP than was a single early follicular phase serum FSH level. Hot flashes, although common in the late transition, are not predictive of proximity of menopause in the absence of information on amenorrhea and FSH levels.

Limitations of the Stages of Reproductive Aging Workshop Model

The STRAW model, now recognized as the gold standard for staging reproductive aging, are widely applicable to women regardless of age, race/ethnicity, body size, or lifestyle characteristics, including smoking status. However, 3 important gaps remain in the clinical application of the STRAW+10 model:

- Evaluation of reproductive aging in women who have had a hysterectomy or ablation must rely on the STRAW+10 hormonal criteria alone. The Women's Ischemia Syndrome Evaluation study proposed an algorithm based on age, time since last menses, surgery history, and serum hormone values.[32]
- As polycystic ovarian syndrome (PCOS) is characterized by oligomenorrhea, STRAW+10 bleeding criteria cannot be applied to women with this condition. Given higher antral follicle counts and higher AMH levels, and less frequent

cycles,[33] women with PCOS may have enhanced ovarian reserve and a later age at menopause than women without PCOS.[34]

- Distinguishing amenorrhea secondary to chronic illness, including human immunodeficiency virus (HIV),[35,36] cancer and chemotherapy,[37–39] medication use,[35,40] or nutritional compromise or weight loss, from amenorrhea attributable to the MT is challenging. For example, studies have reported lower FSH levels in HIV-infected women, secondary to use of opiates, and elevated E2 among women treated with highly active antiretroviral therapy (HAART).[35]

Menstrual Cycle Patterns Leading to the Menopause Differ Across Women

As clinicians are well aware, bleeding patterns during the transition to menopause can differ markedly in some women from the classic pattern described previously. Characteristics of the MT depend to some extent on the age at menopause, with later age at menopause associated with the experience of longer cycles and greater cycle variability in the 2 years preceding the FMP.[3] Women with later menopause also tend to have had longer cycles throughout their reproductive life[41] and in the 9 years before menopause.[42]

Data on the experience of women who report little change in their menstrual cycles until the FMP are limited. In one clinical study, 12% of women reported sudden amenorrhea,[43] confirming self-reports described in other articles.[44] In the reanalysis of Treloar's[10] data described previously, approximately 15% of women were found to have minimal change in their cycle length before the FMP. In another reanalysis of these same data, approximately 25% of women were classified as having no or minimal change in menstrual cycle variability or mean length before their FMP.[45]

ANOVULATION IS CHARACTERISTIC OF THE MENOPAUSAL TRANSITION

In her early pioneering studies of ovulation across the transition, Metcalf[46] documented that 95% of women aged 40 to 55 with no recent change in menstrual cycle length ovulated consistently, versus only 34% of women who reported a recent history of cycles longer than 35 days. The SWAN Daily Hormone Study (DHS) is one of the few studies that has prospectively evaluated changes in endocrine profiles within a menstrual cycle as women approach their FMP. This study reported not only that very short menstrual cycles, less than 21 days, were common in early perimenopause, but that short and long menstrual cycles are both more likely to be anovulatory.[47] The percentage of menstrual cycles that were ovulatory declined beginning approximately 5 years before the FMP with only 22.8% of cycles within a year of the FMP being ovulatory.[48] Ovulatory cycles in the MT had a mean length of 26 to 27 days, only slightly shorter than that of premenopausal women, and whole cycle hormone levels remained relatively stable until approximately 3 years before menopause (evaluation of cycle length in the SWAN menstrual calendars confirm that although long cycles become longer with the approach of the FMP, median length of cycles changes minimally).[49] Thus, confirming the studies of Metcalf,[46] hormonally normal, ovulatory menstrual cycles become less frequent but continue to occur through the end of reproductive life.

EXCESSIVE FLOW AND PROLONGED BLEEDING ARE COMMON IN THE MENOPAUSAL TRANSITION

Considerably less information is available regarding how menstrual bleeding itself changes with reproductive aging. Although short bleeding and spotting episodes occur more frequently after the onset of the MT,[50] excessive flow and prolonged menstrual bleeding is often a hallmark of women's experience during this phase of reproductive life. Clinical studies as well as cross sectional and longitudinal population-based studies of midlife women document an increased duration and amount of menstrual flow.[51–53] The classic study by Hallberg and colleagues[54] documented that 50-year-old women bled approximately 6 mL more than women aged 20 to 45, with heavy bleeding being most common in this age group: the 90th percentile of blood loss was 133 mL in women aged 50, versus 86 to 88 mL for women aged 30 to 45. In a recent study that quantified blood loss across 2 bleeding episodes, the range of menstrual blood loss was significantly greater among women in the late MT, compared with younger women.[52] Blood loss greater than 200 mL was associated with being in late MT and with cycles being ovulatory with high E2 levels.[22,52] Another population-based prospective diary study found that the MT was associated with increases in the reported variability in length of bleeding episodes and increased reporting of spotting and bleeding episodes that lasted $\geq$10 days.[55] Consistent with this study and studies in reproductive-age women,[56] the SWAN DHS[47] reported heavy bleeding less frequently after anovulatory cycles than after ovulatory cycles in the early transition.

Chronic abnormal uterine bleeding (AUB) is bleeding "that is abnormal in duration, volume, and/or frequency and has been present for the majority of the last 6 months.".[57,58] However, given the nature of changes in menstrual function during the MT, identifying what constitutes abnormal in this reproductive life-stage remains a challenge for women and their health care providers. FIGO (International Federation of Gynecology and Obstetrics) defines the limits of normal menstruation by 4 parameters: frequency, regularity, duration of flow, and volume of blood loss.[57,58] During the MT, frequent (more often than every 24 days over a 6-month period), infrequent (less than every 38 days over a 6-month period), and irregular (variation from cycle to cycle within a woman over a 1-year period of more than 20 days) is expected and normative. Prolonged menstrual flow (>8 days of flow occurring on a regular basis) is experienced by most women at some point during their MT.[59] Heavy menstrual bleeding (blood loss >80 mL) can be difficult to measure quantitatively and thus is considered excessive when it interferes with a woman's quality of life. SWAN is one of the few studies to characterize change in menstrual bleeding duration and flow using prospective menstrual calendars.[59] During the MT, three-quarters of SWAN women had 3 of more episodes of menstrual bleeding lasting 10 or more days, one-quarter of whom reported 3 episodes within 6 months of the first such episode. In addition, one-third of SWAN women had 3 or more heavy bleeding episodes lasting 3 or more days, of whom 40% experienced those episodes within 6 months. Although comparable to data from population-based surveys of reproductive-age women where 10% to 35% report symptoms indicative of heavy menstrual bleeding,[60–63] many women with AUB had had a hysterectomy and were not eligible to participate in SWAN. Clinical case series evaluating women with AUB in the MT have found that up to three-quarters may have no anatomic pathology.[64,65]

HOW LONG DOES THE MENOPAUSAL TRANSITION LAST?

Treloar[10] estimated the median duration of the MT to be 4.8 years. Applying the STRAW criteria to the SWAN menstrual calendar data, the median duration of the MT was found to depend largely on the age at which it began, with later onset associated with a shorter duration.[66] Thus, median duration of the MT ranged from 4.4 to 8.6 years depending on age at onset. A reanalysis of the Treloar data grouped women into 6 categories based on the timing and duration of their early and late transitions.[67]

Four subgroups were found to begin the MT on average near age 40 years, whereas 2 other subgroups began the transition much later, on average at age 46.5 years (based on age inclusion criteria most of the cohort studies of midlife women include only women represented by these latter 2 subgroups who represent only one-third of women). The average duration of the transition for the 2 older age onset subgroups and one of the early age onset subgroups was 6 years, whereas for the other 3 early age onset subgroups, the average duration was 9 to 11 years. In women with no obvious change in menstrual patterns, the MT may be quite short.

ETHNICITY

Evidence suggests that age at onset of the MT differs by ethnicity. The Harvard Study of Moods and Cycles reported that women of color had an earlier entry into perimenopause than did white women.[68] Both POAS[69] and SWAN[66] also found that African American women started the MT earlier than white women. In SWAN, duration of the MT was also longer in African American women. Studies of postmenarchal girls and adult women in the United States suggest racial/ethnic differences in menstrual cycle length and bleeding patterns across reproductive life. In the postmenarchal period, white girls have longer menstrual cycle lengths and longer bleeding episodes on average, but are less likely to report heavy bleeding than African American girls,[70,71] and 2 California studies of adult women reported that menstrual cycles of Asian women were on average approximately 2 days longer than those of white women.[72,73] Similarly, in SWAN, Chinese and Japanese women had longer menstrual cycles during the MT than white women.[49] In the SWAN DHS, probability of ovulation was lower in African American and Hispanic women than in white, Japanese, and Chinese women; however, ethnic differences were not observed in the characteristics of menstrual bleeding episodes after adjustment for body mass index (BMI).[47]

BODY SIZE

BMI and nutritional status influence reproductive function, including menstrual cycle length, amount of flow, and timing of reproductive aging. Data on whether BMI influences age at onset of the MT is contradictory.[66,68,69] Both low and high BMI are associated with longer menstrual cycles.[73–77] In SWAN, menstrual calendar data document that, during the MT, obese women have longer menstrual cycles than nonobese women.[49] BMI also influences bleeding duration and heaviness of flow, with low BMI associated with longer bleeds[70,78,79] and high BMI with shorter bleeds[70,74,80] in most, but not all, studies.[81,82] A population-based survey reported that obesity was associated with a higher frequency of flooding in both premenopausal and perimenopausal women.[55] In the SWAN DHS,[47] obesity was associated with an increased number of heavy bleeding days.

CIGARETTE SMOKING AND ENVIRONMENTAL CHEMICALS

Smoking has been associated with earlier age at menopause[83,84] and an early age at onset and shorter MT.[66,69] It is less clear whether smoking influences menstrual bleeding parameters. The evidence for an impact on menstrual cycle length is contradictory, with some studies suggesting that smokers have shorter cycles[77,85,86] and others not.[72,74,81,87] Smoking has been associated with shorter[86,87] and longer periods[81] and heavier menstrual flows,[87] but not in all studies.[47]

MEDICAL CONDITIONS

Although data are limited, medical conditions, their treatment, or their impact on nutritional status can alter or suppress menstrual function. These conditions may be particularly relevant to reproductive aging, as the burden of chronic illness increases in the midlife, but data on the impact of chronic conditions or medication are very limited. In SWAN and other studies, diabetes has been associated with an earlier age at menopause[84,88] and with premature menopause.[89] A few reports suggest that diabetes may be associated with longer menstrual cycles[17,77,90] and longer and heavier bleeding episodes in some[90] but not all studies.[47] In a recent systematic review,[91] type 1 diabetes mellitus was associated with an increased frequency of oligomenorrhea, amenorrhea, and heavy menstrual bleeding throughout reproductive life and may be associated with a shorter reproductive lifespan; however, data on its association with ovarian reserve and age at menopause are limited and inconsistent, and may depend on level of glycemic control. Type 2 diabetes mellitus before or early in the MT has been associated with an earlier age at menopause in prospective studies, but data are inconsistent.

Data are more limited for thyroid disorders. One study reported that women with a history of Graves disease were more likely to report long cycles,[77] whereas another reported that hyperthyroidism was associated with reduced menstrual flow and hypothyroidism with increased frequency of menorrhagia.[92] In SWAN, higher baseline thyroid-stimulating hormone was associated with longer bleed duration in the whole cohort,[93] but self-reported thyroid conditions were not associated with menstrual parameters in the DHS.[47] Data on the impact of uterine leiomyomas on bleeding parameters during the MT are limited, despite their association with AUB and hysterectomy.[94–96] In the SWAN DHS, fibroids were associated with shorter menstrual cycles but longer and heavier bleeding episodes.[47] AUB also may be secondary to use of oral anticoagulants.[40]

CLINICAL IMPLICATIONS

- The classic description of the MT, as a period of increased variability followed by increasingly long cycles until permanent amenorrhea is achieved, describes the experience of many women; however, 15% to 25% of women will have no or minimal change in the regularity of their menstrual cycles before the FMP and little is understood about the transition experience of women with PCOS.
- Short cycles are most frequent early in the transition, whereas long cycles are most frequent late in the transition. Longer menstrual cycles, both during the transition and throughout reproductive life, are associated with having an older age at menopause.
- The length of bleeding episodes is more variable and the amount of blood loss is frequently heavier during the MT, with an increased probability of experiencing 3 or more episodes of prolonged (10 or more days) or excessive blood loss during this reproductive life stage, particularly for obese women and women with leiomyomas. Excessive bleeding is most often associated with ovulatory cycles in this reproductive phase, although spotting and bleeding for longer than 8 days are associated with anovulatory cycles.
- Based on the STRAW+10 model, onset of the early transition is best characterized by a noticeable change in menstrual cycle lengths after age 40, defined as a persistent difference in consecutive menstrual cycles of 7 or more days. The early transition heralds the FMP, on average, 6 to 8 years later. Onset of the late transition is best characterized by a menstrual cycle of 60 or more days, with onset

occurring on average 2 years before the FMP. Identifying onset of the MT and the FMP may be difficult in women with chronic diseases associated with nutritional compromise, or in women using medications that alter hormone profiles (such as HIV-infected women taking HAART).

- Clinicians should pay careful attention to medical factors, including both medical conditions and medical treatments, that may increase menstrual blood loss or alter menstrual cycle characteristics sufficiently to obscure the onset of the MT or the FMP when treating women in the midlife, although scientific data to guide clinical practice are limited.
- Finally, although ovulation and hormonally normal menstrual cycles become rarer as women approach the FMP, such cycles continue to occur up until the FMP, with their concomitant risk of unintended pregnancy.

ACKNOWLEDGMENTS

SDH gratefully acknowledge use of the services and facilities of the Population Studies Center at the University of Michigan, funded by NICHD Center Grant R24 HD041028.

The Study of Women's Health Across the Nation (SWAN) has grant support from the National Institutes of Health (NIH), DHHS, through the National Institute on Aging (NIA), the National Institute of Nursing Research (NINR) and the NIH Office of Research on Women's Health (ORWH) (Grants U01NR004061; U01AG012505, U01AG012535, U01AG012531, U01AG012539, U01AG012546, U01AG012553, U01AG012554, U01AG012495). The content of this article is solely the responsibility of the authors and does not necessarily represent the official views of the NIA, NINR, ORWH or the NIH.

Clinical Centers: *University of Michigan, Ann Arbor – Siobán Harlow, PI 2011 – present, MaryFran Sowers, PI 1994-2011; Massachusetts General Hospital, Boston, MA – Joel Finkelstein, PI 1999 – present; Robert Neer, PI 1994 – 1999; Rush University, Rush University Medical Center, Chicago, IL – Howard Kravitz, PI 2009 – present; Lynda Powell, PI 1994 – 2009; University of California, Davis/Kaiser – Ellen Gold, PI; University of California, Los Angeles – Gail Greendale, PI; Albert Einstein College of Medicine, Bronx, NY – Carol Derby, PI 2011 – present, Rachel Wildman, PI 2010 – 2011; Nanette Santoro, PI 2004 – 2010; University of Medicine and Dentistry – New Jersey Medical School, Newark – Gerson Weiss, PI 1994 – 2004;* and the *University of Pittsburgh, Pittsburgh, PA – Karen Matthews, PI.*

NIH Program Office: *National Institute on Aging, Bethesda, MD – Chhanda Dutta 2016- present; Winifred Rossi 2012–2016; Sherry Sherman 1994 – 2012; Marcia Ory 1994 – 2001; National Institute of Nursing Research, Bethesda, MD – Program Officers.*

Central Laboratory: *University of Michigan, Ann Arbor – Daniel McConnell* (Central Ligand Assay Satellite Services).

SWAN Repository: *University of Michigan, Ann Arbor – Siobán Harlow 2013 - Present; Dan McConnell 2011 - 2013; MaryFran Sowers 2000 – 2011.*

Coordinating Center: *University of Pittsburgh, Pittsburgh, PA – Maria Mori Brooks, PI 2012 - present; Kim Sutton-Tyrrell, PI 2001 – 2012; New England Research Institutes, Watertown, MA - Sonja McKinlay, PI 1995 – 2001.*

Steering Committee: Susan Johnson, Current Chair; Chris Gallagher, Former Chair

We thank the study staff at each site and all the women who participated in SWAN.

REFERENCES

1. Vollman RF. The degree of variability of the length of the menstrual cycle in correlation with age of woman. Gynaecologia 1956;142:310–4.

2. Treloar AE, Boynton RE, Behn BG, et al. Variation of the human menstrual cycle through reproductive life. Int J Fertil 1067;12:77–120.
3. Wallace RB, Sherman BM, Bean JA, et al. Probability of menopause with increasing duration of amenorrhea in middle-aged women. Am J Obstet Gynecol 1979;135:1021–4.
4. Sowers M, Crawford S, Sternfeld B, et al. SWAN: a multicenter, multiethnic, community-based cohort study of women and the MT. In: Lobo RA, Kelsey J, Marcus R, editors. Menopause: biology and pathobiology. San Diego (CA): Academic Press; 2000. p. 175–88.
5. McKinlay SM, Brambilla DJ, Posner JG. The normal menopause transition. Am J Hum Biol 1992;4:37–46.
6. Szoeke C, Coulson M, Campbell S, Dennerstein L and the WHAP Investigators. Cohort profile: women's healthy ageing project (WHAP)—a longitudinal prospective study of Australian women since 1990. Womens Midlife Health 2016;2:5.
7. Woods NF, Mitchell ES. The Seattle Midlife Women's Health Study: a longitudinal prospective study of women during the MT and early postmenopause. Womens Midlife Health 2016;2:6.
8. Freeman E, Sammel MD. Methods in a longitudinal cohort study of late reproductive age women: the Penn Ovarian Aging Study (POAS). Womens Midlife Health 2016;2:1.
9. Taffe JR, Dennerstein L. Menstrual patterns leading to the final menstrual period. Menopause 2002;9:32–40.
10. Treloar AE. Menstrual cyclicity and the pre-menopause. Maturitas 1981;3:249–64.
11. Soules MR, Sherman S, Parrott E, et al. Executive summary: stages of reproductive aging workshop (STRAW). Fertil Steril 2001;76:874–8.
12. Harlow SD, Crawford S, Dennerstein L, et al. Recommendations from a multi-study evaluation of proposed criteria for staging reproductive aging. Climacteric 2007;10:112–9.
13. Harlow SD, Gass M, Hall JE, et al. Executive summary of the stages of reproductive aging workshop + 10: addressing the unfinished agenda of staging reproductive aging. J Clin Endocrinol Metab 2012;97:1159–68.
14. Harlow SD, Gass M, Hall JE, et al. Executive summary of the stages of reproductive aging workshop + 10: addressing the unfinished agenda of staging reproductive aging. Menopause 2012;19:387–95.
15. Harlow SD, Gass M, Hall JE, et al. Executive summary of the stages of reproductive aging workshop + 10: addressing the unfinished agenda of staging reproductive aging. Fertil Steril 2012;97:843–51.
16. Harlow SD, Gass M, Hall JE, et al. Executive summary of the stages of reproductive aging workshop + 10: addressing the unfinished agenda of staging reproductive aging. Climacteric 2012;15:105–14.
17. Mitchell ES, Woods NF, Mariella A. Three stages of the MT from the Seattle Midlife Women's Health Study: toward a more precise definition. Menopause 2000;7:334–49.
18. Harlow SD, Mitchell ES, Crawford S, et al. The ReSTAGE collaboration: defining optimal bleeding criteria for onset of early MT. Fertil Steril 2008;89:129–40.
19. Randolph JF Jr, Zheng H, Sowers MR, et al. Change in follicle-stimulating hormone and estradiol across the MT: effect of age at the final menstrual period. J Clin Endocrinol Metab 2011;96:746–54.
20. Sowers MR, Zheng H, McConnell D, et al. Follicle stimulating hormone and its rate of change in defining menopause transition stages. J Clin Endocrinol Metab 2008;93:3958–64.

21. Burger HG, Hale GE, Dennerstein L, et al. Cycle and hormone changes during perimenopause: the key role of ovarian function. Menopause 2008;15:603–12.

22. Hale GE, Zhao X, Hughes CL, et al. Endocrine features of menstrual cycles in middle and late reproductive age and the MT classified according to the Staging of Reproductive Aging Workshop (STRAW) staging system. J Clin Endocrinol Metab 2007;92:3060–7.

23. Landgren BM, Collins A, Csemiczky G, et al. Menopause transition: annual changes in serum hormonal patterns over the menstrual cycle in women during a nine-year period prior to menopause. J Clin Endocrinol Metab 2004;89:2763–9.

24. Sowers MR, Eyvazzadeh AD, McConnell D, et al. Anti-Mullerian hormone and inhibin B in the definition of ovarian aging and the menopause transition. J Clin Endocrinol Metab 2008;03:3178–83.

25. Burger HG, Dudley E, Mamers P, et al. Early follicular phase serum FSH as a function of age: the roles of inhibin B, inhibin A and estradiol. Climacteric 2000;3: 17–24.

26. Robertson DM. Anti-Mullerian hormone as a marker of ovarian reserve: an update. Womens Health (Lond) 2008;4:137–41.

27. Brambilla DJ, McKinlay SM, Johannes CB. Defining the perimenopause for application in epidemiologic investigations. Am J Epidemiol 1994;140:1091–5.

28. Lisabeth LD, Harlow SD, Gillespie B, et al. Staging reproductive aging: a comparison of proposed bleeding criteria for the MT. Menopause 2004;11:186–97.

29. Harlow SD, Cain K, Crawford S, et al. Evaluation of four proposed bleeding criteria for the onset of late MT. J Clin Endocrinol Metab 2006;91:3432–8.

30. Randolph JF Jr, Crawford S, Dennerstein L, et al. The value of follicle-stimulating hormone concentration and clinical findings as markers of the late menopausal transition. J Clin Endocrinol Metab 2006;91:3034–40.

31. Taffe JR, Cain KC, Mitchell ES, et al. "Persistence" improves the 60-day amenorrhea marker of entry to late-stage MT for women aged 40 to 44 years. Menopause 2010;17:191–3.

32. Johnson BD, Merz CN, Braunstein GD, et al. Determination of menopausal status in women: the NHLBI-sponsored Women's Ischemia Syndrome Evaluation (WISE) Study. J Womens Health (Larchmt) 2004;13:872–87.

33. Hudecova M, Holte J, Olovsson M, et al. Long-term follow-up of patients with polycystic ovary syndrome: reproductive outcome and ovarian reserve. Hum Reprod 2009;24:1176–83.

34. Tehrani FR, Solaymani-Dodaran M, Hedayati M, et al. Is polycystic ovary syndrome an exception for reproductive aging? Hum Reprod 2010;25:1775–81.

35. Santoro N, Arnsten JH, Buono D, et al. Impact of street drug use, HIV infection, and highly active antiretroviral therapy on reproductive hormones in middle-aged women. J Womens Health (Larchmt) 2005;14:898–905.

36. Santoro N, Lo Y, Moskaleva G, et al. Factors affecting reproductive hormones in HIV-infected, substance-using middle-aged women. Menopause 2007;14: 859–65.

37. Su HI, Sammel MD, Green J, et al. Antimullerian hormone and inhibin B are hormone measures of ovarian function in late reproductive-aged breast cancer survivors. Cancer 2010;116:592–9.

38. Su HI, Sammel MD, Velders L, et al. Association of cyclophosphamide drug-metabolizing enzyme polymorphisms and chemotherapy-related ovarian failure in breast cancer survivors. Fertil Steril 2009;94:645–54.

39. Sukumvanich P, Case LD, Van Zee K, et al. Incidence and time course of bleeding after long-term amenorrhoa after breast cancer treatment: a prospective study. Cancer 2010;116:3102–11.

40. Sjalander A, Friberg B, Svensson P, et al. Menorrhagia and minor bleeding symptoms in women on oral anticoagulation. J Thromb Thrombolysis 2007;24:39–41.

41. Lisabeth L, Harlow S, Qaqish B. A new statistical approach demonstrated menstrual patterns during the MT did not vary by age at menopause. J Clin Epidemiol 2004;57:484–96.

42. den Tonkelaar I, te Velde ER, Looman CW. Menstrual cycle length preceding menopause in relation to age at menopause. Maturitas 1998;29:115–23.

43. Seltzer VL, Benjamin F, Deutsch S. Perimenopausal bleeding patterns and pathologic findings. J Am Med Womens Assoc 1990;45:132–4.

44. Mansfield PK, Carey M, Anderson A, et al. Staging the MT: data from the TREMIN research program on women's health. Womens Health Issues 2004;14:220–6.

45. Gorrindo T, Lu Y, Pincus S, et al. Lifelong menstrual histories are typically erratic and trending: a taxonomy. Menopause 2007;14:74–88.

46. Metcalf MG. Incidence of ovulatory cycles in women approaching the menopause. J Biosoc Sci 1979;11:39–48.

47. Van Voorhis BJ, Santoro N, Harlow S, et al. The relationship of bleeding patterns to daily reproductive hormones in women approaching menopause. Obstet Gynecol 2008;112:101–8.

48. Santoro N, Crawford SL, El Khoudary SR, et al. Menstrual cycle hormone changes in women traversing menopause: study of women's health across the nation. J Clin Endocrinol Metab 2017;102:2218–29.

49. Paramsothy P, Harlow SD, Elliott MR, et al. Influence of race/ethnicity, body mass index, and proximity of menopause on menstrual cycle patterns in the MT: the Study of Women's Health Across the Nation. Menopause 2015;22:159–65.

50. Johannes CB, Crawford SL, Longcope C, et al. Bleeding patterns and changes in the perimenopause: a longitudinal characterization of menstrual cycles. Clinical Consultations in Obstetrics and Gynecology 1996;8(1):9–20.

51. Ballinger CB, Browning MC, Smith AH. Hormone profiles and psychological symptoms in peri-menopausal women. Maturitas 1987;9:235–51.

52. Hale GE, Manconi F, Luscombe G, et al. Quantitative measurements of menstrual blood loss in ovulatory and anovulatory cycles in middle- and late-reproductive age and the MT. Obstet Gynecol 2010;115:249–56.

53. Mitchell ES, Woods NF. Symptom experiences of midlife women: observations from the Seattle Midlife Women's Health Study. Maturitas 1996;25:1–10.

54. Hallberg L, Hogdahl AM, Nilsson L, et al. Menstrual blood loss: a population study. Variation at different ages and attempts to define normality. Acta Obstet Gynecol Scand 1966;45:320–51.

55. Astrup K, Olivarius Nde F, Moller S, et al. Menstrual bleeding patterns in pre- and perimenopausal women: a population-based prospective diary study. Acta Obstet Gynecol Scand 2004;83:197–202.

56. Dasharathy SS, Mumford SL, Pollack AZ, et al. Menstrual bleeding patterns among regularly menstruating women. Am J Epidemiol 2012;175(6):536–45.

57. Fraser IS, Critchley HO, Broder M, et al. The FIGO recommendations on terminologies and definitions for normal and abnormal uterine bleeding. Semin Reprod Med 2011;29:383–90.

58. Munro MG, Critchley HO, Fraser IS. The FIGO systems for nomenclature and classification of causes of abnormal uterine bleeding in the reproductive years: who needs them? Am J Obstet Gynecol 2012;207:259–65.

59. Paramsothy P, Harlow SD, Greendale GA, et al. Bleeding patterns during the MT in the multi-ethnic Study of Women's Health Across the Nation (SWAN): a prospective cohort study. BJOG 2014;121:1564–73.
60. Z1 Liu, Doan QV, Blumenthal P, et al. A systematic review evaluating health-related quality of life, work impairment, and health-care costs and utilization in abnormal uterine bleeding. Value Health 2007;10:183–94.
61. Fraser IS, Mansour D, Breymann C, et al. Prevalence of heavy menstrual bleeding and experiences of affected women in a European patient survey. Int J Gynaecol Obstet 2015;128:196–200.
62. Santer M, Warner P, Wykec SA. Scottish postal survey suggested that the prevailing clinical preoccupation with heavy periods does not reflect the epidemiology of reported symptoms and problems. J Clin Epidemiol 2005;58:1206–10.
63. Santos IS, Minten GC, Valle NC, et al. Menstrual bleeding patterns: a community-based cross-sectional study among women aged 18-45 years in Southern Brazil. BMC Womens Health 2011;11:26.
64. Rezk M, Masood A, Dawood R. Perimenopausal bleeding: patterns, pathology, response to progestins and clinical outcome. J Obstet Gynaecol 2015;35:517–21.
65. Goldstein SR. Modern evaluation of the endometrium. Obstet Gynecol 2010;116:168–76.
66. Paramsothy P, Harlow SD, Nan B. Duration of the MT is longer in women with young age at onset: the multiethnic Study of Women's Health Across the Nation. Menopause 2017;24:142–9.
67. Huang X, Harlow SD, Elliott MR. Distinguishing six population subgroups by timing of and bleeding patterns during the MT. Am J Epidemiol 2012;175:74–83.
68. Wise LA, Krieger N, Zierler S, et al. Lifetime socioeconomic position in relation to onset of perimenopause. J Epidemiol Community Health 2002;56:851–60.
69. Sammel MD, Freeman EW, Liu Z, et al. Factors that influence entry into stages of the MT. Menopause 2009;16:1218–27.
70. Harlow SD, Campbell B. Ethnic differences in the duration and amount of menstrual bleeding during the postmenarcheal period. Am J Epidemiol 1996;144:980–8.
71. Harlow SD, Campbell B, Lin X, et al. Ethnic differences in the length of the menstrual cycle during the postmenarcheal period. Am J Epidemiol 1997;146:572–80.
72. Liu Y, Gold EB, Lasley BL, et al. Factors affecting menstrual cycle characteristics. Am J Epidemiol 2004;160:131–40.
73. Waller K, Swan SH, Windham GC, et al. Use of urine biomarkers to evaluate menstrual function in healthy premenopausal women. Am J Epidemiol 1998;147:1071–80.
74. Cooper GS, Sandler DP, Whelan EA, et al. Association of physical and behavioral characteristics with menstrual cycle patterns in women age 29–31 years. Epidemiology 1996;7:624–8.
75. Symons JP, Sowers MF, Harlow SD. Relationship of body composition measures and menstrual cycle length. Ann Hum Biol 1997;24:107–16.
76. Harlow SD, Matanoski GM. The association between weight, physical activity, and stress and variation in the length of the menstrual cycle. Am J Epidemiol 1991;133:38–49.
77. Rowland AS, Baird DD, Long S, et al. Influence of medical conditions and lifestyle factors on the menstrual cycle. Epidemiology 2002;13:668–74.

78. Harlow SD, Campbell BC. Host factors that influence the duration of menstrual blooding. Epidemiology 1994,5.352–5.
79. Cooper GS, Klebanoff MA, Promislow J, et al. Polychlorinated biphenyls and menstrual cycle characteristics. Epidemiology 2005;16:191–200.
80. Belsey EM, d'Arcangues C, Carlson N. Determinants of menstrual bleeding patterns among women using natural and hormonal methods of contraception. II. The influence of individual characteristics. Contraception 1988;38:243–57.
81. Sternfeld B, Jacobs MK, Quesenberry CP Jr, et al. Physical activity and menstrual cycle characteristics in two prospective cohorts. Am J Epidemiol 2002;156: 402–9.
82. Santoro N, Lasley B, McConnell D, et al. Body size and ethnicity are associated with menstrual cycle alterations in women in the early MT: the Study of Women's Health across the Nation (SWAN) Daily Hormone Study. J Clin Endocrinol Metab 2004;89:2622–31.
83. Santoro N, Brockwell S, Johnston J, et al. Helping midlife women predict the onset of the final menses: SWAN, the Study of Women's Health Across the Nation. Menopause 2007;14:415–24.
84. Gold EB, Bromberger J, Crawford S, et al. Factors associated with age at natural menopause in a multiethnic sample of midlife women. Am J Epidemiol 2001;153: 865–74.
85. Kato I, Toniolo P, Koenig KL, et al. Epidemiologic correlates with menstrual cycle length in middle aged women. Eur J Epidemiol 1999;15:809–14.
86. Windham GC, Elkin EP, Swan SH, et al. Cigarette smoking and effects on menstrual function. Obstet Gynecol 1999;93:59–65.
87. Hornsby PP, Wilcox AJ, Weinberg CR. Cigarette smoking and disturbance of menstrual function. Epidemiology 1998;9:193–8.
88. Dorman JS, Steenkiste AR, Foley TP, et al. Menopause in type 1 diabetic women: is it premature? Diabetes 2001;50:1857–62.
89. Luborsky JL, Meyer P, Sowers MF, et al. Premature menopause in a multi-ethnic population study of the menopause transition. Hum Reprod 2003;18:199–206.
90. Strotmeyer ES, Steenkiste AR, Foley TP Jr, et al. Menstrual cycle differences between women with type 1 diabetes and women without diabetes. Diabetes Care 2003;26:1016–21.
91. Wellons MF, Matthews JJ, Kim C. Ovarian aging in women with diabetes: an overview. Maturitas 2017;96:109–13.
92. Benson RC, Dailey ME. The menstrual pattern in hyperthyroidism and subsequent posttherapy hypothyroidism. Surg Gynecol Obstet 1955;100:19–26.
93. Sowers M, Luborsky J, Perdue C, et al. Thyroid stimulating hormone (TSH) concentrations and menopausal status in women at the mid-life: SWAN. Clin Endocrinol (Oxf) 2003;58:340–7.
94. DeWaay DJ, Syrop CH, Nygaard IE, et al. Natural history of uterine polyps and leiomyomata. Obstet Gynecol 2002;100:3–7.
95. Marino JL, Eskenazi B, Warner M, et al. Uterine leiomyoma and menstrual cycle characteristics in a population-based cohort study. Hum Reprod 2004;19: 2350–5.
96. Wegienka G, Baird DD, Hertz-Picciotto I, et al. Self-reported heavy bleeding associated with uterine leiomyomata. Obstet Gynecol 2003;101:431–7.

Menstrual Cycle Hormone Changes Associated with Reproductive Aging and How They May Relate to Symptoms

Amanda Allshouse, MS[a], Jelena Pavlovic, MD, PhD[b],
Nanette Santoro, MD[c],*

KEYWORDS

- Reproductive aging • Perimenopause • Gonadotropins • Folliculogenesis

KEY POINTS

- As opposed to midreproductive life, perimenopausal cycles have less predictable physiologic features such as ovulation, and more variability in reproductive hormones over time.
- Intensive, longitudinal study designs provide the clearest picture of the transition, but not all women seen by clinicians are represented in these samples.
- Symptoms such as headache and trouble sleeping vary across the menstrual cycle, but others, such as hot flashes, are related to increased longer-term hormone variability.

INTRODUCTION

For most women, the unpredictable menstrual and hormonal events of the perimenopause follow decades of predictable cycles and hormone patterns. By a median age of 47 years, both the outward evidence of "normal" reproductive function—a menstrual period every 25 to 35 days—and the internal hormonal milieu begin to demonstrate marked variability.[1] These changes cause disruption, which can be emotional/psychological, or can involve more somatic symptoms that are related to specific hormonal events or patterns. This article reviews the hormonal changes within menstrual cycles and discusses within and between-cycle individual hormonal patterns that relate to changes in sleep, mood, and headache.

Disclosure Statement: Dr N. Santoro is a consultant for Ogeda/Astellas Pharmaceuticals and has stock options with Menogenix, Inc.

[a] Department of Biostatistics, Colorado School of Public Health, 13001 E 17th Place, Aurora, CO 80045, USA; [b] Department of Neurology, Albert Einstein College of Medicine, 1300 Morris Park Avenue, Bronx, NY 10461, USA; [c] Department of Obstetrics and Gynecology, University of Colorado School of Medicine, 12631 East 17th Avenue, Mail Stop B-198, Aurora, CO 80045, USA
* Corresponding author.
E-mail address: Nanette.Santoro@ucdenver.edu

Obstet Gynecol Clin N Am 45 (2018) 613–628
https://doi.org/10.1016/j.ogc.2018.07.004
0889-8545/18/© 2018 Elsevier Inc. All rights reserved.

obgyn.theclinics.com

STUDYING SEX HORMONES DURING THE MENOPAUSAL TRANSITION
Types of Studies

Challenges in studying sex hormones in perimenopausal women include study design, measurement, participant burden, and incomplete knowledge around theoretic models, time, money, and complexities of statistical analysis. As such, large-scale efforts to characterize hormones in the research setting are infrequent. Studies that are interview/survey only without biological sampling can describe what women are experiencing, thinking, or feeling, but preclude linking that information to mechanistic evidence about hormonal levels or changes that are part of the experience. Designs that include one instance of biologic sampling allow for a snapshot of hormones and symptoms and their correlation. Sampling of women annually or at other intervals allows for a within-person picture of a trend over time. Both cross-sectional and longitudinal biospecimen sampling must indicate the phase of a menstrual cycle during which the sampling occurred, and this must be consistent for all women in the study protocol. Daily biologic sampling for an entire menstrual cycle allows for the fullest description of sex hormones. Herein the authors discuss major contributing design features of studies that have informed the current knowledge of sex hormones during the years preceding menopause.

Longitudinal Biologic Sampling

A longitudinal study design includes the same person at multiple points over time. The Rotterdam study (described in later discussion) enrolled multiple cohorts over time, so although all participants are followed longitudinally, some participants have been followed longer than others. In contrast, in a cross-sectional study, information from each participant is obtained only once. Although cross-sectional studies are easier to operationalize and analyze, the data from such a study would not be useful in the study of sex hormones among women approaching menopause for several reasons. Sex hormones change within a person more consistently than across women: if averaging across women, the change over time could be obscured by between-women differences. In order to characterize a biologic sample measured on (for instance) the fourth to sixth day of a menstrual cycle by how far it precedes the final menstrual period (FMP), longitudinal follow-up is required, because it is not yet possible to know the time to FMP until a year after it has happened. Chronologic age cannot substitute for reproductive age, because women reach menopause at different ages.

A commonly used way to characterize sex hormone change over time can be achieved with annual sampling of the same woman. Annual serum sampling per study protocol occurs early in the follicular phase for each study described. This timing will miss the large midcycle spikes in estradiol, luteinizing hormone (LH), and follicle-stimulating hormone (FSH) that prompt ovulation. Sampling during the luteal phase of the cycle would be challenging to coordinate, because timing would require knowledge of when ovulation occurred, a far less obvious event than the start of a menstrual cycle. Luteal phase biologic sampling is necessary, however, to reliably characterize events like progesterone production, and the secondary estrogen surge.

Longitudinal biologic sampling is essential for full-cycle characterization of hormones measured in urine, such as in the Study of Women's Health Across the Nation (SWAN) Daily Hormone Study (DHS, described in later discussion). The steepness with which hormones rise and fall can only be characterized when biologic sampling is obtained every day from the same woman during one cycle. How to best characterize hormones within a cycle is an evolving area of research (eg, whole-cycle average, absolute peak, difference between peak and trough, percent change in days following peak). Characterizing (or parameterizing) sex hormones in a clinically meaningful manner requires pairing with other health information from the same individual, because the DHS, which included a daily diary during the month urine was collected, allowed researchers to do so.

Statistical analysis of data collected in a longitudinal study can be carried out using only one observation per person. To fully use the longitudinal nature of the data, sophisticated statistical methods are required; consideration of the impact of missing data due to dropout or other reasons is critical.

Longitudinal, Epidemiologic Studies of Reproductive Hormones Across the Menopause Transition

In the 1960s and 1970s, clinicians were informed by their experience in practice, rather than population-based data, which was not yet available. By the 1980s, available studies of midlife women largely focused on alleviating symptoms rather than cultivating an understanding of the in vivo patterns and mechanisms of reproductive aging.[2] Methodological problems common to many, but not all, of these studies included an absence of baseline data, retrospective reporting, absent or inaccurate measurement of endogenous hormones, absence of appropriate control groups for studies of hormone therapy, and lack of diversity of study participants.[2]

The Rotterdam Study

The Rotterdam Study began in 1990 as a prospective study of men and women to determine causes of late-life diseases.[3] Recruitment occurred in 4 phases: 1990, 2000 (both of age 55 and older), and 2006 (age 45–54); by 2008, 14,926 persons were included. In 2016, a new cohort was added of persons aged 40 to 55, with plans to enroll an additional 4000 by 2019. Additional inclusion criteria included residence in particular districts within the Netherlands. As part of the genomics, biomarker, and microbiome studies, biological samples have been banked. As part of a Reproductive Traits study, age at menopause and sex hormones measured in serum will be investigated for their impact on health later in life. The Rotterdam Study remains open and revisits participants in all cohorts around every 4 to 5 years.

The Melbourne Women's Midlife Health Project

Melbourne was a community-based study of Australian-born women, started in 1991, with 9 years of annual interviews of participants aged 45 to 55 at enrollment, all of whom had menstruated in the previous 3 months and were not using hormone therapy.[4] This study was the first to follow women annually, establish patterns of change in cardinal reproductive hormones (FSH, estradiol, inhibins A and B, sex hormone binding globulin, testosterone, free testosterone index, and dehydroepiandrosterone), and to link them to symptoms. Of the 438 women initially enrolled, 88% were retained in the ninth year; only 8% were not yet menopausal at the end of follow-up. Blood was sampled between days 4 and 8 of the menstrual cycle to standardize them to the follicular phase of the menstrual cycle, and other measures included interviews, menstrual calendars, quality of life, and measures of bone density.

The Seattle Midlife Women's Health Study

The Seattle Midlife Women's Health Study began enrollment in 1990 and was designed to illuminate women's symptom experience during the menopausal transition.[5] In its second and third phases, a urinary hormone assay component was included. The Seattle study was community based, screening 1428 women and following 390 longitudinally in all phases. Age upon enrollment was 35 to 55 years, and follow-up continued for 23 years. For a subset, first morning voided urine was collected on the sixth day of the cycle (follicular phase) at monthly intervals between July 1996 and 2001, quarterly between 2001 and 2005, and annually through 2006. Urine was assayed for estrone glucuronide, the chief urinary metabolite of estradiol, FSH, total testosterone, cortisol, epinephrine, and norepinephrine (NE). Other measures included yearly health questionnaires, health diaries, menstrual calendars, and buccal smears. Follow-up for each participant ended up to 5 years after menopause, with 2013 the final year of follow-up for the study.

The Penn Ovarian Aging Study

The Penn Ovarian Aging Study (POAS)[6] is a longitudinal cohort study of women recruited in Philadelphia County, Pennsylvania. Eligible women had at least one ovary, a uterus, at least one menstrual period within the previous 3 months, a cycle duration of 22 to 35 days, and age between 35 and 47 years. Exclusions included some medications, medical conditions that might affect hormones, pregnancy, or non-English fluency. Of 1426 women aged 35 to 47 screened, 436 of 578 eligible were enrolled over 18 months in 1996 and 1997. Enrolled women were of either black or white race. Blood samples were collected in the early follicular phase of the menstrual cycle (days 2–6) during all 28 study visits over 14 years, spaced as 2 visits one menstrual cycle apart, occurring every 9 months for the first 5 years of the study and then annually for years 6 to 15. After 14 years of follow-up, 67% of participants remained active. Phone-only interviews were done in years 15 to 17, with a full follow-up in year 18 (final year). A unique feature of the POAS design is back-to-back monthly samples, and 9-month spacing of the paired visits in the first 5 years.

The Study of Women's Health Across the Nation and the Daily Hormone Study

SWAN[7] used a prospective, multicenter design, initiated to characterize the natural history of the menopausal transition. A screening interview of 16,065 US women during 1995 to 1996 constituted the sampling frame for the longitudinal study. Sites in Pittsburgh, Pennsylvania, Boston, Massachusetts, Detroit, Michigan area, Chicago, Illinois, Los Angeles, California, Oakland, California area, and Newark, New Jersey recruited women of black and white races, and Japanese, Chinese, and Hispanic ethnicities.[8] Upon enrollment, women were aged 40 to 55 years; follow-up is ongoing. SWAN's design allows for investigation of race/ethnicity-, culture-, or geographic region-based differences, or adjustment for these characteristics in other analyses. Sex hormones are available from serum drawn during annual visits. Timing of the fasting blood draw was targeted to the early follicular phase (days 2–5 after menses) among menstruating women, and within 90 days of baseline examination date anniversary.

The DHS included a subset of SWAN participants, with the first DHS visit coinciding with approximately the first annual SWAN follow-up. Eight hundred forty-eight women completed the first DHS visit. Women collected a daily, first-morning-void urine beginning with the start of one menstrual cycle and stopping with onset of the subsequent cycle (or after 50 days in the absence of a second cycle). During collection, a daily diary was used to record mood and menopausal symptoms, and a follicular phase blood draw after the menstrual period that ended the urine collection was done. DHS visits were offset from SWAN visits by half a year: there would be 2 instances of a blood draw from these women in each year of dual-participation, in addition to the urine samples from the DHS. The DHS was designed to continue for up to 10 years, or for a fixed number of days 1 year after the FMP, whichever came first. Whole cycle hormones allow for characterization of a cycle in terms of the timing of presumed ovulation,[9] and parameters within a cycle indicating longer-term patterns of hormonal change.[10]

Limitations of Studies Performed to Date

Exclusions

With the exception of the Rotterdam Study, which does not seek to characterize cycle patterns, all of the studies described above excluded women who did not have at least somewhat regular menstrual cycles. Although this design feature is essential to allow investigators to define the FMP, it eliminates women with irregular or absent menses. Polycystic ovary syndrome (PCOS) is prevalent in up to 20% of women[11] and is diagnosed in part by irregular menses. Treatment of PCOS can involve birth control pills, which is an exclusion criterion for the studies presented herein. Among women aged 35 to 45 years, an estimated 11% have undergone a hysterectomy.[12] Functional hypothalamic amenorrhea[13] is another cause of secondary amenorrhea, present in about 5% of adult women. Premature ovarian failure or insufficiency, the loss of ovarian function before age 40, is found in 1% of adult women.[14] Pregnancy and lactation were also exclusions for most studies, but this likely had a minor impact, as only 0.2% of women between ages 40 and 44 gave birth in 2012.[15] Approximately 11% of women in the United States between ages 40 and 44 use hormonal contraception.[16] Taken together, potentially more than a third of adult women have not contributed data to studies of the menopausal transition to date. It is important to keep this in mind when interpreting the data and applying it to patient care.

Geographic considerations

The Rotterdam, Melbourne, Seattle, and Penn studies included women living in or near the eponymous region. SWAN intentionally expanded and overrecruited multiple underrepresented races and ethnicities in multiple locations. However, the southeast and southwest United States have been missing from all studies, namely Alabama, Arizona, Arkansas, Georgia, Florida, Kentucky, Louisiana, Mississippi, New Mexico, North Carolina, Oklahoma, South Carolina, Tennessee, Texas, Virginia, and West Virginia. As these regions of the country have different weather patterns, cultures, and structures, unmeasured regional differences in hormonal patterns could exist among women who live and are traversing menopause there.

Respondent burden

Collection of urine, completion of lengthy questionnaires, allowing research staff to swab for samples, disclosing personal information, and repeating this process year after year is burdensome for participants. Although the most frequent sampling possible would be ideal for precision of estimation, the less frequently a participant is contacted, the less burdensome their participation, and the more likely they will continue. Ethnic and racial minorities are frequently overrecruited for studies, thereby burdening this population for research more so than their counterparts of white race. Very detailed protocols such as the DHS, in tandem with its parent study, SWAN, could theoretically be used to determine the optimal frequency of sampling to ensure precision while minimizing respondent burden.

In summary, features of what would characterize a gold-standard study of hormones include prospective, longitudinal design, diversity of the cohort, multiple visits in a year, herculean efforts to maximize retention, full-cycle characterization of hormones within a woman, and extensive biological sampling. The DHS is a high-quality source of complete hormone characterization during the final years of reproductive function; however, like most studies designed to characterize midlife women, its strict exclusion criteria precluded a substantial portion of women from participating. As such, and as should be the case with any study, care should be taken in extrapolating results to the appropriate population.

CHANGES IN MENSTRUAL CYCLE PATTERNS AND HORMONES WITH PROGRESSION TO MENOPAUSE

As women age, the follicle cohort shrinks along with the decline in the total oocyte pool[17] (see Molly M. Quinn and Marcelle I. Cedars' article, "Declining Fertility with Reproductive Aging: How to Protect Your Patient's Fertility by Knowing the Milestones," and Clarisa R. Gracia and Ellen W. Freeman's article, "Onset of the Menopause Transition: The Earliest Signs and Symptoms," and Siobán D. Harlow's article, "Menstrual Cycle Changes as Women Approach the Final Menses: What Matters?," in this issue for more detail). Briefly, anti-Müllerian hormone (AMH), a stable product of very small, but growing follicles that reflect the available remaining follicle complement most accurately, declines throughout reproductive life.[18] The decline in AMH may directly release ovarian follicles from inhibition, allowing the less responsive follicles in the ovary to activate and to maintain the ovulatory capacity of the human menstrual cycle in the face of ever-dwindling gametes. Inhibin B, which is produced by later-stage, growing follicles, also declines with reproductive aging, reflecting the reduced follicle cohort size over time. Secondary to these ovarian changes, FSH increases,[19] especially in the early follicular phase.[20] This increase in FSH appears necessary to maintain normal folliculogenesis because the remaining follicles have a higher threshold for activation and stimulation. Finally, ultrasound assessment of small, antral follicles 2 to 9 mm in size (antral follicle count) also provides a measure of ovarian reserve.[21] The process of follicle loss is initially compensated by lower AMH and inhibin B and intermittently rising FSH (STRAW-2: the early transition) and then becomes intermittently uncompensated (STRAW-1, the late transition), until follicle exhaustion is complete at menopause (STRAW stage 0).[1] Investigators from the POAS identified a stage that divides the STRAW Stage-2, the early transition, into a late premenopause (with only one irregular menstrual cycle event) and the early transition (2 or more cycle length changes).[22] Menstrual cycle changes will be briefly reviewed for each of these stages.

The Early Transition (Including Penn Ovarian Aging Study Late Premenopause): Compensated Follicle Failure

This first stage of the menopause transition can be conceptualized as a critical decrease in follicle numbers that causes the first noticeable changes in a woman's menstrual cycle. She then experiences one of 2 events: (a) her cycles become noticeably less regular, or (b) she skips a menstrual cycle, and then resumes her previous pattern. At least a decade of rising FSH and reduced inhibin A and B[23] and AMH precede this event, but these hormonal adjustments are clinically silent, reflecting the compensatory mechanisms invoked to maintain regular cyclicity and potential fertility in the face of follicle loss. These changes are described in **Fig. 1**.

In addition to these changes in circulating hormones, the process of follicle maturation is altered, and there are changes within oocytes. Follicles grow earlier in the cycle than ever before,[24] due to high FSH stimulation, and they grow more rapidly.[25,26] Increased follicular aromatase[27] leads to maintenance of midreproductive, or even higher than midreproductive, estrogen production.[28] Follicle growth becomes dysregulated, in that ovulation occurs earlier in the menstrual cycle[25] and follicle diameter at the time of ovulation is smaller[26] than in midreproductive women's cycles.

Oocytes of reproductively aging women are more prone to meiotic spindle abnormalities[29] and to have a loss of mitochondrial DNA.[30] These deficits likely underlie the propensity for older reproductive aged women to undergo nondisjunction during gametogenesis and to have a greater risk of chromosomal abnormalities in conceived

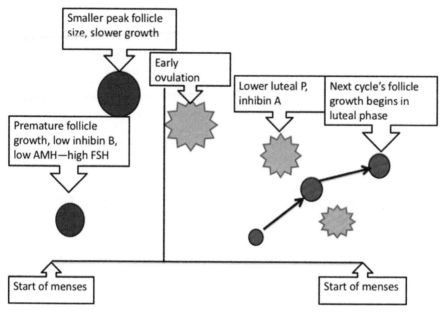

Fig. 1. Summary of the events involved in the "compensated failure" of follicle growth during the menstrual cycle in the early transition. Reduced inhibin B and AMH, reflective of the smaller follicle cohort, remove restraint on follicle activation and growth and allow FSH to increase in the early follicular phase. Elevated FSH and accelerated follicle development lead to earlier ovulation of a smaller follicle. Because the follicle has greater aromatase activity, normal estradiol levels are preserved and may even be higher than midovarian aged women's cycles. The earlier ovulation leads to a greater proportion of the cycle being spent in the luteal phase, and the reduced steroid and protein hormones from the corpus luteum fail to restrain FSH in the luteal phase, leading to recruitment of the next cycle's dominant follicle before menses.

offspring. Whether these defects are correctable is not known, but certainly a topic of active investigation.[31]

The underlying physiologic changes described herein predict a hormonal environment that has more frequent and more variable menstrual periods, more variable hormone production, a lesser likelihood of consistent ovulation, and brief bouts of amenorrhea. Collectively, these changes can destabilize women in several ways.

The Late Transition: Longer Periods of Uncompensated Follicle Failure

As women enter the late transition, they are subject to longer periods of amenorrhea (>60 days). These bouts can contain a variety of patterns of hormone production, but eventually they become more uniformly hypoestrogenic and hypergonadotropic. When cycles do occur, they remain relatively likely to be ovulatory, with robust increases in progesterone production, and therefore potentially fertile.

Menstrual Cycle Patterns Throughout the Transition

The most common type of menstrual cycle observed in women as they transition appears to be an ovulatory cycle. These cycles have evidence of luteal activity (ELA), typically defined as a robust and sustained increase in progesterone or in its metabolite, pregnanediol glucuronide (Pdg), when urinary studies are performed. Cycles that do not have a robust increase in progesterone or Pdg may reflect a failed ovulation, or an inadequate luteal phase. Examples of these cycle types have been described in reproductively aging women.[26] It is important to keep in mind, however, that luteal phase progesterone production occurs across a spectrum, and lesser degrees of progesterone production, even though they might result in a cycle being classified as "anovulatory," may not necessarily reflect a failure of follicle growth and estradiol production. Most studies have not combined hormonal assessments with follicle assessments, and thus, it is impossible to know the sequence of ovarian events. An example of a completely anovulatory cycle accompanied by initially normal follicle growth and a normal menstrual cycle length is provided in **Fig. 2.**

SWAN performed the most comprehensive assessment of menstrual cycles in perimenopausal women to date. In the early phases of the SWAN DHS, the FMP was not known for all participants, and thus cycles could not be organized by proximity to the FMP. However, most cycles (most of which, in retrospect, were from the early transition) had an ovulatory pattern with a robust increase in Pdg (80.9%).[32] As women progressed toward menopause, the amount of Pdg produced in the luteal phase declined,[33] but overall preservation of a robust, ovulatory pattern remained for most participants until about 5 years before the FMP.[34] By the year before the FMP, only 23% of cycles retained this ovulatory pattern. **Fig. 3** indicates the drop off in cycles with an ovulatory pattern as women approached the FMP.

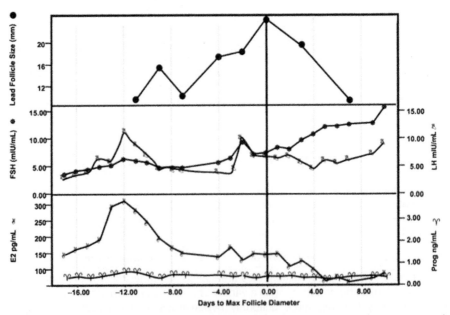

Fig. 2. Follicle growth and estradiol production without ovulation in a perimenopausal woman. The participant had a 28-day intermenstrual interval. Note the early increase in estradiol to 300 pg/mL (1101 nmol/L) without evidence of large follicle growth and no sign of subsequent progesterone production. Peak estradiol production is seen on cycle day 6 (day 12 on the graph), and peak follicle growth to more than 20 mm is apparent by cycle day 18 (day 0 on the graph). (*From* Santoro N, Isaac B, Neal-Perry G, et al. Impaired folliculogenesis and ovulation in older reproductive aged women. J Clin Endocrinol Metab 2003;88(11):5506. By permission of Oxford University Press.)

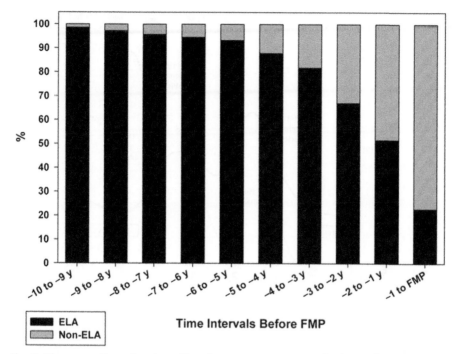

Fig. 3. The proportion of cycles with robust progesterone production, called ELA in the figure, declines as women approach the FMP, but the change is most striking in the latter few years before FMP. (*From* Santoro N, Crawford SL, El Khoudary SR, et al. Menstrual Cycle Hormone Changes in Women Traversing Menopause: Study Of Women's Health Across the Nation. J Clin Endocrinol Metab 2017;102(7):2222. By permission of Oxford University Press.)

The luteal-out-of-phase cycle

Hale and colleagues[35] defined a type of menstrual cycle pattern unique to women in the menopausal transition. The accelerated follicle growth that occurs in older reproductive aged women appears related to abnormally early growth of follicles from the previous luteal phase. The wave of follicles recruited during the luteal phase of the cycle are close to maturation at the time of menses, leading to a very rapid, very early second ovulatory event, hence the name "luteal-out-of-phase" (LOOP) to characterize this cycle type (**Fig. 4**). LOOP events are associated with higher luteal estradiol exposure as well as rapidly successive progesterone excursions.

Cycles without evidence of luteal activity

The non-ELA cycles described in the SWAN DHS[36] do not simply represent cycles without robust estrogen production. Non-ELA cycles may have a robust estrogen increase that mimics nearly exactly the estrogen increase seen in a clearly ovulatory cycle, or there may be an atypically large estrogen increase, or they may be no estrogen production at all. Non-ELA cycles with an estrogen increase may or may not have an accompanying LH surge, and the amount of Pdg produced is variable but insufficient to meet the criteria for an ovulatory cycle. These cycle patterns appear to be associated with differing symptoms. **Table 1** indicates the classification of non-ELA cycles and their associated bleeding patterns. This work is ongoing, and further classifications may emerge.

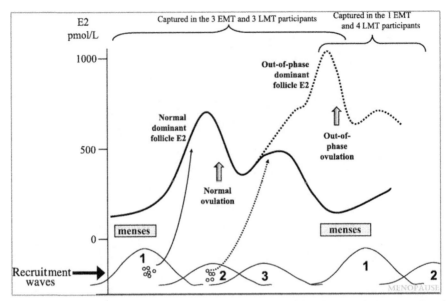

Fig. 4. LOOP cycle and its underlying mechanisms. A wave of follicle growth that is initiated in the prior luteal phase causes very early ovulation immediately after or concurrent with menses from the prior cycle. Higher estradiol levels and rapid reexposure to progesterone result. E2, estradiol. EMT, early menopausal transition; LMT, late menopausal transition. (*From* Hale GE, Hughes CL, Burger HG, et al. Atypical estradiol secretion and ovulation patterns caused by luteal out-of-phase (LOOP) events underlying irregular ovulatory menstrual cycles in the menopausal transition. Menopause 2009;16(1):56; with permission.)

LINKING HORMONES TO SYMPTOMS

The menopausal transition has long been associated with luteal-out-of-phase symptoms, with vasomotor symptoms (VMS) recognized as the cardinal menopausal symptom (see Clarisa R. Gracia and Ellen W. Freeman's article, "Onset of the Menopause Transition: The Earliest Signs and Symptoms," in this issue). Although other symptoms such as mood disorders, sleep disturbances, and headaches have been long recognized to significantly affect quality of life in menopause, their recognition as being specifically related to reproductive hormones during the transition remains controversial. This controversy is due, in part, to a lack of studies targeting midlife women with nonVMS and conflicting methodologies for characterizing reproductive staging. There is also a scarcity of longitudinal studies including both hormone and symptoms data. Many studies relating hormones to changes in symptoms across the menopausal

Table 1
Cycles without luteal activity identified in the Study of Women's Health Across the Nation Daily Hormone Study and their hormonal and expected menstrual correlates

Hormonal Pattern	LH Surge	Pdg Pattern	Bleeding Pattern
Estrogen rise	+	Variable but low	Menses when estrogen falls
Estrogen rise	–	Variable but low	Menses when estrogen falls
No estrogen rise	N/A	None	No menses

Abbreviation: N/A, not applicable.

transition use only a single point of hormone and symptom assessment performed no more than annually. The prevailing hypothesis is that the erratic fluctuations in hormones (estrogen in particular) result in susceptibility to symptoms (mood changes, sleep disturbance, headache) and ultimately syndrome (depression, insomnia, migraine) presentation, but the knowledge of precise hormonal change and resulting biological mechanisms remains limited. The hormone and daily symptom diary data used by the SWAN DHS can provide information on trajectories of both hormonal and symptom changes (hot flashes, mood, headache, and others) across and within women.

Mood

Most women of perimenopausal age endorse symptoms of depression in cross-sectional studies (see Joyce T. Bromberger and C. Neill Epperson's article, "Depression During and After the Perimenopause: Impact of Hormones, Genetics, and Environmental Determinants of Disease," in this issue, for more details on mood and the perimenopause). A 1.5- to 3-fold increased risk of depressive symptoms has been seen in longitudinal studies of menopausal transition.[37] The effects of changing estrogen on perimenopausal mood reflect the prevailing opinion that, as the levels of estrogen vary widely and decline, susceptibility to mood symptoms and major depression increases.[38] Estrogen has long been implicated in the activity of neurotransmitters involved in depressive symptoms, namely serotonin (5-HT) and norepinephrine (NE). Estrogen exerts antidepressant properties by regulating the synthesis, metabolism, and receptor activity of 5-HT and NE. Wider fluctuations in estradiol levels and FSH are associated with worse mood symptoms.[37] Long-term trajectories of mood symptoms have also been examined in SWAN, but day-to-day changes in mood in association with menstrual cycles have not yet been reported.

Four distinct trajectories of depressive symptoms were identified in the Australian Longitudinal Study of Women's Health over a 15-year follow-up, with 80% of women having low scores, 9% with increasing scores, 8.5% with decreasing depression scores, and 2.5% of women with stable high depression scores. A recent study used a mathematical model (latent class analyses) to group women going through the different stages of menopause into one of 6 symptom classes.[39] Women in the highest symptom class (LC1) reported a high intensity of most symptoms, including physical and psychological symptoms such as depression and anxiety, followed by women with moderate intensity of most symptoms (LC2). Lower symptom classes included women with moderate intensity of a subset of symptoms (VMS, pain, fatigue, sleep disturbances, and physical health symptoms), women with numerous milder symptoms (LC3–LC5), and women who were relatively asymptomatic (LC6). In premenopause, 10% of women were classified in LC1, 16% in LC2, 14% in LC3, 26% in LC4, 14% in LC5, and 20% in LC6, and most women remained in the same latent class while transitioning through menopause, further supporting the need to study individual hormonal and symptom fingerprints of women by examining multiple years of follow-up.[40]

Sleep

Poor sleep quality and sleep disruption are frequently observed in the menopause transition[41] and have most typically been attributed to VMS, which have been seen as the primary risk factor for sleep disruption in midlife women[42,43] (see Howard M. Kravitz and colleagues' article, "Sleep, Health, and Metabolism in Midlife Women and Menopause: Food for Thought," in this issue, for more information on sleep and perimenopause). However, fluctuations in hormones have been associated with sleep disturbance during the menopausal transition independent of VMS, suggesting that not all perimenopausal sleep disturbances are explained by night sweats and that menopausal transition–related hormonal changes can independently lead to sleep disturbance.[44–46] When day-to-day menstrual cycle hormones were assessed along with daily self-reported trouble sleeping, the periovulatory phase of the cycle was associated with the least trouble sleeping.[42] This implies that daily hormonal exposures influence sleep. Independent of VMS, night-time awakenings and difficulty falling and staying asleep during the menopausal transition and after menopause have been associated with lower estradiol.[41,47] Difficulty falling asleep and remaining asleep has been associated with higher levels of FSH,[48] and more rapidly increasing levels of FSH.[41] In contrast to SWAN, there was no consistent change in estradiol, testosterone, and FSH in relation to sleep disruption in the POAS cohort.[49]

Headaches and Pain

Pain symptoms are generally perceived as a common symptom of aging and not specifically transition related, although women are at greater risk for developing pain disorders and exhibit greater sensitivity to noxious stimuli compared with men. Past studies suggest that perimenopause is associated with increased prevalence of some pain disorders, such as headache,[50,51] and musculoskeletal pain[52]; however, the effect of the stage of the menopausal transition on the frequency of subjective pain complaints has not been completely explored. Postmenopausal women report greater musculoskeletal pain than premenopausal women,[52] but this was a study limited to a single annual follow-up and based on a one-time retrospective assessment of musculoskeletal pain complaints over the prior 4 weeks, rather than a daily, prospective assessment. Bodily pain (aches, joint pain, and stiffness) have been associated with estradiol variability in the POAS.[53] In contrast, joint pain and back pain were not associated with urinary levels of estrone or FSH in the Seattle Midlife Women's Health Study.[54]

Although migraine headache has long been recognized to be hormonally regulated in women, no study to date has focused on specific sex hormone changes over the menopausal transition. Overall, stable and increasing estrogen levels, such as seen in pregnancy, have been associated with fewer attacks of migraine, while rapidly changing estrogen levels such as seen in perimenopause have been associated with more frequent migraine attacks. Migraine affects close to a quarter of perimenopausal aged women and is a priority for further study using adequate methodology. The SWAN DHS substudy has been the only study to date to compare within-woman change in hormones in migraineurs compared with controls. Women with history of migraine had a faster urinary E1c decline over the 2 days following the luteal peak than controls; this finding was independent of headache occurrence in the cycle of study, suggesting an endogenous difference in estrogen processing in women with migraine as compared with women without history of migraine.[10] DHS data are currently being used to further examine the day-to-day occurrence of headache in relation to daily hormone changes in women with migraine.

SUMMARY

Current data from several longitudinal studies of perimenopausal women are being used to describe how reproductive hormone change over time affects women's symptom experience. In addition to characterization of cycles and their eventual breakdown, longitudinal day-to-day sampling indicates that both sleep and headache vary in relation to specific hormone patterns. Overall, hormonal instability appears to be associated with worse symptoms, but more research is needed. A better understanding of how hormone patterns may cause symptoms in midlife women will inform appropriate approaches to treatment.

ACKNOWLEDGMENTS

The Study of Women's Health Across the Nation (SWAN) has grant support from the National Institutes of Health (NIH), DHHS, through the National Institute on Aging (NIA), the National Institute of Nursing Research (NINR) and the NIH Office of Research on Women's Health (ORWH) (Grants U01NR004061, U01AG012505, U01AG012535, U01AG012531, U01AG012539, U01AG012546, U01AG012553, U01AG012554, U01AG012495). The content of this article is solely the responsibility of the authors and does not necessarily represent the official views of the NIA, NINR, ORWH, or the NIH.

REFERENCES

1. Harlow SD, Gass M, Hall JE, et al. Executive summary of the Stages of Reproductive Aging Workshop + 10: addressing the unfinished agenda of staging reproductive aging. J Clin Endocrinol Metab 2012;97:1159–68.
2. Rostosky SS, Travis CB. Menopause research and the dominance of the biomedical model 1984–1994. Psychol Women Q 1996;20:285–312.
3. Ikram MA, Brusselle GGO, Murad SD, et al. The Rotterdam Study: 2018 update on objectives, design and main results. Eur J Epidemiol 2017;32:807–50.
4. Guthrie JR, Dennerstein L, Taffe JR, et al. The menopausal transition: a 9-year prospective population-based study. The Melbourne Women's Midlife Health Project. Climacteric 2004;7:375–89.
5. Woods NF, Mitchell ES. The Seattle Midlife Women's Health Study: a longitudinal prospective study of women during the menopausal transition and early postmenopause. Womens Midlife Health 2016;2:6.
6. Freeman EW, Sammel MD. Methods in a longitudinal cohort study of late reproductive age women: the Penn Ovarian Aging Study (POAS). Womens Midlife Health 2016;2:1.
7. Lobo RA, Kelsey J, Marcus R. Menopause: biology and pathobiology. San Diego (CA): Elsevier Science; 2000.
8. Sommer B, Avis N, Meyer P, et al. Attitudes toward menopause and aging across ethnic/racial groups. Psychosom Med 1999;61:868–75.
9. Santoro N, Crawford SL, Allsworth JE, et al. Assessing menstrual cycles with urinary hormone assays. Am J Physiol Endocrinol Metab 2003;284:E521–30.
10. Pavlovic JM, Allshouse AA, Santoro NF, et al. Sex hormones in women with and without migraine: Evidence of migraine-specific hormone profiles. Neurology 2016;87:49–56.
11. Sirmans SM, Pate KA. Epidemiology, diagnosis, and management of polycystic ovary syndrome. Clin Epidemiol 2014;6:1–13.
12. Shuster LT, Rhodes DJ, Gostout BS, et al. Premature menopause or early menopause: long-term health consequences. Maturitas 2010;65:161–6.
13. Meczekalski B, Katulski K, Czyzyk A, et al. Functional hypothalamic amenorrhea and its influence on women's health. J Endocrinol Invest 2014;37:1049–56.
14. Murray A, Schoemaker MJ, Bennett CE, et al. Population-based estimates of the prevalence of FMR1 expansion mutations in women with early menopause and primary ovarian insufficiency. Genet Med 2014;16:19–24.

15. Matthews TJ, Hamilton BE. First births to older women continue to rise. NCHS Data Brief 2014;(152):1–8.

16. Allen RH, Cwiak CA, Kaunitz AM. Contraception in women over 40 years of age. CMAJ 2013;185:565–73.

17. Hansen KR, Knowlton NS, Thyer AC, et al. A new model of reproductive aging: the decline in ovarian non-growing follicle number from birth to menopause. Hum Reprod 2008;23:699–708.

18. Kelsey TW, Wright P, Nelson SM, et al. A validated model of serum anti-mullerian hormone from conception to menopause. PLoS One 2011;6:e22024.

19. Ahmed Ebbiary NA, Lenton EA, Cooke ID. Hypothalamic-pituitary ageing: progressive increase in FSH and LH concentrations throughout the reproductive life in regularly menstruating women. Clin Endocrinol (Oxf) 1994;41:100 206.

20. Burger HG, Dudley EC, Robertson DM, et al. Hormonal changes in the menopause transition. Recent Prog Horm Res 2002;57:257–75.

21. Hansen KR, Craig LB, Zavy MT, et al. Ovarian primordial and nongrowing follicle counts according to the Stages of Reproductive Aging Workshop (STRAW) staging system. Menopause 2012;19:164–71.

22. Gracia CR, Sammel MD, Freeman EW, et al. Defining menopause status: creation of a new definition to identify the early changes of the menopausal transition. Menopause 2005;12:128–35.

23. Welt CK, McNicholl DJ, Taylor AE, et al. Female reproductive aging is marked by decreased secretion of dimeric inhibin. J Clin Endocrinol Metab 1999;84:105–11.

24. Klein NA, Harper AJ, Houmard BS, et al. Is the short follicular phase in older women secondary to advanced or accelerated dominant follicle development? J Clin Endocrinol Metab 2002;87:5746–50.

25. Klein NA, Battaglia DE, Fujimoto VY, et al. Reproductive aging: accelerated ovarian follicular development associated with a monotropic follicle-stimulating hormone rise in normal older women. J Clin Endocrinol Metab 1996;81:1038–45.

26. Santoro N, Isaac B, Neal-Perry G, et al. Impaired folliculogenesis and ovulation in older reproductive aged women. J Clin Endocrinol Metab 2003;88:5502–9.

27. Shaw ND, Srouji SS, Welt CK, et al. Compensatory increase in ovarian aromatase in older regularly cycling women. J Clin Endocrinol Metab 2015;100:3539–47.

28. Santoro N, Brown JR, Adel T, et al. Characterization of reproductive hormonal dynamics in the perimenopause. J Clin Endocrinol Metab 1996;81:1495–501.

29. Battaglia DE, Goodwin P, Klein NA, et al. Influence of maternal age on meiotic spindle assembly in oocytes from naturally cycling women. Hum Reprod 1996;11:2217–22.

30. Keefe DL, Niven-Fairchild T, Powell S, et al. Mitochondrial deoxyribonucleic acid deletions in oocytes and reproductive aging in women. Fertil Steril 1995;64:577–83.

31. Bentov Y, Casper RF. The aging oocyte–can mitochondrial function be improved? Fertil Steril 2013;99:18–22.

32. Santoro N, Lasley B, McConnell D, et al. Body size and ethnicity are associated with menstrual cycle alterations in women in the early menopausal transition: The Study of Women's Health across the Nation (SWAN) Daily Hormone Study. J Clin Endocrinol Metab 2004;89:2622–31.

33. Santoro N, Crawford SL, Lasley WL, et al. Factors related to declining luteal function in women during the menopausal transition. J Clin Endocrinol Metab 2008;93:1711–21.

34. Santoro N, Crawford SL, El Khoudary SR, et al. Menstrual cycle hormone changes in women traversing the menopause: study of women's health across the nation. J Clin Endocrinol Metab 2017;102(7):2218–29.

35. Hale GE, Hughes CL, Burger HG, et al. Atypical estradiol secretion and ovulation patterns caused by luteal out-of-phase (LOOP) events underlying irregular ovulatory menstrual cycles in the menopausal transition. Menopause 2009;16:50–9.

36. Weiss G, Skurnick JH, Goldsmith LT, et al. Menopause and hypothalamic-pituitary sensitivity to estrogen. JAMA 2004;292:2991–6.

37. Soares CN. Mood disorders in midlife women: understanding the critical window and its clinical implications. Menopause 2014;21:198–206.

38. Freeman EW, Sammel MD, Lin H, et al. Associations of hormones and menopausal status with depressed mood in women with no history of depression. Arch Gen Psychiatry 2006;63:375–82.

39. Harlow SD, Karvonen-Gutierrez C, Elliott MR, et al. It is not just menopause: symptom clustering in the Study of Women's Health Across the Nation. Womens Midlife Health 2017;3 [pii:2].

40. Bromberger JT, Kravitz HM, Youk A, et al. Patterns of depressive disorders across 13 years and their determinants among midlife women: SWAN mental health study. J Affect Disord 2016;206:31–40.

41. Kravitz HM, Zhao X, Bromberger JT, et al. Sleep disturbance during the menopausal transition in a multi-ethnic community sample of women. Sleep 2008;31: 979–90.

42. Kravitz HM, Janssen I, Santoro N, et al. Relationship of day-to-day reproductive hormone levels to sleep in midlife women. Arch Intern Med 2005;165:2370–6.

43. Joffe H, Crawford S, Economou N, et al. A gonadotropin-releasing hormone agonist model demonstrates that nocturnal hot flashes interrupt objective sleep. Sleep 2013;36:1977–85.

44. Freeman EW, Sammel MD, Gross SA, et al. Poor sleep in relation to natural menopause: a population-based 14-year follow-up of midlife women. Menopause 2015;22:719–26.

45. Kravitz HM, Joffe H. Sleep during the perimenopause: a SWAN story. Obstet Gynecol Clin North Am 2011;38:567–86.

46. Kravitz HM, Janssen I, Bromberger JT, et al. Sleep trajectories before and after the final menstrual period in the Study of Women's Health Across the Nation (SWAN). Curr Sleep Med Rep 2017;3:235–50.

47. Woods NF, Mitchell ES. Sleep symptoms during the menopausal transition and early postmenopause: observations from the Seattle Midlife Women's Health Study. Sleep 2010;33:539–49.

48. de Zambotti M, Colrain IM, Baker FC. Interaction between reproductive hormones and physiological sleep in women. J Clin Endocrinol Metab 2015;100:1426–33.

49. Pien GW, Sammel MD, Freeman EW, et al. Predictors of sleep quality in women in the menopausal transition. Sleep 2008;31:991–9.

50. Wang SJ, Fuh JL, Lu SR, et al. Migraine prevalence during menopausal transition. Headache 2003;43:470–8.

51. Martin VT, Pavlovic J, Fanning KM, et al. Perimenopause and menopause are associated with high frequency headache in women with migraine: results of the American migraine prevalence and prevention study. Headache 2016;56: 292–305.

52. Dugan SA, Powell LH, Kravitz HM, et al. Musculoskeletal pain and menopausal status. Clin J Pain 2006;22:325–31.

53. Freeman EW, Sammel MD, Lin H, et al. Symptoms associated with menopausal transition and reproductive hormones in midlife women. Obstet Gynecol 2007; 110:230–40.

54. Mitchell ES, Woods NF. Pain symptoms during the menopausal transition and early postmenopause. Climacteric 2010;13:467–78.

Vasomotor Symptoms Across the Menopause Transition

Differences Among Women

Nancy E. Avis, PhD[a],*, Sybil L. Crawford, PhD[b], Robin Green, PsyD[c]

KEYWORDS

- Menopause • Hot flashes • Night sweats • Vasomotor symptoms

KEY POINTS

- Vasomotor symptoms (VMS) occur in up to 80% of women during the menopausal transition, peaking near the final menstrual period.
- On average, VMS last approximately 10 years, with a longer duration for women with an earlier onset.
- Black (or African American) and Hispanic women tend to report more hot flashes, whereas Asian women report fewer hot flashes compared with non-Hispanic white women.
- Cigarette smoking, higher levels of anxiety and depression, lower educational attainment, and premenstrual symptoms are risk factors for VMS. Data on physical activity, alcohol, and diet are inconsistent.
- Women show several different patterns of timing and frequency of VMS.

VASOMOTOR SYMPTOMS: PRIMARY SYMPTOMS ASSOCIATED WITH MENOPAUSE

Vasomotor symptoms (VMS), or hot flashes and night sweats, are hallmarks of the menopausal transition (MT) and can significantly affect quality of life.[1–4] Up to 80% of women experience VMS during menopause,[5,6] and most women rate them as moderate to severe.[7] Recent research from the Study of Women's Health Across the Nation (SWAN) found that frequent VMS last a median of 7.4 years, which is longer than previously thought.[8] The Penn Ovarian Aging Study has shown that the mean duration for *any* VMS is about 10 years.[9] VMS are one of the chief menopause-related complaints for which US women seek medical treatment.[10,11] VMS are also

National Institute on Aging (U01AG012535) and (U01AG01253).

[a] Department of Social Sciences and Health Policy, Wake Forest School of Medicine, Medical Center Boulevard, Winston-Salem, NC 27157, USA; [b] Graduate School of Nursing, University of Massachusetts Medical School, 55 Lake Avenue, S1-853, Worcester, MA 01655, USA; [c] The Saul R. Korey Department of Neurology, Albert Einstein College of Medicine, Jack and Pearl Resnick Campus, 1300 Morris Park Avenue Block, Room 316, Bronx, NY 10461, USA
* Corresponding author.
E-mail address: navis@wakehealth.edu

independently associated with multiple indicators of elevated cardiovascular risk,[12,13] greater bone loss,[14] and higher bone turnover.[14]

The cause of hot flashes is not fully understood and is likely multifactorial. It is generally thought that hot flashes result from a narrowing of the thermoneutral zone in perimenopausal women.[15] Reproductive hormones play an important role in this narrowing, given that the onset of VMS corresponds to changes in reproductive hormones at the MT and the therapeutic effect of exogenous estrogen. Although lower levels of estrogen and higher follicle-stimulating hormone (FSH) are associated with VMS reporting, not all women who experience hormonal changes have VMS.[16] Longitudinal analyses from SWAN found that FSH is more strongly associated with VMS than estradiol (E2).[17] SWAN further found that neither hormone levels nor bleeding changes entirely explained VMS prevalence or frequency, thus, suggesting the importance of other factors, such as lifestyle and psychosocial characteristics.

Although symptoms, such as depression, difficulty concentrating, and moodiness, are often thought to be associated with menopause, VMS are the only symptom clearly and directly associated with menopause.[18,19] Research using large lists of symptoms to look at how symptoms aggregate has found that hot flashes and night sweats do not track with these other symptoms.[18,20,21] Further, the Stages of Reproductive Aging Workshop (STRAW) also concluded that these other symptoms do not track closely with menstrual cycle or endocrine changes during the MT.[19] This finding was later confirmed in a follow-up consensus workshop referred to as STRAW+10 (**Table 1**).[22]

PREVALENCE, FREQUENCY, AND SEVERITY

VMS occur during the MT for up to 80% of US women,[16,23] but the daily frequency varies. On average, women report 4 to 5 hot flashes per day,[24,25] although some women have as many as 20 per day.[26] One in 4 women report having VMS every day.[24] Daytime hot flashes are reported more often than night sweats,[24–27] although this may reflect difficulty in perceiving or recording nighttime symptoms.[28] Night sweats are generally considered more bothersome than daytime symptoms.[24,26] Greater frequency of VMS is also linked to higher bother.[26] Overall, about half of symptomatic women report only mild severity or bother.[26,29]

For women undergoing a natural MT, not due to hysterectomy/oophorectomy or other medical intervention, the occurrence of VMS varies widely by MT stage.[5–7,24,30] Occurrence is lowest before entering the MT, increasing in the early transition and higher still in the late transition near the final menstrual period (FMP).[5] After menopause, VMS occur in as many as 3 out of 4 women in the first 2 years after FMP and decline slowly afterward, taking 8 to 10 years to return to pre-FMP levels (**Fig. 1**).[7,31] Patterns for severe VMS, defined variously across studies in terms of higher frequency, severity, or bother, are generally similar, with a peak prevalence of 50% near the FMP.[6,7,25,31]

Table 1	
Prevalence of vasomotor symptoms by stage of menopausal transition	
Stages of Menopause Transition as Defined by the STRAW +10 Staging System[22]	**VMS Prevalence Estimates[5] (%)**
Late reproductive stage: possible subtle changes in menstrual cycle length or flow	6–13
Early MT: change in menstrual cycle regularity	4–46
Late MT: skipped menstrual periods	33–63
Postmenopause: 1 y+ with no menstrual flow	41–79

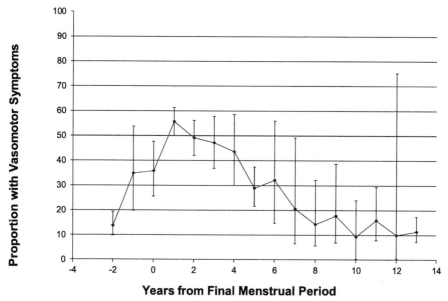

Fig. 1. Pooled estimates from 6 studies of proportion of VMS by years to/from FMP. One study was longitudinal, and 5 were cross-sectional. (*From* Politi MC, Schleinitz MD, Col NF. Revisiting the duration of vasomotor symptoms of menopause: a meta-analysis. J Gen Intern Med 2008;23(9):1510; with permission.)

Although menopausal hormone therapy (HT) is a highly effective treatment of VMS,[32] VMS often recur after HT discontinuation.[33–38] In one recent study, more than 90% of women discontinuing HT had a recurrence, with severe VMS in two-thirds of women.[38] Recurrence after HT discontinuation is more common in women with VMS before HT initiation[33,35] and in women who initiated HT for symptom relief,[33] although even previously asymptomatic women may have new VMS after HT discontinuation, estimated in one study at 7%.[34] VMS recurrence also is more likely in younger women.[37]

HOW LONG DO THEY LAST?

Despite their pervasiveness, negative influence on quality of life, and association with adverse health indicators, we have lacked robust estimates of how long VMS last. In part this is because, until recently, few studies had sufficient follow-up of individual participants, and thus within-woman duration was inferred indirectly by comparing different women at varying stages of the MT. Previous clinical guidelines suggested a typical duration of VMS between 6 months and 2 years.[39] Recent findings, however, indicate that VMS last much longer. Any VMS, that is, regardless of frequency or severity, have been found to last a total of 10.2 years on average; the average duration after the FMP is 4.9 years among those who continue to have symptoms.[7] Average or median durations for frequent or moderate/severe VMS are somewhat shorter at 7.4 to 8.8 years in total and 4.5 to 4.6 years after the FMP.[7,8] VMS last longer in women whose symptoms begin earlier in the MT. Frequent or moderate/severe VMS have a median duration of approximately 3.5 years in women whose symptoms begin after menopause, compared with more than 11.5 years in women with an onset of VMS near the start of the MT.[7,8]

RISK FACTORS FOR VASOMOTOR SYMPTOMS

Many studies have identified characteristics of women who are most likely to get hot flashes (**Box 1**). Researchers have looked at health behaviors, psychosocial characteristics, and sociodemographic factors. Studies have also looked at racial and ethnic differences, and these are discussed in a separate section.

An early myth about hot flashes is that being overweight can be protective. Early observations from postmenopausal women found that greater estrone production in peripheral fat from aromatization of androstenedione was associated with less symptom reporting.[40,41] Later longitudinal and cross-sectional studies of women during the MT indicated that greater body mass index (BMI) was associated with *worse* VMS.[6,30,42] Recent data from SWAN have helped address this apparent contradiction.[43] SWAN data show that, although greater BMI is related to less frequent VMS in late menopause, BMI is positively related to VMS in early menopause.[43] Thus, BMI seems to have a different relationship with VMS before and after menopause.

Smoking is the primary health behavior that has been associated with VMS. SWAN has shown that both active smoking and passive smoke exposure are related to a greater likelihood of VMS.[44] Current smokers have more than a 60% increased likelihood of reporting VMS, even adjusting for confounding factors, such as education and race/ethnicity.[6] Although it has been hypothesized that this relationship is due to the antiestrogenic effects of cigarette smoking, differences in endogenous E2 levels do not account for this association in SWAN.[44]

Physical activity, diet, and alcohol consumption are other health behaviors people have studied; but these results are weak and inconsistent. About half of the observational studies report no association between physical activity and VMS (eg,[6,45,46]), whereas others report a protective association (eg,[47,48]). In a randomized aerobic exercise intervention trial, the Menopause Strategies: Finding Lasting Answers for Symptoms and Health (MsFLASH) study, found no benefit of exercise on the frequency or bothersome level of VMS.[49]

Although alcohol can serve as a trigger for hot flashes, research has shown that alcohol consumption and VMS have either no[44,50] or modest association.[51] SWAN found that *less* alcohol consumption was related to more frequent VMS in unadjusted analyses and showed no relationship when analyses controlled for other variables.[6]

Box 1
Risk factors for hot flashes

Good evidence for

- Menopause status
- Anxiety or depression before menopause
- Generally more sensitive to symptoms
- Black race
- Smoking
- Antiendocrine (estrogen or androgen) therapy

Mixed or no evidence

- Physical activity
- Diet
- Alcohol consumption

Similar to physical activity and alcohol, research has not found a consistent relationship between diet and VMS. Phytoestrogens, a group of plant-derived chemicals found in foods, such as soy, red clover, and alfalfa, have been thought to be protective against VMS because of their structural resemblance to E2 and the lower prevalence of VMS among Asian women. However, a meta-analysis of randomized studies found no indication that phytoestrogens show a beneficial effect on VMS.[52] In SWAN, baseline genistein (one type of phytoestrogen) intake was not related longitudinally to VMS and did not account for reduced symptom reporting in Asian women.[6]

In contrast to the inconsistent role of lifestyle factors, studies have shown that psychosocial factors, such as anxiety and depression, are more consistently associated with VMS.[5,6,53,54] Although in cross-sectional studies it is not possible to determine whether VMS or psychosocial distress comes first, longitudinal studies suggest that psychological factors may impact subsequent VMS. The Penn Ovarian Aging Study found that anxiety and depression preceded hot flashes.[54,55] In SWAN, depressive symptoms and anxiety at the first visit with frequent VMS were related to longer duration of VMS.[8] SWAN has also shown that stress and generally being sensitive to symptoms are related to longer duration of VMS.[8] Pathways connecting negative affective factors and VMS are likely complex and bidirectional.[26,56,57] A direct physiologic link, through the hypothalamic-pituitary-gonadal axis, between negative affect and VMS has been proposed[58] but is not well tested.

Research has also shown that older age,[6] lower education level,[6,23,50] and premenstrual symptoms[6] are related to VMS. The association between lower educational attainment and VMS does not seem to be explained by confounding factors, such as smoking, higher BMI, higher perceived stress, or higher negative affect.[6]

Most studies investigating the time course of VMS and the risk factors for VMS focus on population averages and do not consider variation in VMS patterns. However, not all women experience the same pattern of VMS. The Australian Longitudinal Study on Women's Health (ALSWH) followed 695 white women over 14 years and identified 4 patterns of VMS severity over the MT.[59] Most women (42%) had moderate symptoms, peaking at menopause. Other women had early and severe VMS that began before menopause but steadily declined after menopause (11% of women), whereas some had late and severe VMS (28%) or late moderate VMS (18%) that peaked after menopause and slowly declined but continued for more than a decade.

SWAN followed 1455 women from 5 racial/ethnic groups who experienced natural menopause over 15 years and also found 4 distinct trajectories of VMS frequency (**Fig. 2**).[60] Similar to the ALSWH study, SWAN found a group (18.4%) that had an early onset of VMS 11 years before the FMP, with later decline. A larger group had a later onset nearer the FMP with later decline (29%). However, somewhat different from the ALSWH study, SWAN found groups with persistently high frequency (25.6%) and persistently low frequency of VMS (29.0%). These differences could be due to racial/ethnic compositions of samples or other sample differences. In SWAN, women who had either persistently high or early onset VMS had higher baseline anxiety and depressive symptoms relative to women with persistently low frequency of VMS. SWAN also found that black women were overrepresented in the late-onset and high VMS groups. There was a trend for the consistently high groups to have low levels of E2 across the MT. However, the dynamics of E2 and VMS were correlated but not perfectly consistent, reinforcing the evidence that E2 alone is not the complete mechanistic explanation for VMS.[61,62]

Two groups of women deserve special attention: those who undergo a hysterectomy or oophorectomy and those who experience VMS as a result of breast cancer treatment. VMS are more likely in women with a hysterectomy, even with ovarian

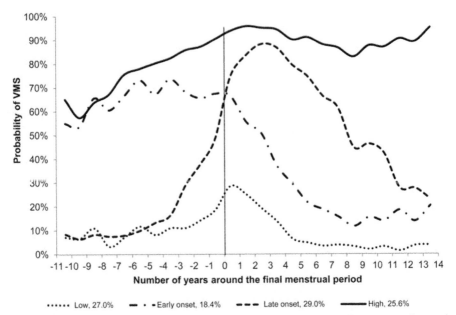

Fig. 2. Trajectories of VMS over the MT. Probability of VMS represents the average observed probability of VMS at each time point within each trajectory subgroup. No factors were included in the model. (*From* Tepper PG, Brooks MM, Randolph JF, et al. Characterizing the trajectories of vasomotor symptoms across the menopausal transition. Menopause 2016;23(10):1070; with permission.)

conservation, than in women with a natural menopause,[25,63,64] possibly because of disruption of blood flow to the ovaries (which in turn affects hormone levels) from abdominal surgery. Bilateral salpingo ovariectomy without concurrent exogenous HT is also linked to more frequent and severe VMS compared with a natural menopause.[65–67] This link may be due to a more abrupt decline in gonadal steroids, which prevents a downward regulation of hormone receptors in the hypothalamus.[68]

VMS are a particular problem for breast cancer survivors.[69,70] Hot flashes affect approximately 65% of women following treatment of breast cancer,[69,71,72] with many women rating them as severe.[71,72] Hot flashes are even more prevalent among tamoxifen users, women taking aromatase inhibitors, or those who experience treatment-induced menopause.[73–75] Among premenopausal women who receive both chemotherapy and antiestrogen endocrine therapy, the prevalence of VMS is as high as 90%[76] and may lead to discontinuation of endocrine therapy. Nonadherence to endocrine therapy has been reported to range from 25% to 55%, with the development of adverse effects being the primary reason for nonadherence.[77] Relief from hot flashes is a common request from breast cancer survivors.[78]

RACIAL/ETHNIC AND CROSS-CULTURAL DIFFERENCES
Racial/Ethnic

Several studies have shown that black, or African American, women experience more hot flashes compared with white women.[6,18,30,51,79] Longitudinal data from SWAN show that a higher percentage of African American women reported both any and frequent VMS across all stages of the MT compared with other racial/ethnic groups.[6] For example, in the transition from early to late perimenopause, approximately 80% of

African American women reported any hot flashes compared with about 65% of white women. Research suggests that the higher rates among African Americans may in part be due to lower levels of E2 and a higher BMI.[51,79] However, racial differences may also be due to differences in perception and tolerance of temperature change. Several experimental studies have shown that African Americans have lower levels of tolerance to cold[80] and heat[81,82] than whites and that more African Americans than whites rate heat as being unpleasant.[81]

VMS symptom reporting has also been shown to vary by ethnicity.[6,18,51,83] SWAN found that Hispanic women as a group tend to report somewhat more hot flashes compared with white women.[6] This finding was also found in a study conducted in Texas.[84] Multivariable analyses in SWAN suggest that the higher occurrence of VMS in Hispanics compared with non-Hispanic whites is largely due to factors such as education, anxiety, and depression.[6] Additional SWAN analyses, however, have shown a marked variation across Hispanics of a different origin.[85] These analyses found that Central American women had the highest rates of VMS reporting and that Cuban women had the lowest rates relative to non-Hispanic Caucasians.[85] These results suggest that, despite a shared language, Hispanic/Latina women from diverse racial/ethnic and cultural groups should not be considered a single group. These groups vary in terms of education, financial strain, health habits, and acculturation, all of which have been related to VMS.[6]

Women of Asian ethnicity consistently report fewer hot flashes and a shorter duration of VMS than other groups.[30,51,86,87] SWAN data show that Chinese and Japanese women are the least likely to report any VMS or report them as bothersome when compared with other racial/ethnic groups.[6,26,88] Some studies have suggested that higher soy intake among Asian women might account for these differences,[89] but this was not the case in SWAN.[6,44] Reasons for these differences are not fully understood and likely result from a combination of factors, including lifestyle, genetics, psychosocial, and perceptual.

Cross-Cultural

VMS reporting varies widely across different countries and cultures, with the lowest reporting in Asian countries and the highest in Europe and the United States.[90] Despite the variation in prevalence, VMS are linked to the stage of the MT consistently across numerous racial/ethnic and cultural groups.[18,91] So what accounts for these differences? They seem to stem from both biological factors, which likely affect the *occurrence* of VMS, and nonbiological factors, which likely affect *perception or reporting* of VMS.[92] Examples of biological factors related to both VMS and culture include

- Estrogen levels and genes involved in estrogen metabolism and receptors
- Lifestyle behaviors, such as smoking, diet (including phytoestrogens), and body composition
- Gynecologic surgeries, such as tubal ligation, hysterectomy, and oophorectomy

Examples of relevant nonbiological factors include

- Socioeconomic status indicators, such as education
- Symptom sensitivity
- Attitudes toward menopause and VMS, for example, natural versus bothersome or requiring medical intervention
- Language and acculturation, which may affect specific words used for VMS
- Conversational norms or acceptability of the topic

Comparisons of VMS across multiple cultures should be done based on consistent measurement methods, ideally within the same study. The changing racial and ethnic composition of the US population requires greater awareness of ethnic diversities and variations in VMS reporting for optimal health care delivery.

SUMMARY

VMS are the primary menopausal symptom, peaking around the FMP and occurring in up to 80% of women during the MT. On average, they last for 10 years, with a longer duration in women with an earlier onset of symptoms. However, women show different patterns of experiencing VMS in terms of timing of onset and frequency level. Compared with non-Hispanic white women, black and Hispanic women are more likely and Asian women are less likely to report VMS, perhaps reflecting racial/differences in characteristics, such as weight, smoking, and gynecologic surgeries. Additional risk factors for VMS include body composition, although it seems to be protective in later stages of the MT, as well as smoking, prior and concurrent anxiety and depression, sensitivity to symptoms, premenstrual syndrome, education, and medical treatments, such as hysterectomy, bilateral oophorectomy, and use of breast cancer–related endocrine therapies. It is important to keep in mind that although VMS are common during the MT, their patterns over time and within higher-risk subgroups are heterogeneous.

REFERENCES

1. Avis NE, Ory M, Matthews KA, et al. Health-related quality of life in a multiethnic sample of middle-aged women: study of Women's Health Across the Nation (SWAN). Med Care 2003;41(11):1262–76.
2. Avis NE, Colvin A, Bromberger JT, et al. Change in health-related quality of life over the menopausal transition in a multiethnic cohort of middle-aged women: study of Women's Health Across the Nation. Menopause 2009;16(5):860–9.
3. Blumel JE, Chedraui P, Baron G, et al. A large multinational study of vasomotor symptom prevalence, duration, and impact on quality of life in middle-aged women. Menopause 2011;18(7):778–85.
4. Williams RE, Levine KB, Kalilani L, et al. Menopause-specific questionnaire assessment in US population-based study shows negative impact on health-related quality of life. Maturitas 2009;62(2):153–9.
5. Woods NF, Mitchell ES. Symptoms during the perimenopause: prevalence, severity, trajectory, and significance in women's lives. Am J Med 2005; 118(Suppl 12B):14–24.
6. Gold EB, Colvin A, Avis N, et al. Longitudinal analysis of the association between vasomotor symptoms and race/ethnicity across the menopausal transition: Study of women's health across the nation. Am J Public Health 2006;96(7):1226–35.
7. Freeman EW, Sammel MD, Sanders RJ. Risk of long-term hot flashes after natural menopause: evidence from the Penn Ovarian Aging Study cohort. Menopause 2014;21(9).
8. Avis NE, Crawford SL, Greendale G, et al. Duration of menopausal vasomotor symptoms over the menopause transition. JAMA Intern Med 2015;175(4):531–9.
9. Freeman EW, Sammel MD, Lin H, et al. Duration of menopausal hot flushes and associated risk factors. Obstet Gynecol 2011;117(5):1095–104.
10. Williams RE, Kalilani L, DiBenedetti DB, et al. Healthcare seeking and treatment for menopausal symptoms in the United States. Maturitas 2007;58(4):348–58.

11. Nicholson WK, Ellison SA, Grason H, et al. Patterns of ambulatory care use for gynecologic conditions: a national study. Am J Obstet Gynecol 2001;184(4): 523–30.

12. Thurston RC, Sowers MR, Sternfeld B, et al. Gains in body fat and vasomotor symptom reporting over the menopausal transition: The Study of Women's Health Across the Nation. Am J Epidemiol 2009;170(6):766–74.

13. Thurston RC, Sutton-Tyrrell K, Everson-Rose SA, et al. Hot flashes and carotid intima media thickness among midlife women. Menopause 2011;18(12):352–8.

14. Crandall CJ, Tseng CH, Crawford SL, et al. Association of menopausal vasomotor symptoms with increased bone turnover during the menopausal transition. J Bone Miner Res 2011;26(4):840–9.

15. Freedman RR, Krell W. Reduced thermoregulatory null zone in postmenopausal women with hot flashes. Am J Obstet Gynecol 1999;181(1):66–70.

16. Kronenberg F. Hot flashes: epidemiology and physiology. Ann N Y Acad Sci 1990; 592:52–86.

17. Randolph JF Jr, Sowers M, Bondarenko I, et al. The relationship of longitudinal change in reproductive hormones and vasomotor symptoms during the menopausal transition. J Clin Endocrinol Metab 2005;90(11):6106–12.

18. Avis NE, Stellato R, Crawford S, et al. Is there a menopausal syndrome? Menopausal status and symptoms across racial/ethnic groups. Soc Sci Med 2001; 52(3):345–56.

19. Soules MR, Sherman S, Parrott E, et al. Executive summary: Stages of Reproductive Aging Workshop (STRAW). Fertil Steril 2001;76:874–8.

20. Harlow SD, Karvonen-Gutierrez C, Elliott MR, et al. It is not just menopause: symptom clustering in the Study of Women's Health Across the Nation. Womens Midlife Health 2017;3(2):1–13.

21. Cray LA, Woods NF, Herting JR, et al. Symptom clusters during the late reproductive stage through the early postmenopause: observations from the Seattle Midlife Women's Health Study. Menopause 2012;19(8):864–9.

22. Harlow SD, Gass M, Hall JE, et al. Executive summary of the stages of reproductive aging workshop + 10: addressing the unfinished agenda of staging reproductive aging. Fertil Steril 2012;97(4):843–51.

23. Avis NE, Crawford SL, McKinlay SM. Psychosocial, behavioral, and health factors related to menopause symptomatology. Womens Health 1997;3(2):103–20.

24. Williams RE, Kalilani L, DiBenedetti DB, et al. Frequency and severity of vasomotor symptoms among peri- and postmenopausal women in the United States. Climacteric 2008;11(1):32–43.

25. Hunter M, Gentry-Maharaj A, Ryan A, et al. Prevalence, frequency and problem rating of hot flushes persist in older postmenopausal women: impact of age, body mass index, hysterectomy, hormone therapy use, lifestyle and mood in a cross-sectional cohort study of 10 418 British women aged 54-65. BJOG 2012; 119(1):40–50.

26. Thurston RC, Bromberger JT, Joffe H, et al. Beyond frequency: who is most bothered by vasomotor symptoms? Menopause 2008;15(5):841–7.

27. Sievert L, Makhlouf Obermeyer C, Price K. Determinants of hot flashes and night sweats. Ann Hum Biol 2006;33(1):4–16.

28. Sievert LL. Subjective and objective measures of hot flashes. Am J Hum Biol 2013;25(5):573–80.

29. Whiteley J, Wagner J-S, Bushmakin A, et al. Impact of the severity of vasomotor symptoms on health status, resource use, and productivity. Menopause 2013; 20(5):1.

30. Gold EB, Sternfeld B, Kelsey JL, et al. The relation of demographic and lifestyle factors to symptoms in a multi-racial/ethnic population of women 40-55 years of age. Am J Epidemiol 2000;152:463–73.

31. Politi MC, Schleinitz MD. Col NF revisiting the duration of vasomotor symptoms of menopause: a meta-analysis. J Gen Intern Med 2008;23(9):1507–13.

32. North American Menopause Society. The 2017 hormone therapy position statement of The North American Menopause Society. Menopause 2017;24(7):728–53.

33. Grady D, Ettinger B, Tosteson ANA, et al. Predictors of difficulty when discontinuing postmenopausal hormone therapy. Obstet Gynecol 2003;102(6):1233–9.

34. Brunner RL, Aragaki A, Barnabei V, et al. Menopausal symptom experience before and after stopping estrogen therapy in the Women's Health Initiative randomized, placebo-controlled trial. Menopause 2010;17(5):946–54.

35. Ockene JK, Barad DH, Cochrane BB, et al. Symptom experience after discontinuing use of estrogen plus progestin. J Am Med Assoc 2005;294(2):183–93.

36. Espen Gjelsvik B, Straand J, Hunskaar S, et al. Use and discontinued use of menopausal hormone therapy by healthy women in Norway: the Hordaland Women's Cohort study. Menopause 2014;21(5):459–68.

37. Ness J, Aronow WS, Beck G. Menopausal symptoms after cessation of hormone replacement therapy. Maturitas 2006;53(3):356–61.

38. Gentry-Maharaj A, Karpinskyj C, Glazer C, et al. Use and perceived efficacy of complementary and alternative medicines after discontinuation of hormone therapy: a nested United Kingdom Collaborative Trial of Ovarian Cancer Screening cohort study. Menopause 2015;22(4):384–90.

39. American College of Obstetricians and Gynecologists Practice Bulletin No. 141: management of menopausal symptoms. Obstet Gynecol 2014;123(1):202–16.

40. Soules MR, Bremner WJ. The menopause and climacteric: endocrinologic basis and associated symptomatology. J Am Geriatr Soc 1982;30(9):547–61.

41. Nimrod A, Ryan KJ. Aromatization of androgens by human abdominal and breast fat tissue. J Clin Endocrinol Metab 1975;40(3):367–72.

42. Herber-Gast G, Mishra GD, van der Schouw YT, et al. Risk factors for night sweats and hot flushes in midlife: results from a prospective cohort study. Menopause 2013;20(9):953–9.

43. Gold EB, Crawford SL, Shelton JF, et al. Longitudinal analysis of changes in weight and waist circumference in relation to incident vasomotor symptoms: the Study of Women's Health Across the Nation (SWAN). Menopause 2017;24(1):9–26.

44. Gold EB, Block G, Crawford S, et al. Lifestyle and demographic factors in relation to vasomotor symptoms: Baseline results from the Study of Women's Health Across the Nation. Am J Epidemiol 2004;159(12):1189–99.

45. Guthrie JR, Smith AM, Dennerstein L, et al. Physical activity and the menopause experience: a cross-sectional study. Maturitas 1994;20:71–80.

46. Sternfeld B, Quesenberry CP, Husson G. Habitual physical activity and menopausal symptoms: a case-control study. J Womens Health 1999;8(1):115–23.

47. Elavsky S, McAuley E. Physical activity, symptoms, esteem, and life satisfaction during menopause. Maturitas 2005;52(3–4):374–85.

48. Moilanen J, Aalto A-M, Hemminki E, et al. Prevalence of menopause symptoms and their association with lifestyle among Finnish middle-aged women. Maturitas 2010;67(4):368–74.

49. Sternfeld B, Guthrie KA, Ensrud KE, et al. Efficacy of exercise for menopausal symptoms: a randomized controlled trial. Menopause 2014;21(4):330–8.

50. Schwingl P, Hulka B, Harlow S. Risk factors for menopausal hot flashes. Obstet Gynecol 1994;84(1):29–34.

51. Freeman EW, Sammel MD, Grisso JA, et al. Hot flashes in the late reproductive years: Risk factors for African American and Caucasian women. J Womens Health Gend Based Med 2001;10(1):67–76.
52. Lethaby A, Marjoribanks J, Kronenberg F, et al. Phytoestrogens for vasomotor menopausal symptoms. Cochrane Database Syst Rev 2007;17(4):CD001395.
53. Lermer MA, Morra A, Moineddin R, et al. Somatic and affective anxiety symptoms and menopausal hot flashes. Menopause 2011;18(2):129–32.
54. Freeman EW, Sammel MD, Lin H, et al. The role of anxiety and hormonal changes in menopausal hot flashes. Menopause 2005;12(3):258–66.
55. Freeman EW, Sammel MD, Lin H. Temporal associations of hot flashes and depression in the transition to menopause. Menopause 2009;16(4):728–34.
56. Hunter MS, Chilcot J. Testing a cognitive model of menopausal hot flushes and night sweats. J Psychosom Res 2013;74(4):307–12.
57. Thurston RC, Blumenthal JA, Babyak MA, et al. Emotional antecedents of hot flashes during daily life. Psychosom Med 2005;67(1):137–46.
58. Hanisch LJ, Hantsoo L, Freeman EW, et al. Hot flashes and panic attacks: a comparison of symptomatology, neurobiology, treatment, and a role for cognition. Psychol Bull 2008;134(2):247–69.
59. Mishra GD, Dobson AJ. Using longitudinal profiles to characterize women's symptoms through midlife: results from a large prospective study. Menopause 2012;19(5):549–55.
60. Tepper PG, Brooks MM, Randolph JF, et al. Characterizing the trajectories of vasomotor symptoms across the menopausal transition. Menopause 2016; 23(10):1067–74.
61. Lasley BL, Santoro N, Randolf JF, et al. The relationship of circulating dehydroepiandrosterone, testosterone, and estradiol to stages of the menopausal transition and ethnicity. J Clin Endocrinol Metab 2002;87(8):3760–7.
62. Lasley BL, Chen J, Stanczyk FZ, et al. Androstenediol complements estrogenic bioactivity during the menopausal transition. Menopause 2012;19(6):650–7.
63. Wilson LF, Pandeya N, Byles J, et al. Hot flushes and night sweats symptom profiles over a 17-year period in mid-aged women: the role of hysterectomy with ovarian conservation. Maturitas 2016;91:1–7.
64. Zeleke BM, Bell RJ, Billah B, et al. Vasomotor and sexual symptoms in older Australian women: a cross-sectional study. Fertil Steril 2016;105(1):149–55.
65. Benshushan A, Rojansky N, Chaviv M, et al. Climacteric symptoms in women undergoing risk-reducing bilateral salpingo-oophorectomy. Climacteric 2009;12(5):404–9.
66. Özdemir S, Çelik Ç, Görkemli H, et al. Compared effects of surgical and natural menopause on climacteric symptoms, osteoporosis, and metabolic syndrome. Int J Gynaecol Obstet 2009;106(1):57–61.
67. Hendrix SL. Bilateral oophorectomy and premature menopause. Am J Med 2005; 118(12):131–5.
68. Bachmann GA. Vasomotor flushes in menopausal women. Am J Obstet Gynecol 1999;180:S312–6.
69. Mom CH, Buijs C, Willemse PH, et al. Hot flushes in breast cancer patients. Crit Rev Oncol Hematol 2006;57(1):63–77.
70. Davis SR, Panjari M, Robinson PJ, et al. Menopausal symptoms in breast cancer survivors nearly 6 years after diagnosis. Menopause 2014;21(10):1075–81.
71. Couzi RJ, Helzlsouer KJ, Fetting JH. Prevalence of menopausal symptoms among women with a history of breast cancer and attitudes toward estrogen replacement therapy. J Clin Oncol 1995;13(11):2737–44.

72. Carpenter JS, Andrykowski MA, Cordova M, et al. Hot flashes in postmenopausal women treated for breast carcinoma: prevalence, severity, correlates, management, and relation to quality of life. Cancer 1998;82:1682–91.

73. Vincent AJ, Ranasinha S, Sayakhot P, et al. Sleep difficulty mediates effects of vasomotor symptoms on mood in younger breast cancer survivors. Climacteric 2014;17(5):598–604.

74. Olin JL, St PM. Aromatase inhibitors in breast cancer prevention. Ann Pharmacother 2014;48(12):1605–10.

75. Maunsell E, Goss PE, Chlebowski RT, et al. Quality of life in MAP.3 (Mammary Prevention 3): a randomized, placebo-controlled trial evaluating exemestane for prevention of breast cancer. J Clin Oncol 2014;32(14):1427–36.

76. Riglia N, Cozzarella M, Cacciari F, et al. Menopause after breast cancer: a survey on breast cancer survivors. Maturitas 2003;45(1):29–38.

77. Cella D, Fallowfield LJ. Recognition and management of treatment-related side effects for breast cancer patients receiving adjuvant endocrine therapy. Breast Cancer Res Treat 2007;107(2):167–80.

78. Hickey M, Saunders CM, Stuckey BG. Management of menopausal symptoms in patients with breast cancer: an evidence-based approach. Lancet Oncol 2005; 6(9):687–95.

79. Miller SR, Gallicchio LM, Lewis LM, et al. Association between race and hot flashes in midlife women. Maturitas 2006;54(3):260–9.

80. Walsh NE, Schoenfeld L, Ramamurthy S, et al. Normative model for cold pressor test. Am J Phys Med Rehabil 1989;68(1):6–11.

81. Edwards RR, Fillingim RB. Ethnic differences in thermal pain responses. Psychosom Med 1999;61(3):346–54.

82. Chapman WP, Jones CM. Variations in cutaneous and visceral pain sensitivity in normal subjects. J Clin Invest 1944;23(1):81–91.

83. Adler SR, Fosket JR, Kagawa-Singer M, et al. Conceptualizing menopause and midlife: Chinese American and Chinese women in the US. Maturitas 2000; 35(0378–5122):11–23.

84. Simpkins JW, Brown K, Bae S, et al. Role of ethnicity in the expression of features of hot flashes. Maturitas 2009;63(4):341–6.

85. Green R, Polotsky AJ, Wildman RP, et al. Menopausal symptoms within a Hispanic cohort: SWAN, the Study of Women's Health Across the Nation. Climacteric 2010;13(4):376–84.

86. Avis NE, Kaufert PA, Lock M, et al. The evolution of menopausal symptoms. Baillieres Clin Endocrinol Metab 1993;7(1):17–32.

87. Haines CJ, Chung TK, Leung DH. A prospective study of the frequency of acute menopausal symptoms in Hong Kong Chinese women. Maturitas 1994;18(3): 175–81.

88. Green R, Santoro N. Menopausal symptoms and ethnicity: The Study of Women's Health across the Nation. Womens Health 2009;5(2):127–33.

89. Reed SD, Lampe JW, Qu C, et al. Premenopausal vasomotor symptoms in an ethnically diverse population. Menopause 2014;21(2):153–8.

90. Obermeyer CM. Menopause across cultures: a review of the evidence. Menopause 2000;7(3):184–92.

91. Obermeyer CM, Reher D, Saliba M. Symptoms, menopause status, and country differences: a comparative analysis from DAMES. Menopause 2007;14(4): 788–97.

92. Crawford SL. The roles of biologic and nonbiologic factors in cultural differences in vasomotor symptoms measured by surveys. Menopause 2007;14(4):725–33.

Cardiovascular Implications of the Menopause Transition
Endogenous Sex Hormones and Vasomotor Symptoms

Samar R. El Khoudary, PhD, MPH[a],*, Rebecca C. Thurston, PhD[b]

KEYWORDS

- Estradiol • Follicle-stimulating hormone • Hot flashes • Subclinical atherosclerosis
- Menopause • Vasomotor symptoms

KEY POINTS

- The menopause transition is a critical period of women's lives, marked by changes in sex hormones, body composition/fat distribution, lipids/lipoproteins, and vascular remodeling.
- Patterns of hormone change over the course of midlife are more informative than a single measurement at 1 time point before or after menopause.
- Growing evidence supports the notion that follicle-stimulating hormone has implications on body tissues other than gonads, independent of estradiol.
- Studies support a relationship between vasomotor symptoms and cardiovascular disease (CVD) risk factors and subclinical CVD, associations not explained by sex hormones.

INTRODUCTION

Cardiovascular disease (CVD) remains the leading cause of death in women, claiming the lives of 399,028 US women in 2014.[1] This number is similar to the number of female deaths from cancer, chronic lower respiratory disease, and diabetes combined.[1] The incidence of coronary heart disease (CHD) in women lags behind men by almost 10 years,[1] with noticeable risk increase postmenopausally.[1,2] Therefore, the menopause

Disclosure: Dr S.R. El Khoudary is supported by the coordinating center of the Study of Women's Health Across the Nation (SWAN); U01 AG012553-20; NIA; and receives grant support from the National Heart, Lung, and Blood Institute (R21: R21HL140011). Dr R.C. Thurston receives grant support from the NIH via the National Heart, Lung, and Blood Institute (K24HL123565, R01HL105647) and the National Institute of Aging (RF1AG053504), and consulting fees from Guidepoint and MAS Innovations.
^a Department of Epidemiology, Graduate School of Public Health, Epidemiology Data Center, University of Pittsburgh, 4420 Bayard Street, Suite 600, Pittsburgh, PA 15260, USA; ^b Departments of Psychiatry and Epidemiology, School of Medicine, Graduate School of Public Health, University of Pittsburgh, 3811 O'Hara Street, Pittsburgh, PA 15213, USA
* Corresponding author.
E-mail address: elkhoudarys@edc.pitt.edu

Obstet Gynecol Clin N Am 45 (2018) 641–661
https://doi.org/10.1016/j.ogc.2018.07.006
0889-8545/18/© 2018 Elsevier Inc. All rights reserved.

obgyn.theclinics.com

transition (MT) is hypothesized to contribute to this increase in CVD risk. Over the past 2 decades, observational studies of women transitioning through menopause have contributed significantly to the understanding of the MT and its relationship with CVD risk, and have allowed investigators to disentangle chronologic aging from reproductive aging in relation to disease. This article focuses on 2 features of the MT:

1. Endogenous sex hormones that dramatically change over the MT (estradiol [E2] and follicle-stimulating hormone [FSH])
2. Vasomotor symptoms (VMS), the cardinal symptom of the MT

The article highlights novel research concerning the relationship of menopause to CVD risk, describes the natural history of hormonal alterations and VMS over the MT, and concisely reviews research linking endogenous sex hormones and VMS with several CVD risk indicators.

MENOPAUSE AND CARDIOVASCULAR DISEASE RISK
Lipids

Significant increases in total cholesterol, triglycerides, apolipoprotein B, and low-density lipoprotein cholesterol (LDL-C) levels are reported at midlife around menopause.[3–5] The Study of Women's Health Across the Nation (SWAN), which assessed lipid changes in relation to years since the final menstrual period (FMP), has provided the strongest evidence that the MT is linked to worse lipid profiles[5]; total cholesterol, LDL-C, and apolipoprotein B levels increase substantially within a 1-year interval surrounding the FMP, independent of age.[5] The accelerated increases in LDL-C around the FMP have been related to greater likelihood of carotid plaque presence after menopause.[6]

Change in high-density lipoprotein cholesterol (HDL-C) over the MT is less straightforward,[7] with studies reporting a significant reduction,[8,9] an increase around menopause,[3,4] or no change.[10,11] Not only is the direction of HDL-C change over the MT inconsistent, so is its assumed cardioprotective role.[7] In contrast with epidemiologic studies supporting a correlation between higher levels of HDL-C and reduced CVD risk,[12] studies in midlife women have cumulatively reported higher HDL-C levels associated with increased CVD risk.[7] A switch in the direction of the association between HDL-C and atherosclerotic risk has been described over the MT.[13] In SWAN, greater increases in HDL-C, mainly before menopause, were significantly associated with smaller carotid intima media thickness (cIMT), a measure of vascular health and remodeling, whereas increased HDL-C after menopause was associated with larger cIMT.[13] These findings suggest that the quality of HDL particles changes over the MT.[7] Notably, although higher concentrations of large HDL particles have been correlated with a greater ability of HDL to promote cholesterol efflux (the main process by which HDL removes cholesterol from peripheral cells), this correlation was stronger before than after menopause.[14]

Other Traditional Cardiovascular Disease Risk Factors and the Metabolic Syndrome

Weight gain is common during midlife, likely driven more by aging than by menopause.[15,16] However, there also seem to be changes in body composition and fat distribution,[17–20] particularly a shift from lean mass to fat mass with reproductive as well as chronologic aging.[17] Results from several cross-sectional and a few longitudinal studies showed that postmenopausal women had greater central adiposity than premenopausal women.[18–20]

Studies following women over the MT have not supported a strong impact of menopause on other traditional CVD risk factors, including blood pressure, insulin, and glucose.[5,21,22] However, the MT may contribute to the development of the metabolic syndrome,[23,24] a constellation of metabolic risk factors including hypertension, dyslipidemia, impaired glucose metabolism, and central abdominal obesity.[25] Notably, the MT seems more associated with the clustering of metabolic syndrome components than worsening of a single component alone.[26]

Heart Fat

Heart fat depots, including epicardial adipose tissue (EAT; ie, directly covering the heart between the outer wall of the myocardium and the visceral layer of the pericardium) and paracardial adipose tissue (PAT; ie, located anterior to EAT, outside the parietal layer of the pericardium) have emerged as novel CHD risk factors.[27,28] They have more detrimental impact than visceral fat, given their closer anatomic location.[29] Among 456 midlife women in the SWAN cardiovascular fat ancillary study, late perimenopausal/postmenopausal women had 9.9% more EAT and 20.7% more PAT volumes than premenopausal/early premenopausal women. Greater PAT volume, but not EAT, was associated with reduced E2 independent of potential confounders.[30] In addition, postmenopausal women with more PAT had greater CHD risk compared with premenopausal women independent of age.[31] Thus, PAT may be a novel, menopause-specific CHD risk marker. Racial differences exist in heart fat depots and their associations with adiposity measures. Although midlife African American women have less heart fat (both EAT and PAT) than white women, their propensity to accumulate EAT seems to be higher at higher levels of visceral abdominal fat than that of white women.[32]

Subclinical Cardiovascular Disease

Subclinical CVD measures predict mortality and incident CVD events. They include cIMT,[33] coronary artery calcification (CAC),[34] aortic calcification (AC),[35] aortic pulse wave velocity (a measure of vascular stiffness),[36] and flow-mediated dilatation (FMD; a marker of endothelial function).[37]

The MT is associated with adverse vascular remodeling (changes in cIMT and carotid adventitial diameter).[38–40] Late perimenopausal and postmenopausal women have significantly larger carotid adventitial diameter but not cIMT.[38] However, women who rapidly transition through menopause have greater cIMT progression than women with a slower transition.[39] The late perimenopause stage is marked by increases in cIMT and carotid adventitial diameter,[40] a time when both lipid levels and risk of metabolic syndrome worsen. Emerging evidence suggest a link between the MT and risk of endothelial dysfunction and arterial stiffness.[41–43]

Cardiovascular Disease Events, Stroke, and Related Mortality

Earlier age at menopause has been independently associated with higher risk of CVD, heart failure, ischemic stroke, and total and ischemic heart disease mortality[44–47] but not with atrial fibrillation.[48,49] Two recent meta-analyses confirmed that earlier age at menopause or premature menopause is associated with greater risk of CHD and CHD mortality but not with stroke or stroke mortality.[50,51] However, the relationship between age at menopause and CVD events may be bidirectional: a worse premenopausal CVD profile may predict an earlier age at menopause.[52] Further, age at menopause may have a U-shaped relationship with CVD/mortality risk,[44,46,53] with later menopause (>52 or >55 years old) also linked to CVD risk,[54,55] but findings are mixed.[46] Several methodological issues should be considered in interpreting findings, including definitions of early versus late menopausal age, whether oophorectomy or hormone therapy (HT) use was considered, and method of menopausal age assessment.

ENDOGENOUS SEX HORMONES AND VASOMOTOR SYMPTOMS ACROSS THE MENOPAUSE TRANSITION
Cardinal Hormonal Alterations of the Menopause Transition

The MT is characterized by alterations in E2 and FSH. Early findings from SWAN and the Melbourne Women's Midlife Health Project showed that E2 levels begin to decline about 2 years before the FMP, whereas FSH levels start to increase as early as 6 years before the FMP.[56,57]

A potential increase in E2 levels before the FMP has been observed, particularly during the early phase of the MT,[58] suggesting that the widely believed uniform pattern of progressive E2 decline across the MT[56,57] is not universal. SWAN shows that midlife women experience distinct patterns of E2 decline over the MT (**Fig. 1A**).[59] A significant increase in E2 level as early as 5.5 years before the FMP was observed in 44.5% of women (n = 1316, over a mean follow-up time of 9.5 ± 1.6 years), with a steep early decline in E2 level almost 1 year before the FMP in 71% of these women (E2 increase–early decline), and a late E2 level decline after the FMP (E2 increase–late decline) reported among the rest. Almost 55.5% of the women followed either a slow-decline (26.9%) or flat pattern (28.6%), **Fig. 1A**. For FSH level increase, 3 patterns were observed across the MT with various degrees of increase (**Fig. 1B**).[59]

Race/ethnicity and premenopausal body mass index (BMI) are important predictors of which hormonal pattern a midlife woman will follow.[59] In SWAN, the pattern of E2 level increase before the FMP was mainly observed among nonobese women of all racial/ethnic groups, whereas the flat E2 and low-increase FSH patterns were more pronounced among obese women regardless of race/ethnicity. African American women were more likely to experience a flat E2 pattern unrelated to BMI.[59]

Vasomotor Symptoms

VMS, reported by more than 70% of women at some point during the MT, are considered the classic menopause symptoms.[60] In contrast with earlier data that VMS last for a few years around the FMP, newer data indicate that moderate-severe or frequent VMS persist for an average of 7 to 10 years, and, for many women, longer.[61,62]

As with FSH and E2 levels, VMS follow 4 distinct trajectories over time.[63,64] For a sizable number of women, VMS start in their late reproductive or early perimenopausal years, and stop around the time of their FMP. For others, VMS begin in the early postmenopause and persist for several years thereafter. Other women have no/mild VMS that largely occur around the FMP, and still other women have VMS that begin in their early perimenopausal years and persist well into the postmenopause. Approximately equal proportions of women are in these groups (**Fig. 2**).[63] These patterns were confirmed in another cohort from Australia, with mild and late-occurring VMS profiles most common.[64]

In the United States, racial/ethnic differences in VMS are striking. African American women are most affected, with the earliest onset, most persistent, and bothersome VMS of all racial/ethnic groups.[60,63,65] Women in lower socioeconomic positions are more likely to report VMS than more advantaged women, independent of race/ethnicity.[60]

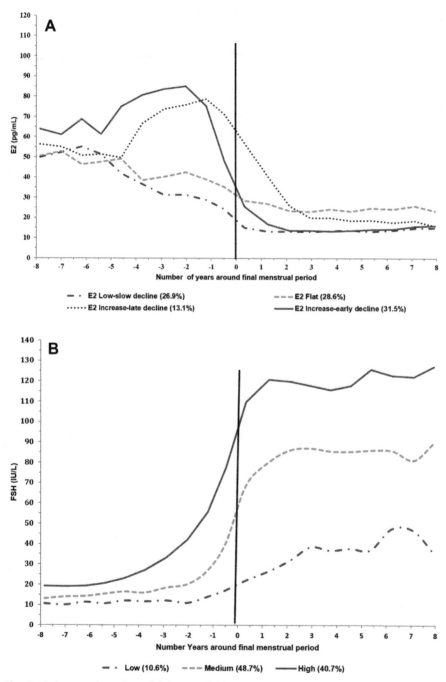

Fig. 1. Trajectory clustering of (*A*) E2 and (*B*) FSH across the FMP. (*A*) E2 levels were the average observed serum E2 levels at each time point. (*B*) FSH levels were the average observed serum FSH levels at each time point. (*Adapted from* Tepper PG, Randolph JF Jr, McConnell DS, et al. Trajectory clustering of estradiol and follicle-stimulating hormone during the menopausal transition among women in the Study of Women's Health across the Nation (SWAN). J Clin Endocrinol Metab 2012;97(8):2872–80; By permission of Oxford University Press.)

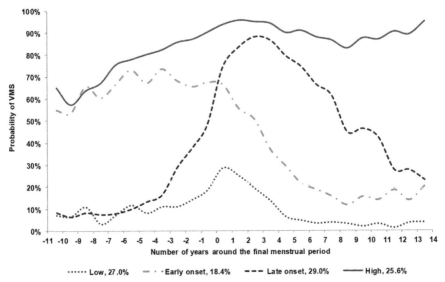

Fig. 2. Trajectory clustering of VMS across the FMP. Probability of VMS: average observed probability of VMS at each time point without including any covariates. (*Adapted from* Tepper PG, Brooks MM, Randolph JF Jr, et al. Characterizing the trajectories of vasomotor symptoms across the menopausal transition. Menopause 2016;23(10):1067–74; with permission.)

ENDOGENOUS SEX HORMONES AND VASOMOTOR SYMPTOMS IN RELATION TO CARDIOVASCULAR DISEASE RISK
Endogenous Sex Hormones and Cardiovascular Disease Risk

Endogenous sex hormones and traditional and novel cardiovascular disease risk factors

Adiposity Associations between E2 and obesity are complex and potentially bidirectional.[66,67] Earlier reports from SWAN among premenopausal and early perimenopausal women showed inverse associations of E2 level with BMI and waist circumference.[68] Later, associations seemed to be bidirectional and differed by menopause status.[56,66,67] Among premenopausal/early perimenopausal women, greater waist circumference predicted lower future E2 level. In contrast, during late perimenopause/postmenopause, greater waist circumference predicted higher future E2 level. In both the early and later transition, higher E2 level was associated with slightly smaller future waist circumference.[66]

Several studies have shown that FSH level is lower in midlife obese women than in nonobese.[56,57,59,66,67] Unlike E2, waist circumference predicted (lower) future FSH level but not vice versa,[66] particularly among postmenopausal women.[67] FSH may also play a more direct role in controlling obesity; in animal model, FSH receptor blockade reduced adiposity and increased mitochondria-rich, Ucp-1 (uncoupling-protein-1) thermogenic adipose tissue.[69]

Lipids Despite improvements in lipids observed after exogenous estrogen use,[70,71] results linking endogenous estrogens with lipids are contradictory. Some studies show no associations between lipids and endogenous E2 after adjusting for BMI and other confounders,[72,73] others show protective associations[68,74] and some report proatherogenic associations.[75,76] This lack of agreement could be attributed to different study populations (premenopausal/early perimenopausal vs postmenopausal women) and/or not accounting for menopause status or E2 measurement timing within the menstrual cycle.[77] These data are based on cross sectional analyses, longitudinal studies are needed.

Similarly, associations between FSH and lipids are inconsistent. Higher FSH level was associated with lower triglyceride and higher HDL-C and apolipoprotein A-1 levels among healthy postmenopausal women not using HT.[75] In contrast, higher FSH level was associated with higher total cholesterol level among premenopausal and early perimenopausal women[68] and higher total cholesterol and LDL-C levels among postmenopausal women.[78] FSH may reduce hepatocyte low-density lipoprotein (LDL) receptor activity and thus increase LDL-C as suggested from animal studies.[78] In an ovariectomized mouse model using gonadotropin-releasing hormone agonist with or without exogenous FSH, mice with experimentally induced high serum FSH and lipid levels had reduced hepatic LDL receptor expression.[78]

Blood pressure In cross-sectional studies of premenopausal/perimenopausal[68] or postmenopausal women,[75] E2 level is not related to systolic blood pressure (BP), diastolic BP, or diastolic arterial pressure. However, in longitudinal research among postmenopausal women who were normotensive at baseline,[79] higher baseline E2 level was associated with greater risk of hypertension and increases in BP levels over 5 years; this association was largely attenuated after adjustment for BMI.[79]

For FSH, research among premenopausal/early perimenopausal women finds no associations between FSH and BP,[68] but, in other work in postmenopausal women, higher FSH level was associated with lower diastolic arterial pressure.[75]

Insulin resistance/glucose/diabetes Associations between E2 and diabetes/diabetes-related risk factors seem to depend on menopause status. Cross-sectional studies of premenopausal/early perimenopausal women do not show a relationship between E2 level and fasting insulin, glucose, or HOMA-IR (homeostatic model assessment, insulin resistance; an indicator of insulin resistance) levels,[68,80] but, in postmenopausal women, higher E2 level seems associated with higher fasting glucose, insulin, HOMA-IR levels, and a higher prevalence of type 2 diabetes mellitus.[75,81] Prospective studies generally agree with cross-sectional studies in postmenopausal women; a recent meta-analysis of 13 studies confirmed an independent association between higher postmenopausal E2 level and incident diabetes.[82–84]

A burgeoning literature suggests that higher FSH is associated with a salubrious diabetes-related risk profile independent of E2.[84–87] Higher FSH level was associated with lower fasting glucose level, hemoglobin A1c level, and risk of diabetes in postmenopausal women, but associations were explained by waist circumference and HOMA-IR.[86] In addition, postmenopausal women with baseline FSH level greater than 50 IU/L had approximately half the risk of developing type 2 diabetes mellitus over 7 to 9 years of follow-up than women with lower FSH level, independent of other sex hormones and risk factors.[87] Further, a faster increase in FSH level in the early, but not late, transition was significantly associated with lower diabetes risk.[85] Because obesity influences both diabetes risk and sex hormones, midlife obesity control is important to postmenopausal diabetes prevention.[85]

Inflammatory/hemostatic markers Endogenous E2 has been linked to multiple inflammatory/hemostatic markers. In postmenopausal women (but not premenopausal/early perimenopausal women[68,80,88]), higher E2 level was positively associated with higher C-reactive protein (CRP) level, adjusting for adiposity.[89,90] Endogenous estrogens were also positively related to coagulation factors (eg, fibrinogen) in postmenopausal women[90,91] (but not premenopausal/early perimenopausal women[68,80,88]). In contrast, premenopausal/perimenopausal E2 level was negatively associated with fibrinolytic markers (eg, plasminogen activator inhibitor-1, tissue plasminogen activator) in cross-sectional and longitudinal studies.[80,88]

Although limited data exist for FSH, studies of premenopausal/early perimeno-pausal women typically do not find relationships between FSH and inflammatory/he-mostatic markers.[68,80] However, one longitudinal study observed higher FSH levels associated with lower fibrinogen and CRP levels and higher PAI and factor VII-C levels.[88] Further longitudinal studies with repeated measurements of sex hormones and inflammatory/hemostatic markers are warranted.

Endogenous sex hormones and subclinical cardiovascular disease
Studies assessing associations between sex hormones and subclinical CVD mea-sures[38,41,92–105] have been mainly cross-sectional[38,92–102] with most evaluating only postmenopausal women.[95–102]

Estradiol Potential associations between endogenous E2 and subclinical CVD are observed in some studies including women at different stages of the MT[38,41] and in the few longitudinal studies that assessed the relationship of sex hormone variability across the MT with subclinical CVD.[103–105] Cross-sectional studies including only postmenopausal women have not shown any association except for a few, inconsis-tent findings.[97,101,102] In postmenopausal women, lower E2 level was not related to cIMT,[96] CAC,[96] AC,[100] or carotid distensibility[97] (a measure of arterial stiffness) but was related to a wider carotid diameter, a marker of vascular remodeling and vulner-ability.[97] Another cross-sectional study of postmenopausal women showed lower E2 level associated with reduced CAC risk.[101] Notably, these studies are limited by use of E2 assays with poor precision for the low levels of circulating E2 postmenopausally.[106] Among 32 older postmenopausal women (mean age, 70 years) for whom E2 was measured using state-of-the-art liquid chromatography tandem mass spectrom-etry,[107] higher postmenopausal estrogens were related to greater cIMT.[102] Results from women at different stages of the MT have not been consistent.[38,41,92–94,108]

Longitudinal associations between E2 and carotid atherosclerotic measures over up to 9 years of follow-up among SWAN participants showed lower E2 level associated with a wider carotid adventitial diameter.[103] This study assumed a universal E2 decline over the MT.[58] Recently, the authors evaluated in SWAN the relationship of hormonal trajectories over 9.6 years across the MT to atherosclerosis risk after menopause.[104] Women with higher E2 levels before the FMP but lower levels thereafter were 43% less likely to have carotid plaque after menopause than women with consistently low E2 levels across the MT. In contrast, women with a flat E2 pattern (medium E2 levels before the FMP but stable and high postmenopausal E2 levels; see **Fig. 1**A) had greater cIMT than women with low E2 levels across the MT. The conflicting effects of E2 patterns over the MT on carotid atherosclerosis suggest a potential shift in the cardioprotective role of endogenous E2 as women traverse menopause, highlighting the importance of assessing patterns of hormonal changes over time.

Follicle-stimulating hormone Less research has reported on associations between FSH and subclinical CVD,[38,41,92,93,95,103,104] with most cross-sectional study designs including women at different stages of the MT.[38,41,92,93] Although not all have shown a link between FSH and subclinical CVD,[38] studies that found significant associations were consistent. Higher FSH levels in midlife women were related to thicker cIMT,[93] lower brachial artery FMD,[41] and greater number of aortic plaques (but this last rela-tionship was explained by CVD risk factors).[92] In 2 longitudinal reports from SWAN assessing the dynamic changes or trajectories in increased FSH level over the MT in relation to carotid atherosclerosis,[103,104] lower FSH level over the MT or a lower FSH trajectory increase after menopause was independently associated with lower cIMT over the MT[103] or after menopause.[104] The impact and molecular mechanisms of FSH in different cell types of the cardiovascular system should be further explored.

Endogenous sex hormones and cardiovascular disease events/death

Cardiovascular disease events/death Studies assessing associations between endogenous estrogen and CVD events[109–119] show conflicting results, with some reporting null findings[109,112,114,115,119] and others showing inconsistent associations.[110,111,113,116–118] None have assessed repeated measures of E2 over the MT. Understanding how the dynamic changes in E2 level or the declining pattern of E2 trajectories[58] over the MT are related to CVD events later in life is urgently needed. SWAN will be able to contribute to this question in the near future.[120]

Most studies linking endogenous E2 to CVD events have assessed postmenopausal E2 level using insufficiently sensitive assays. Some studies show postmenopausal E2 not associated with prevalent CVD[111,112] or atrial fibrillation.[119] In contrast, a series of other studies of postmenopausal women show increased estrogen synthesis–associated with prevalent CVD,[110] higher E2 level related to prevalent myocardial infarction,[111] higher E2 level associated with no-reflow outcome among women with myocardial infarction,[118] and higher total and bioavailable E2 levels associated with increased ischemic arterial disease risk independent of traditional risk factors.[116] Some work shows that the relationship of E2 level to ischemic arterial disease depends on genetic variations in estrogen receptor 1.[121]

Harmful associations between endogenous E2 and CVD have not been shown in studies evaluating E2 from women at different MT stages.[113–115] A prospective study of 4600 women (76% postmenopausal) followed for less than or equal to 30 years found women with baseline E2 level less than the fifth percentile, compared with the 10th and 89th percentile, at 44% higher risk of developing ischemic heart disease, adjusting for confounders.[113] No association between E2 level and incident ischemic stroke or venous thromboembolism was observed.[114,115]

E2 was not associated with mortality risk in 2 longitudinal studies assessing this relationship, regardless of menopausal status.[113,122]

VASOMOTOR SYMPTOMS AND CARDIOVASCULAR DISEASE RISK
Vasomotor Symptoms and Traditional and Novel Cardiovascular Disease Risk Factors

VMS have been associated with CVD risk factors, which have been conceptualized as risk factors for, cofactors with, or potential sequelae of VMS. Although links between VMS and CVD risk factors are not universally consistent,[123] a 2015 meta-analysis[124] supports VMS associated with an adverse CVD risk profile. In the case of BP, VMS reporting has been associated with higher BP cross-sectionally[125] and longitudinally.[126] In SWAN, women reporting frequent VMS were more likely to develop subsequent hypertension.[126] Using ambulatory BP monitoring,[127] acute increases in BP were observed with VMS; others[128] found increased systolic BP with severe overnight VMS, and still others[129] showed increased wake and sleep systolic BP among women with VMS relative to those without VMS. VMS have also been linked to lipids. Over 8 years of follow-up, VMS reporting was associated with higher LDL-C, apolipoprotein B, and triglyceride levels, and higher HDL-C and apolipoprotein A-1 levels, controlling for BMI and other CVD risk factors.[130] Other studies have similarly associated VMS with higher total cholesterol level,[131] higher LDL-C level,[132] and a poorer metabolic profile. VMS may be associated with a more insulin-resistant profile, controlling for risk factors such as adiposity,[133] and VMS early in the transition with increased diabetes risk over 15 years.[134] Among 150,007 women, VMS reported at enrollment (presence, severity, longer duration of VMS) were associated with greater subsequent diabetes risk, independent of obesity.[135] Thus, VMS have been linked to standard CVD risk factors, including BP, lipids, insulin resistance, and diabetes.

VMS are also linked to novel CVD risk factors. Greater hot flash severity was associated with higher interleukin (IL)-8 and tumor necrosis factor alpha, controlling for covariates such as obesity.[136,137] Moreover, hot flash severity was the strongest predictor of p-selectin levels of all covariates examined in a study of 120 midlife women.[138] Further, greater VMS bother was independently linked to higher IL-6 level.[139] In addition, in 3199 women followed for 8 years, greater VMS frequency was independently associated with a more procoagulant profile (higher tissue plasminogen activator antigen and factor VII-C levels).[140] Thus, VMS seem to be associated with a more proinflammatory or procoagulant profile, although further longitudinal research is needed.

Vasomotor Symptoms and Subclinical Cardiovascular Disease

Endothelial function In one of the earliest studies on the relationship of VMS to endothelial function,[141] midlife women reporting VMS had poorer FMD than women not reporting VMS, associations were not explained by CVD risk factors or E2. Other studies[142,143] similarly found VMS associated with poorer FMD among women earlier in the MT. Several studies show a modifying effect of age in these relationships. In a study using physiologic VMS monitoring,[144] among the younger midlife women, more frequent physiologic VMS were associated with poorer endothelial function controlling for risk factors and E2. In other work, women who recalled first having their VMS before age 42 years had poorer endothelial function.[145] Although links between VMS and poorer endothelial function are not universal,[146] findings as a whole support relationships between VMS and poorer endothelial function, particularly for frequent VMS occurring at younger ages in midlife.

Carotid intima media thickness and plaque In SWAN, women with more frequent VMS had greater cIMT than those without VMS, after appropriate adjustments.[147] Findings were most pronounced among overweight or obese women. In other work, more frequent or severe VMS were associated with greater cIMT.[148,149] An exception to this pattern of findings was a study of women with low CVD risk factors.[150] In studies using physiologic VMS measures,[151] a higher frequency of reported or physiologically assessed VMS was associated with greater cIMT and carotid plaque, controlling for covariates including E2. Physiologically assessed VMS accounted for more variance in cIMT than any of the CVD risk factors. In SWAN, the 4 trajectories of VMS were examined in relation to later cIMT.[152] Both persistent and early-onset VMS (see **Fig. 2**) were related to higher subsequent cIMT in unadjusted analyses. When controlling for demographic and CVD risk factors, only early-onset VMS remained associated with cIMT. Thus, VMS seem to be associated with greater cIMT and plaque, particularly when occurring early in the transition.

Coronary and aortic calcification In SWAN, VMS were associated with both AC and CAC[141]; however, only associations between VMS and AC withstood multivariable adjustment (as in other studies in midlife women,[153] CAC was low). In research among hysterectomized women,[154] the retrospective recall of VMS before and up to the time of enrollment was associated with lower odds of CAC; associations approached the null with adjustment for duration of HT use. In other longitudinal work, among HT users, a longer duration of VMS reporting was associated with higher AC.[155] Thus, there is some evidence of associations between VMS and AC, but associations may be modified by HT use.

Vascular stiffness and hemodynamic Increased VMS severity has been independently associated with vascular stiffness (pulse wave velocity).[156] In a cross-sectional analysis of midlife women who underwent a laboratory stress protocol,[139] greater VMS bother was associated with lower cardiac output, lower stroke volume index, and higher vascular resistance (a poorer hemodynamic profile). Other analyses[146,148] have produced more mixed findings. Thus, there is mixed evidence for relationships between VMS and vascular stiffness and hemodynamic measures, although the number and quality of studies are limited.

Vasomotor Symptoms and Cardiovascular Disease Events

The methodologic challenges to examining VMS in relation to clinical CVD events are substantial, given the long follow-up times required for prospective evaluation of VMS, which most commonly occur at midlife, and clinical CVD events, which typically begin in women's sixth and seventh decades of life. Therefore, most studies investigating VMS and clinical CVD have used largely retrospective VMS reports, limited by known biases in VMS reporting.[157]

Symptoms of flushing and sweats (assessed via a variety of questions) were associated with CHD events in more than 10,000 midlife women followed over 10 years, with the finding that sweats, but not flushing, were associated with increased incident CHD risk; associations were attenuated after adjustment for CVD risk factors and were most pronounced among women who had not used HT.[158] Among 11,725 midlife women, those reporting frequent VMS had 2-fold odds of CHD over the subsequent 14 years relative to women without symptoms.[159] In an analysis of postmenopausal women,[160] those reporting both hot flashes and night sweats had lower CVD mortality over 12 years, but associations were accounted for by covariates such as BMI and smoking.

Other evidence indicates the importance of VMS timing for CVD events. In the women's health initiative (WHI) observational study of more than 60,000 women,[161] VMS recalled from around the time of menopause (approximately 15 years earlier) were not associated with CVD risk, but VMS reported within the 4 weeks of enrollment (when women were on average 63 years old) were associated with increased incident CHD and all-cause mortality over the subsequent 10 years, independent of CVD risk factors. In other work, women recalling their VMS beginning before age 42 years had higher CVD mortality over 9 years relative to women with no or later-onset VMS.[145] A 2016 meta-analysis of relationships between VMS and clinical CVD concluded that "VMS and other menopausal symptoms are associated with increased risk of CHD, stroke, or CVD."[162] Despite sparse data of variable quality, there is some evidence of an association between VMS and clinical CVD or CVD mortality.

SUMMARY AND IMPLICATIONS

The MT is marked by dramatic changes in sex hormone levels and adverse changes in body fat deposition, lipid and lipoprotein levels, and vascular remodeling that can collectively increase women's risk of CVD later in life. Emerging findings have pointed out new potential CVD risk markers/issues relevant to menopause and unique to women. One is heart fat, which is at greater levels in postmenopausal women and related to lower E2 level. Future studies should assess whether HT affects heart fat and the related CHD risk in postmenopausal women. A second emerging issue is higher HDL-C level, which is not consistently cardioprotective in postmenopausal women. Longitudinal studies of other HDL metrics over the MT are important to understanding the complex association between menopause and HDL.

Associations between endogenous E2 level and CVD risk are not completely understood and have been limited by cross-sectional study design, an overemphasis on postmenopausal women, and technical challenges in detecting very low postmenopausal levels of E2. Considering dynamic changes of both E2 and FSH levels over the MT is also critical. A growing body of literature suggests that there may be a shift in the role of E2 after menopause, with higher postmenopausal E2 levels linked to detrimental cardiovascular effects. FSH may have a role in controlling fat deposition, insulin resistance, diabetes development, lipid metabolism, and atherosclerosis.

Studies support a relationship between VMS and CVD risk that transcends potential confounders, including endogenous sex hormones. VMS have variously been considered a cofactor, a marker of, or directly involved in the pathophysiology of CVD. The authors conceptualize VMS as a marker of underlying vascular risk that manifests during the MT. VMS are typically assessed with brief questionnaires inquiring about a range of aspects of VMS that are not interchangeable (eg, bother, severity, frequency) and about VMS recalled over long time periods. These reports are subject to memory and other biases, which increase as the frame of recall increases.[157,163] Greater methodologic rigor, prospective VMS assessments, and studies of CVD events are needed to advance the understanding of the relationships between VMS and CVD risk.

Together, findings underscore the importance of the MT as a time of accelerating CVD risk. Sex hormones and VMS may contribute to and reveal those women at greatest risk. Findings emphasize the importance of monitoring women's health during midlife, a critical window for applying early intervention and prevention strategies to reduce CVD risk as women age.

REFERENCES

1. Benjamin EJ, Blaha MJ, Chiuve SE, et al. Heart disease and stroke statistics-2017 update: a report from the American Heart Association. Circulation 2017; 135:e146–603.
2. Gorodeski GI. Impact of the menopause on the epidemiology and risk factors of coronary artery heart disease in women. Exp Gerontol 1994;29:357–75.
3. Derby CA, Crawford SL, Pasternak RC, et al. Lipid changes during the menopause transition in relation to age and weight: the Study of Women's Health Across the Nation. Am J Epidemiol 2009;169:1352–61.
4. de Kat AC, Dam V, Onland-Moret NC, et al. Unraveling the associations of age and menopause with cardiovascular risk factors in a large population-based study. BMC Med 2017;15:2.
5. Matthews KA, Crawford SL, Chae CU, et al. Are changes in cardiovascular disease risk factors in midlife women due to chronological aging or to the menopausal transition? J Am Coll Cardiol 2009;54:2366–73.
6. Matthews KA, El Khoudary SR, Brooks MM, et al. Lipid changes around the final menstrual period predict carotid subclinical disease in postmenopausal women. Stroke 2017;48:70–6.
7. El Khoudary SR. HDL and the menopause. Curr Opin Lipidol 2017;28:328–36.
8. Anagnostis P, Stevenson JC, Crook D, et al. Effects of menopause, gender and age on lipids and high-density lipoprotein cholesterol subfractions. Maturitas 2015;81:62–8.
9. Carr MC, Kim KH, Zambon A, et al. Changes in LDL density across the menopausal transition. J Investig Med 2000;48:245–50.

10. Choi Y, Chang Y, Kim BK, et al. Menopausal stages and serum lipid and lipoprotein abnormalities in middle-aged women. Maturitas 2015;80:399–405.

11. Swiger KJ, Martin SS, Blaha MJ, et al. Narrowing sex differences in lipoprotein cholesterol subclasses following mid-life: the very large database of lipids (VLDL-10B). J Am Heart Assoc 2014;3:e000851.

12. Castelli WP, Garrison RJ, Wilson PW, et al. Incidence of coronary heart disease and lipoprotein cholesterol levels: the Framingham Study. JAMA 1986;256: 2835–8.

13. El Khoudary SR, Wang L, Brooks MM, et al. Increase HDL-C level over the menopausal transition is associated with greater atherosclerotic progression. J Clin Lipidol 2016;10:962–9.

14. El Khoudary SR, Hutchins PM, Matthews KA, et al. Cholesterol efflux capacity and subclasses of HDL particles in healthy women transitioning through menopause. J Clin Endocrinol Metab 2016;101:3419–28.

15. Sternfeld B, Wang H, Quesenberry CP Jr, et al. Physical activity and changes in weight and waist circumference in midlife women: findings from the Study of Women's Health across the Nation. Am J Epidemiol 2004;160:912–22.

16. Matthews KA, Abrams B, Crawford S, et al. Body mass index in mid-life women: relative influence of menopause, hormone use, and ethnicity. Int J Obes Relat Metab Disord 2001;25:863–73.

17. Sowers M, Zheng H, Tomey K, et al. Changes in body composition in women over 6 years at midlife: ovarian and chronological aging. J Clin Endocrinol Metab 2007;92:895–901.

18. Abdulnour J, Doucet E, Brochu M. The effect of the menopausal transition on body composition and cardiometabolic risk factors: a Montreal-Ottawa New Emerging Team group study. Menopause 2012;19:760–7.

19. Lovejoy JC, Champagne CM, de Jonge L, et al. Increased visceral fat and decreased energy expenditure during the menopausal transition. Int J Obes (Lond) 2008;32:949–58.

20. Guthrie JR, Dennerstein L, Taffe JR, et al. The menopausal transition: a 9-year prospective population-based study. The Melbourne Women's Midlife Health Project. Climacteric 2004;7:375–89.

21. Do KA, Green A, Guthrie JR, et al. Longitudinal study of risk factors for coronary heart disease across the menopausal transition. Am J Epidemiol 2000;151: 584–93.

22. Guthrie JR, Ball M, Dudley EC, et al. Impaired fasting glycaemia in middle-aged women: a prospective study. Int J Obes Relat Metab Disord 2001;25:646–51.

23. Gurka MJ, Vishnu A, Santen RJ, et al. Progression of metabolic syndrome severity during the menopausal transition. J Am Heart Assoc 2016;5(8) [pii: e003609].

24. Janssen I, Powell LH, Crawford S, et al. Menopause and the metabolic syndrome: the Study of Women's Health Across the Nation. Arch Intern Med 2008;168:1568–75.

25. Grundy SM. Metabolic syndrome: a multiplex cardiovascular risk factor. J Clin Endocrinol Metab 2007;92:399–404.

26. Lejsková M, Alušík S, Valenta Z, et al. Natural postmenopause is associated with an increase in combined cardiovascular risk factors. Physiol Res 2012;61: 587–96.

27. Rosito GA, Massaro JM, Hoffmann U, et al. Pericardial fat, visceral abdominal fat, cardiovascular disease risk factors, and vascular calcification in a community-based sample: the Framingham Heart Study. Circulation 2008;117:605–13.

28. Lehman SJ, Massaro JM, Schlett CL, et al. Peri-aortic fat, cardiovascular disease risk factors, and aortic calcification: the Framingham Heart Study. Atherosclerosis 2010;210:656–61.

29. Iacobellis G, Gao YJ, Sharma AM. Do cardiac and perivascular adipose tissue play a role in atherosclerosis? Curr Diab Rep 2008;8:20–4.

30. El Khoudary SR, Shields KJ, Janssen I, et al. Cardiovascular fat, menopause, and sex hormones in women: the SWAN cardiovascular fat ancillary study. J Clin Endocrinol Metab 2015;100:3304–12.

31. El Khoudary SR, Shields KJ, Janssen I, et al. Postmenopausal women with greater paracardial fat have more coronary artery calcification than premenopausal women: the Study of Women's Health Across the Nation (SWAN) cardiovascular fat ancillary study. J Am Heart Assoc 2017;6(2) [pii:e004545].

32. Hanley C, Matthews KA, Brooks MM, et al. Cardiovascular fat in women at midlife: effects of race, overall adiposity, and central adiposity. The SWAN Cardiovascular Fat Study. Menopause 2018;25:38–45.

33. Chambless LE, Heiss G, Folsom AR, et al. Association of coronary heart disease incidence with carotid arterial wall thickness and major risk factors: the Atherosclerosis Risk in Communities (ARIC) study, 1987-1993. Am J Epidemiol 1997; 146:483–94.

34. Arad Y, Spadaro LA, Goodman K, et al. Predictive value of electron beam computed tomography of the coronary arteries. 19-month follow-up of 1173 asymptomatic subjects. Circulation 1996;93:1951–3.

35. Witteman JC, Kannel WB, Wolf PA, et al. Aortic calcified plaques and cardiovascular disease (the Framingham Study). Am J Cardiol 1990;66:1060–4.

36. Sutton-Tyrrell K, Najjar SS, Boudreau RM, et al. Elevated aortic pulse wave velocity, a marker of arterial stiffness, predicts cardiovascular events in well-functioning older adults. Circulation 2005;111:3384–90.

37. Halcox JP, Schenke WH, Zalos G, et al. Prognostic value of coronary vascular endothelial dysfunction. Circulation 2002;106:653–8.

38. Wildman RP, Colvin AB, Powell LH, et al. Association of endogenous sex hormones with the vasculature in menopausal women: the Study of Women's Health Across the Nation (SWAN). Menopause 2008;15:414–25.

39. Johnson BD, Dwyer KM, Stanczyk FZ, et al. The relationship of menopausal status and rapid menopausal transition with carotid intima-media thickness progression in women: a report from the Los Angeles Atherosclerosis Study. J Clin Endocrinol Metab 2010;95:4432–40.

40. El Khoudary SR, Wildman RP, Matthews K, et al. Progression rates of carotid intima-media thickness and adventitial diameter during the menopausal transition. Menopause 2013;20:8–14.

41. Moreau KL, Hildreth KL, Meditz AL, et al. Endothelial function is impaired across the stages of the menopause transition in healthy women. J Clin Endocrinol Metab 2012;97:4692–700.

42. Tsai SS, Lin YS, Hwang JS, et al. Vital roles of age and metabolic syndrome-associated risk factors in sex-specific arterial stiffness across nearly lifelong ages: possible implication of menopause and andropause. Atherosclerosis 2017;258:26–33.

43. Samargandy S, Matthews K, Janssen I, et al. Central arterial stiffness increases within one year-interval of the final menstrual period in midlife women: Study of Women's Health Across the Nation (SWAN) heart. Circulation 2018; 137:AP362.

44. Jacobsen BK, Knutsen SF, Fraser GE. Age at natural menopause and total mortality and mortality from ischemic heart disease: the Adventist Health Study. J Clin Epidemiol 1999;52:303–7.

45. Lisabeth LD, Beiser AS, Brown DL, et al. Age at natural menopause and risk of ischemic stroke: the Framingham Heart Study. Stroke 2009;40:1044–9.

46. Appiah D, Schreiner PJ, Demerath EW, et al. Association of age at menopause with incident heart failure: a prospective cohort study and meta-analysis. J Am Heart Assoc 2016;5(8) [pii:e003769].

47. Atsma F, Bartelink ML, Grobbee DE, et al. Postmenopausal status and early menopause as independent risk factors for cardiovascular disease: a meta-analysis. Menopause 2006;13(2):265–79.

48. Magnani JW, Moser CB, Murabito JM, et al. Age of natural menopause and atrial fibrillation: the Framingham Heart Study. Am Heart J 2012;163(4):729–34.

49. Wong JA, Rexrode KM, Sandhu RK, et al. Menopausal age, postmenopausal hormone therapy and incident atrial fibrillation. Heart 2017;103:1954–61.

50. Muka T, Oliver-Williams C, Kunutsor S, et al. Association of age at onset of menopause and time since onset of menopause with cardiovascular outcomes, intermediate vascular traits, and all-cause mortality: a systematic review and meta-analysis. JAMA Cardiol 2016;1(7):767–76.

51. Gong D, Sun J, Zhou Y, et al. Early age at natural menopause and risk of cardiovascular and all-cause mortality: a meta-analysis of prospective observational studies. Int J Cardiol 2016;203:115–9.

52. Kok HS, van Asselt KM, van der Schouw YT, et al. Heart disease risk determines menopausal age rather than the reverse. J Am Coll Cardiol 2006;47:1976–83.

53. Canonico M, Plu-Bureau G, O'Sullivan MJ, et al. Age at menopause, reproductive history, and venous thromboembolism risk among postmenopausal women: the Women's Health Initiative Hormone Therapy clinical trials. Menopause 2014; 21:214–20.

54. Tom SE, Cooper R, Wallance RB, et al. Type and timing of menopause and later life mortality among women in the Iowa Established Populations for the Epidemiological Study of the Elderly cohort. J Womens Health (Larchmt) 2012;21:10–6.

55. Simon T, Beau Yon de Jonage-Canonico M, Oger E, et al. Indicators of lifetime endogenous estrogen exposure and risk of venous thromboembolism. J Thromb Haemost 2006;4:71–6.

56. Randolph JF Jr, Zheng H, Sowers MR, et al. Change in follicle-stimulating hormone and estradiol across the menopausal transition: effect of age at the final menstrual period. J Clin Endocrinol Metab 2011;96:746–54.

57. Burger HG, Dudley EC, Hopper JL, et al. Prospectively measured levels of serum follicle-stimulating hormone, estradiol, and the dimeric inhibins during the menopausal transition in a population-based cohort of women. J Clin Endocrinol Metab 1999;84:4025–30.

58. El Khoudary SR. Gaps, limitations and new insights on endogenous estrogen and follicle stimulating hormone as related to risk of cardiovascular disease in women traversing the menopause: a narrative review. Maturitas 2017;104:44–53.

59. Tepper PG, Randolph JF Jr, McConnell DS, et al. Trajectory clustering of estradiol and follicle-stimulating hormone during the menopausal transition among women in the Study of Women's Health across the Nation (SWAN). J Clin Endocrinol Metab 2012;97:2872–80.

60. Gold E, Colvin A, Avis N, et al. Longitudinal analysis of vasomotor symptoms and race/ethnicity across the menopausal transition: Study of Women's Health Across the Nation (SWAN). Am J Public Health 2006;96:1226–35.

61. Freeman EW, Sammel MD, Lin H, et al. Duration of menopausal hot flushes and associated risk factors. Obstet Gynecol 2011;117:1095–104.

62. Avis NE, Crawford SL, Greendale G, et al. Duration of menopausal vasomotor symptoms over the menopause transition. JAMA Intern Med 2015;175:531–9.

63. Tepper PG, Brooks MM, Randolph JF Jr, et al. Trajectory patterns of vasomotor symptoms over the menopausal transition in the Study of Women's Health Across the Nation. Menopause 2016;23:1067–74.

64. Mishra GD, Dobson AJ. Using longitudinal profiles to characterize women's symptoms through midlife: results from a large prospective study. Menopause 2012;19:549–55.

65. Thurston RC, Bromberger JT, Joffe H, et al. Beyond frequency: who is most bothered by vasomotor symptoms? Menopause 2008;15:841–7.

66. Wildman RP, Tepper PG, Crawford S, et al. Do changes in sex steroid hormones precede or follow increases in body weight during the menopause transition? Results from the Study of Women's Health Across the Nation. J Clin Endocrinol Metab 2012;97:E1695–704.

67. Freeman EW, Sammel MD, Lin H, et al. Obesity and reproductive hormone levels in the transition to menopause. Menopause 2010;17:718–26.

68. Sutton-Tyrrell K, Wildman RP, Matthews KA, et al. Sex-hormone-binding globulin and the free androgen index are related to cardiovascular risk factors in multi-ethnic premenopausal and perimenopausal women enrolled in the Study of Women Across the Nation (SWAN). Circulation 2005;111:1242–9.

69. Liu P, Ji Y, Yuen T, et al. Blocking FSH induces thermogenic adipose tissue and reduces body fat. Nature 2017;546:107–12.

70. Miller V. Effects of estrogen or estrogen/progestin regimens on heart disease risk factors in postmenopausal women: the Postmenopausal Estrogen/Progestin Interventions (PEPI) trial. JAMA 1995;273:199–208.

71. Stevenson JC, Crook D, Godsland IF, et al. Hormone replacement therapy and the cardiovascular system. Nonlipid effects. Drugs 1994;47(Suppl 2):35–41.

72. Shelley JM, Green A, Smith AM, et al. Relationship of endogenous sex hormones to lipids and blood pressure in mid-aged women. Ann Epidemiol 1998;8:39–45.

73. Worsley R, Robinson PJ, Bell RJ, et al. Endogenous estrogen and androgen levels are not independent predictors of lipid levels in postmenopausal women. Menopause 2013;20:640–5.

74. Berg G, Mesch V, Boero L, et al. Lipid and lipoprotein profile in menopausal transition. Effects of hormones, age and fat distribution. Horm Metab Res 2004;36:215–20.

75. Lambrinoudaki I, Christodoulakos G, Rizos D, et al. Endogenous sex hormones and risk factors for atherosclerosis in healthy Greek postmenopausal women. Eur J Endocrinol 2006;154:907–16.

76. Mudali S, Dobs AS, Ding J, et al. Endogenous postmenopausal hormones and serum lipids: the Atherosclerosis Risk in Communities study. J Clin Endocrinol Metab 2005;90:1202–9.

77. Santoro N, Randolph JF Jr. Reproductive hormones and the menopause transition. Obstet Gynecol Clin North Am 2011;38:455–66.

78. Song Y, Wang ES, Xing LL, et al. Follicle-stimulating hormone induces postmenopausal dyslipidemia through inhibiting hepatic cholesterol metabolism. J Clin Endocrinol Metab 2016;101:254–63.

79. Wang L, Szklo M, Folsom AR, et al. Endogenous sex hormones, blood pressure change, and risk of hypertension in postmenopausal women: the Multi-Ethnic Study of Atherosclerosis. Atherosclerosis 2012;224:228–34.

80. Sowers M, Derby C, Jannausch ML, et al. Insulin resistance, hemostatic factors, and hormone interactions in pre- and perimenopausal women: SWAN. J Clin Endocrinol Metab 2003;88:4904–10.
81. Golden SH, Dobs AS, Vaidya D, et al. Endogenous sex hormones and glucose tolerance status in postmenopausal women. J Clin Endocrinol Metab 2007;92: 1289–95.
82. Kalyani RR, Franco M, Dobs AS, et al. The association of endogenous sex hormones, adiposity, and insulin resistance with incident diabetes in postmenopausal women. J Clin Endocrinol Metab 2009;94:4127–35.
83. Stefanska A, Ponikowska I, Cwiklinska-Jurkowska M, et al. Association of FSH with metabolic syndrome in postmenopausal women: a comparison with CRP, adiponectin and leptin. Biomark Med 2014;8:921–30.
84. Muka T, Nano J, Jaspers L, et al. Associations of steroid sex hormones and sex hormone-binding globulin with the risk of type 2 diabetes in women: a population-based cohort study and meta-analysis. Diabetes 2017;66:577–86.
85. Park SK, Harlow SD, Zheng H, et al. Association between changes in oestradiol and follicle-stimulating hormone levels during the menopausal transition and risk of diabetes. Diabet Med 2017;34:531–8.
86. Wang N, Kuang L, Han B, et al. Follicle-stimulating hormone associates with prediabetes and diabetes in postmenopausal women. Acta Diabetol 2016;53: 227–36.
87. Bertone-Johnson ER, Virtanen JK, Niskanen L, et al. Association of follicle-stimulating hormone levels and risk of type 2 diabetes in older postmenopausal women. Menopause 2017;24:796–802.
88. Sowers MR, Matthews KA, Jannausch M, et al. Hemostatic factors and estrogen during the menopausal transition. J Clin Endocrinol Metab 2005;90:5942–8.
89. Störk S, Bots ML, Grobbee DE, et al. Endogenous sex hormones and C-reactive protein in healthy postmenopausal women. J Intern Med 2008;264:245–53.
90. Williams MS, Cushman M, Ouyang P, et al. Association of serum sex hormones with hemostatic factors in women on and off hormone therapy: the multiethnic study of atherosclerosis. J Womens Health (Larchmt) 2016;25:166–72.
91. Canonico M, Brailly-Tabard S, Gaussem P, et al. Endogenous oestradiol as a positive correlate of plasma fibrinogen among older postmenopausal women: a population-based study (the Three-City cohort study). Clin Endocrinol (Oxf) 2012;77:905–10.
92. Munir JA, Wu H, Bauer K, et al. The perimenopausal atherosclerosis transition: relationships between calcified and noncalcified coronary, aortic, and carotid atherosclerosis and risk factors and hormone levels. Menopause 2012;19:10–5.
93. Celestino Catão Da Silva D, Nogueira De Almeida Vasconcelos A, Cleto Maria Cerqueira J, et al. Endogenous sex hormones are not associated with subclinical atherosclerosis in menopausal women. Minerva Ginecol 2013;65:297–302.
94. El Khoudary SR, Wildman RP, Matthews K, et al. Effect modification of obesity on associations between endogenous steroid sex hormones and arterial calcification in women at midlife. Menopause 2011;18:906–14.
95. Creatsa M, Armeni E, Stamatelopoulos K, et al. Circulating androgen levels are associated with subclinical atherosclerosis and arterial stiffness in healthy recently menopausal women. Metabolism 2012;61:193–201.
96. Ouyang P, Vaidya D, Dobs A, et al. Sex hormone levels and subclinical atherosclerosis in postmenopausal women: the Multi-Ethnic Study of Atherosclerosis. Atherosclerosis 2009;204:255–61.

97. Vaidya D, Golden SH, Haq N, et al. Association of sex hormones with carotid artery distensibility in men and postmenopausal women: Multi-Ethnic Study of Atherosclerosis. Hypertension 2015;65:1020–5.

98. Golden SH, Maguire A, Ding J, et al. Endogenous postmenopausal hormones and carotid atherosclerosis: a case-control study of the Atherosclerosis Risk in Communities cohort. Am J Epidemiol 2002;155:437–45.

99. Maturana MA, Franz RF, Metzdorf M, et al. Subclinical cardiovascular disease in postmenopausal women with low/medium cardiovascular risk by the Framingham Risk Score. Maturitas 2015;81:311–6.

100. Michos ED, Vaidya D, Gapstur SM, et al. Sex hormones, sex hormone binding globulin, and abdominal aortic calcification in women and men in the Multi-Ethnic Study of Atherosclerosis (MESA). Atherosclerosis 2008;200:432–8.

101. Jeon GH, Kim SH, Yun SC, et al. Association between serum octradiol level and coronary artery calcification in postmenopausal women. Menopause 2010;17: 902–7.

102. Naessen T, Bergquist J, Lind L, et al. Higher endogenous estrogen levels in 70-year-old women and men: an endogenous response to counteract developing atherosclerosis? Menopause 2012;19:1322–8.

103. El Khoudary SR, Wildman RP, Matthews K, et al. Endogenous sex hormones impact the progression of subclinical atherosclerosis in women during the menopausal transition. Atherosclerosis 2012;225(1):180–6.

104. El Khoudary SR, Santoro N, Chen HY, et al. Trajectories of estradiol and follicle-stimulating hormone over the menopause transition and early markers of atherosclerosis after menopause. Eur J Prev Cardiol 2016;23:694–703.

105. Karim R, Hodis HN, Stanczyk FZ, et al. Relationship between serum levels of sex hormones and progression of subclinical atherosclerosis in postmenopausal women. J Clin Endocrinol Metab 2008;93:131–8.

106. Stanczyk FZ, Cho MM, Endres DB, et al. Limitations of direct estradiol and testosterone immunoassay kits. Steroids 2003;68:1173–8.

107. Nelson RE, Grebe SK, OK DJ, et al. Liquid chromatography-tandem mass spectrometry assay for simultaneous measurement of estradiol and estrone in human plasma. Clin Chem 2004;50:373–84.

108. Thurston RC, Bhasin S, Chang Y, et al. Reproductive hormones and subclinical cardiovascular disease in midlife women. J Clin Endocrinol Metab 2018. https://doi.org/10.1210/jc.2018-00579.

109. Merz CN, Johnson BD, Berga SL, et al. Total estrogen time and obstructive coronary disease in women: insights from the NHLBI-sponsored Women's Ischemia Syndrome Evaluation (WISE). J Womens Health (Larchmt) 2009;18: 1315–22.

110. Naessen T, Sjogren U, Bergquist J, et al. Endogenous steroids measured by high-specificity liquid chromatography-tandem mass spectrometry and prevalent cardiovascular disease in 70-year-old men and women. J Clin Endocrinol Metab 2010;95:1889–97.

111. Dong M, Guo F, Yang J, et al. Detrimental effects of endogenous oestrogens on primary acute myocardial infarction among postmenopausal women. Neth Heart J 2013;21:175–80.

112. Rexrode KM, Manson JE, Lee IM, et al. Sex hormone levels and risk of cardiovascular events in postmenopausal women. Circulation 2003;108:1688–93.

113. Benn M, Voss SS, Holmegard HN, et al. Extreme concentrations of endogenous sex hormones, ischemic heart disease, and death in women. Arterioscler Thromb Vasc Biol 2015;35:471–7.

114. Holmegard HN, Nordestgaard BG, Jensen GB, et al. Sex hormones and ischemic stroke: a prospective cohort study and meta-analyses. J Clin Endocrinol Metab 2016;101:69–78.
115. Holmegard HN, Nordestgaard BG, Schnohr P, et al. Endogenous sex hormones and risk of venous thromboembolism in women and men. J Thromb Haemost 2014;12:297–305.
116. Scarabin-Carre V, Canonico M, Brailly-Tabard S, et al. High level of plasma estradiol as a new predictor of ischemic arterial disease in older postmenopausal women: the three-city cohort study. J Am Heart Assoc 2012;1:e001388.
117. Chen Y, Zeleniuch-Jacquotte A, Arslan AA, et al. Endogenous hormones and coronary heart disease in postmenopausal women. Atherosclerosis 2011;216: 414–9.
118. Dong M, Mu N, Ren F, et al. Prospective study of effects of endogenous estrogens on myocardial no-reflow risk in postmenopausal women with acute myocardial infarction. J Interv Cardiol 2014;27:437–43.
119. O'Neal WT, Nazarian S, Alonso A, et al. Sex hormones and the risk of atrial fibrillation: The Multi-Ethnic Study of Atherosclerosis (MESA). Endocrine 2017;58: 91–6.
120. Sowers M, Crawford S, Sternfeld B, et al. SWAN: a multi-center, multi-ethnic, community-based cohort study of women and the menopausal transition. In: Lobo RA, Kelsey J, Marcus R, editors. Menopause: biology and pathobiology. San Diego (CA): Academic Press; 2000. p. 175–88.
121. Scarabin-Carré V, Brailly-Tabard S, Ancelin ML, et al. Plasma estrogen levels, estrogen receptor gene variation, and ischemic arterial disease in postmenopausal women: the three-city prospective cohort study. J Clin Endocrinol Metab 2014;99:E1539–46.
122. Barrett-Connor E, Goodman-Gruen D. Prospective study of endogenous sex hormones and fatal cardiovascular disease in postmenopausal women. BMJ 1995;311:1193–6.
123. Hitchcock CL, Elliott TG, Norman EG, et al. Hot flushes and night sweats differ in associations with cardiovascular markers in healthy early postmenopausal women. Menopause 2012;19:1208–14.
124. Franco OH, Muka T, Colpani V, et al. Vasomotor symptoms in women and cardiovascular risk markers: Systematic review and meta-analysis. Maturitas 2015;81: 353–61.
125. Gast GC, Grobbee DE, Pop VJ, et al. Menopausal complaints are associated with cardiovascular risk factors. Hypertension 2008;51:1492–8.
126. Jackson EA, El Khoudary SR, Crawford SL, et al. Hot flash frequency and blood pressure: data from the Study of Women's Health Across the Nation. J Womens Health 2016;25:1204–9.
127. Brown DE, Sievert LL, Morrison LA, et al. Relationship between hot flashes and ambulatory blood pressure: the Hilo Women's Health Study. Psychosom Med 2011;73:166–72.
128. Tuomikoski P, Haapalahti P, Ylikorkala O, et al. Vasomotor hot flushes and 24-hour ambulatory blood pressure in recently post-menopausal women. Ann Med 2010;42:216–22.
129. Gerber LM, Sievert LL, Warren K, et al. Hot flashes are associated with increased ambulatory systolic blood pressure. Menopause 2007;14:308–15.
130. Thurston RC, El Khoudary SR, Sutton-Tyrrell K, et al. Vasomotor symptoms and lipid profiles in women transitioning through menopause. Obstet Gynecol 2012; 119:753–61.

131. Gast GC, Samsioe GN, Grobbee DE, et al. Vasomotor symptoms, estradiol levels and cardiovascular risk profile in women. Maturitas 2010;66:285–90.

132. Cagnacci A, Palma F, Romani C, et al. Are climacteric complaints associated with risk factors of cardiovascular disease in peri-menopausal women? Gynecol Endocrinol 2015;31:359–62.

133. Thurston RC, El Khoudary SR, Sutton-Tyrrell K, et al. Vasomotor symptoms and insulin resistance in the Study of Women's Health Across the Nation. J Clin Endocrinol Metab 2012;97:3487–94.

134. Herber-Gast GC, Mishra GD. Early severe vasomotor menopausal symptoms are associated with diabetes. Menopause 2014;21:855–60.

135. Gray KE, Katon JG, LeBlanc ES, et al. Vasomotor symptom characteristics: are they risk factors for incident diabetes? Menopause 2018;25(5):520–30.

136. Huang WY, Hsin IL, Chen DR, et al. Circulating interleukin-8 and tumor necrosis factor-alpha are associated with hot flashes in healthy postmenopausal women. PLoS One 2017;12:e0184011.

137. Yasui T, Uemura H, Tomita J, et al. Association of interleukin-8 with hot flashes in premenopausal, perimenopausal, and postmenopausal women and bilateral oophorectomized women. J Clin Endocrinol Metab 2006;91:4805–8.

138. Bechlioulis A, Naka KK, Kalantaridou SN, et al. Increased vascular inflammation in early menopausal women is associated with hot flush severity. J Clin Endocrinol Metab 2012;97:E760–4.

139. Gordon JL, Rubinow DR, Thurston RC, et al. Cardiovascular, hemodynamic, neuroendocrine, and inflammatory markers in women with and without vasomotor symptoms. Menopause 2016;23:1189–98.

140. Thurston RC, El Khoudary SR, Sutton-Tyrrell K, et al. Are vasomotor symptoms associated with alterations in hemostatic and inflammatory markers? Findings from the Study of Women's Health Across the Nation. Menopause 2011;18: 1044–51.

141. Thurston RC, Sutton-Tyrrell K, Everson-Rose SA, et al. Hot flashes and subclinical cardiovascular disease: findings from the Study of Women's Health Across the Nation Heart Study. Circulation 2008;118:1234–40.

142. Bechlioulis A, Kalantaridou SN, Naka KK, et al. Endothelial function, but not carotid intima-media thickness, is affected early in menopause and is associated with severity of hot flushes. J Clin Endocrinol Metab 2010;95:1199–206.

143. Silveira JS, Clapauch R, Souza M, et al. Hot flashes: emerging cardiovascular risk factors in recent and late postmenopause and their association with higher blood pressure. Menopause 2016;23:846–55.

144. Thurston RC, Chang Y, Barinas-Mitchell E, et al. Physiologically assessed hot flashes and endothelial function among midlife women. Menopause 2017;24: 886–93.

145. Thurston RC, Johnson BD, Shufelt CL, et al. Menopausal symptoms and cardiovascular disease mortality in the Women's Ischemia Syndrome Evaluation (WISE). Menopause 2017;24:126–32.

146. Tuomikoski P, Ebert P, Groop PH, et al. Evidence for a role of hot flushes in vascular function in recently postmenopausal women. Obstet Gynecol 2009; 113:902–8.

147. Thurston RC, Sutton-Tyrrell K, Everson-Rose SA, et al. Hot flashes and carotid intima media thickness among midlife women. Menopause 2011;18:352–8.

148. Lambrinoudaki I, Augoulea A, Armeni E, et al. Menopausal symptoms are associated with subclinical atherosclerosis in healthy recently postmenopausal women. Climacteric 2012;15:350–7.

149. Ozkaya E, Cakir E, Kara F, et al. Impact of hot flashes and night sweats on carotid intima-media thickness and bone mineral density among postmenopausal women. Int J Gynaecol Obstet 2011;113:235–8.
150. Wolff EF, He Y, Black DM, et al. Self-reported menopausal symptoms, coronary artery calcification, and carotid intima-media thickness in recently menopausal women screened for the Kronos Early Estrogen Prevention Study (KEEPS). Fertil Steril 2013;99:1385–91.
151. Thurston RC, Chang Y, Barinas-Mitchell E, et al. Menopausal hot flashes and carotid intima media thickness among midlife women. Stroke 2016;47:2910–5.
152. Thurston RC, El Khoudary SR, Tepper PG, et al. Trajectories of vasomotor symptoms and carotid intima media thickness in the Study of Women's Health Across the Nation. Stroke 2016;47:12–7.
153. McClelland RL, Chung H, Detrano R, et al. Distribution of coronary artery calcium by race, gender, and age: results from the Multi-Ethnic Study of Atherosclerosis (MESA). Circulation 2006;113:30–7.
154. Allison MA, Manson JE, Aragaki A, et al. Vasomotor symptoms and coronary artery calcium in postmenopausal women. Menopause 2010;17:1136–45.
155. Thurston RC, Kuller LH, Edmundowicz D, et al. History of hot flashes and aortic calcification among postmenopausal women. Menopause 2010;17:256–61.
156. Yang R, Zhou Y, Li C, et al. Association between pulse wave velocity and hot flashes/sweats in middle-aged women. Sci Rep 2017;7:13854.
157. Fu PB, Matthews KA, Thurston RC. How well do different measurement modalities estimate the number of vasomotor symptoms? Findings from the Study of Women's Health Across the Nation FLASHES Study. Menopause 2014;21: 124–30.
158. Gast GC, Pop VJ, Samsioe GN, et al. Vasomotor menopausal symptoms are associated with increased risk of coronary heart disease. Menopause 2011; 18:146–51.
159. Herber-Gast G, Brown WJ, Mishra GD. Hot flushes and night sweats are associated with coronary heart disease risk in midlife: a longitudinal study. BJOG 2015;122:1560–7.
160. Svartberg J, von Muhlen D, Kritz-Silverstein D, et al. Vasomotor symptoms and mortality: the Rancho Bernardo Study. Menopause 2009;16:888–91.
161. Szmuilowicz ED, Manson JE, Rossouw JE, et al. Vasomotor symptoms and cardiovascular events in postmenopausal women. Menopause 2011;18:603–10.
162. Muka T, Oliver-Williams C, Colpani V, et al. Association of vasomotor and other menopausal symptoms with risk of cardiovascular disease: a systematic review and meta-analysis. PLoS One 2016;11:e0157417.
163. Erskine A, Morley S, Pearce S. Memory for pain: a review. Pain 1990;41:255–65.

Depression During and After the Perimenopause

Impact of Hormones, Genetics, and Environmental Determinants of Disease

Joyce T. Bromberger, PhD[a,b,]*, Cynthia Neill Epperson, MD[c,d,e]

KEYWORDS

- Depression • Perimenopause • Hormones • Genetics
- Psychosocial and health factors

KEY POINTS

- Longitudinal studies, conducted across the world and in diverse populations, confirm that women are 2 to 5 times more likely to experience a depressive disorder during the perimenopausal versus the late premenopausal years.
- Screening for depressive symptoms or disorder in the primary care setting is recommended and can be accomplished easily with standard patient-rated scales.
- Treatment of depression or depressive symptoms during perimenopause and early postmenopause includes the use of standard antidepressants, hormone therapy, and behavioral modifications to sleep patterns and exercise.
- As current and early life stressors/adversity are often contributing factors, many women may benefit from psychotherapy, cognitive behavioral therapy, or trauma-focused therapy.

Disclosures: Dr C.N. Epperson consults Sage Therapeutics and Shire Pharmaceuticals and has investments in Pfizer, Merck, Johnson and Johnson, Abbott, and Abbvie.

This article has been written with financial support for Dr C.N. Epperson's effort from the NIH Office of Research on Women's Health (P50 MH099910) and NIMH (P50 MH099910) and with financial support for Dr J.T. Bromberger's effort from the NIA (AG012546).

[a] Department of Epidemiology, University of Pittsburgh, 3811 O'Hara Street, Pittsburgh, PA 15213, USA; [b] Department of Psychiatry, University of Pittsburgh, 3811 O'Hara Street, Pittsburgh, PA 15213, USA; [c] Department of Psychiatry, Perelman School of Medicine, University of Pennsylvania, 3535 Market Street, Philadelphia, PA, 19104, USA; [d] Obstetrics and Gynecology, Perelman School of Medicine, University of Pennsylvania, 3535 Market Street, Philadelphia, PA, 19104, USA; [e] Penn PROMOTES Research on Sex and Gender in Health, University of Pennsylvania, 3535 Market Street, Philadelphia, PA, 19104, USA

* Corresponding author. Sterling Plaza, 201 North Craig Street, Suite 200, Pittsburgh, PA 15213.

E-mail address: brombergerjt@upmc.edu

Obstet Gynecol Clin N Am 45 (2018) 663–678

https://doi.org/10.1016/j.ogc.2018.07.007

0889-8545/18/© 2018 Elsevier Inc. All rights reserved.

obgyn.theclinics.com

INTRODUCTION

Epidemiologic research indicates that roughly 1 in 5 women will experience an episode of major depressive disorder (MDD) at some point in their lifetime.[1] Importantly, for some women, depression can present or worsen during periods of dynamic hormonal flux, such as premenstruum, peripartum, and perimenopause.[2,3] Longitudinal research of women from the premenopause to postmenopause stages of reproductive life, indicates that some women demonstrate a greater sensitivity to gonadal steroid shifts with respect to risk for negative mood symptoms such that a history of severe premenstrual mood symptoms is associated with increased risk for perimenopause onset or relapse of MDD.[4] The focus of this article is on the period of a woman's life when her reproductive system and its endocrine activity are changing and in transition (perimenopause) to a relatively hormonally quiescent stage (postmenopause). The authors discuss the evidence that reproductive aging is associated with an increased risk for depression as well as the varied endocrine, genetic, behavioral, and social factors that may explain the association.

DEFINING DEPRESSION

Depression is a generic term used by the media, the general public, and health care professionals to refer to negative mood symptoms that range in severity from unhappy psychological states to MDD. MDD is characterized in the *Diagnostic and Statistical Manual of Mental Disorders*, Fifth Edition (*DSM-5*), by a range of mood and cognitive and behavioral symptoms that lead to clinically meaningful distress or functional impairment.[5] The various symptoms and behaviors included in the *DSM-5* diagnosis for MDD and minor depressive disorder are included in **Table 1**. The term *depression* can also refer to a cluster of negative mood and behavioral symptoms that do not meet the diagnostic criteria for MDD but may be associated with impaired functioning or distress and is likely to be more consistent with the diagnosis of minor depressive disorder.[6] Clinical (major and minor) depression and depressive symptoms are assessed in multiple settings, including primary care, gynecologic, and psychiatric. Depressive symptoms are typically assessed with self-report scales, of which there are many (for example, Center for Epidemiologic Studies of Depression [CES-D][7] and Beck Depression Inventory[8] to name few). Self-report scales are useful to assess the number and severity of current symptoms and to identify individuals who should undergo additional screening but are not diagnostic of major or minor depressive disorder. A standardized structured or semistructured interview conducted by a trained clinician is the gold standard for *DSM-5* differential diagnosis of depressive disorders that include minor depression, dysthymia, premenstrual dysphoric disorder, or bipolar disorder-depressive episode. Clinicians may also use standard questionnaires, such as the PRIME-MD (Primary Care Evaluation of Mental Disorders), both clinician[9] and patient administered,[10] and the Patient's Health Questionnaire (PHQ; 2-item for screening and 9-item for diagnosis).[11] Most epidemiologic studies focusing on depression during perimenopause rely on standardized patient-rated questionnaires to determine the presence and duration of various depressive symptoms to quantify the severity of symptoms and not a formal psychiatric evaluation or standardized interview to assess clinical depression. Therefore, the authors use here the term *depression* or MDD to connote a clinical condition that is evidenced by a standardized interview or the PRIME-MD or PHQ-9, which research has demonstrated to be consistent with a probable diagnosis of MDD. The term *depressive symptoms* refers only to symptom levels or syndromes for which the diagnosis of MDD or minor depression is doubtful or not confirmed.

Table 1
Major versus minor depressive disorder

Characteristics	Major	Minor
Symptoms		
Depressed mood (eg, sad, hopeless)	X	X
Decreased interest or pleasure	X	X
Weight change (>5% of body weight per month) or change in appetite	+/−	+/−
Sleep disturbance (insomnia/hypersomnia)	+/−	+/−
Fatigue	+/−	+/−
Feelings of worthlessness or excessive guilt	+/−	+/−
Difficulty concentrating	+/−	+/−
Psychomotor agitation or slowing	+/−	+/−
Recurrent thoughts of death	+/−	+/−
Number of symptoms	5 or more Most days for at least 2 wk	2–4 Most days for at least 2 wk
Significant distress or impairment in function	X	X
Not attributable to physiologic effect of a substance, medication, or general medical condition	X	X
Does not occur exclusively during a psychotic disorder	X	X

Major and minor depression both require one of the two hallmark symptoms (*italicized font*) of depressed mood or decreased interest or pleasure in all, or almost all, activities. For both diagnoses, symptoms must be present most of the days during a 2-week period; cause clinically meaningful distress or impairment in social, occupational, or other areas of function; and not be solely attributable to another disorder, medical condition, or substance. The other symptoms are listed at ±, as they do not have to be present, though 5 symptoms are required for MDD, whereas only 2 to 4 symptoms are required for minor depressive disorder.

Women interface with their health care providers relatively often during their reproductive years, prefer to be treated for depression in the primary care setting, and should be screened for MDD and for elevated depressive symptoms. Indeed, the US Preventive Services Task Force recommends that all individuals are screened for depression at every contact with their health care provider.[12] Identifying a first episode of depression is critical, as the risk for recurrent episodes and chronicity of symptoms increases with failure to adequately treat patients with MDD. Fifty percent to 75% of individuals have recurring episodes of MDD.[13,14] MDD and depressive symptoms are about twice as common among women as men,[1] highlighting it as an important public health problem that significantly contributes to a bias in disease burden for women.

DEPRESSION AND THE MENOPAUSE TRANSITION
Epidemiology

For many decades, there has been an ongoing debate about whether the menopause transition (MT) and/or postmenopause is associated with an increased risk for depressive symptoms or disorder. Although some studies failed to find a relationship between depression or depressive symptoms risk and the MT,[15,16] 2 well-designed longitudinal studies of clinical depression found a 2- to 5-fold increased risk for

MDD during perimenopause versus late premenopause.[4,17–20] The Study of Women's Health Across the Nation (SWAN)[17,18] used a standardized semistructured interview (Structured Clinical Interview for DSM-IV), and the Penn reproductive aging Study (POAS)[4,19,20] used standardized questionnaires (PRIME-MD and/or PHQ-9) and rating scales' scores demonstrating sufficient severity (eg, CES-D $\geq$25) to confirm probable MDD. A similar increased risk for depressive symptoms was observed in other large, longitudinal studies (eg, the Harvard Study of Midlife Mood and Cycles,[21] the Australian Longitudinal Study of Women's Health [ASWH],[22] and the Seattle Midlife Women's Health Study.[23] In addition to carefully characterizing the level of depressive symptom severity, each of these longitudinal studies used menstrual diaries and/or hormone levels to confirm the menopause stage during which such symptoms were observed. Based on this literature, the authors conclude that there is a subset of women who are vulnerable to depressive disorder or symptoms during the MT and early postmenopause. Importantly, the risk for depression seems to decline 2 to 4 years after the final menstrual period, particularly for those women whose only episode of depression occurred during perimenopause[17,24] indicating that the increase in risk for depression and depressive symptoms during the MT is not due to aging itself.

Psychosocial and Health-Related Factors

Current research is focused on elucidating why some women are more vulnerable to depression and depressive symptoms during perimenopause, a time of changing and unpredictable patterns of gonadal steroid levels and menstrual cycles. A common hypothesis is that endocrine changes driving the MT and affecting numerous tissues and biological systems, including those in the brain, are primarily responsible for unmasking the risk for depression symptoms or disorder in susceptible women. Nevertheless, there are numerous and varied other domains and factors that are associated with depressive disorder and symptoms in general and during perimenopause (**Table 2**) (**Fig. 1**).

Table 2
Psychosocial and health-related risk factors for depression and/or depression symptoms during the menopause transition

Categories of Risk	Domains	Specific Risk Factor
Demographic	Race/ethnicity	Minority status
	Income	Low income
	Education	Low education attainment
	Marital status	Unmarried, divorced, widowed
Psychological	Personality traits	Trait anxiety
	Attitudes toward	Pessimism
	menopause, aging	Rumination
Social/environmental	Adverse life events	Childhood and lifetime adversity, trauma
	Chronic adverse conditions	Current stressful situations
	Social relationships	Poor social supports
Health related	Health behaviors	Smoking, physical inactivity
	Chronic conditions	Sleep disturbance or disorders
	Physical symptoms	Lifetime psychiatric disorders
	Functioning	Comorbid medical conditions
		Chronic pain
		Vasomotor symptoms
		Limitations in functioning due to physical or emotional problems

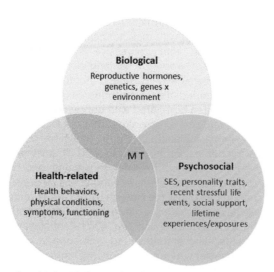

Fig. 1. Intersection of multiple risk factors for depression during the MT. SES, socioeconomic status.

Demographic characteristics

Studies have shown that being unmarried (eg, divorced, single, widowed), having a high school education or less, and experiencing financial hardships are major risk factors for depressive *symptoms* during the MT.[24–27] Results for race/ethnic differences in association with depression symptoms are mixed; most observed differences for black and white women are no longer significant when adjusted for sociodemographic and health factors, such as education, medical conditions, current significant stressors, and financial strain.[28–30]

Psychological characteristics

Personality traits are predispositions that reflect cognitive, affective, or behavioral tendencies that are relatively stable across time and situations. Although there are many such traits, only a small number have been examined in the context of depressive symptoms during midlife: *instrumentality (task/action oriented), pessimism, trait anxiety,* and *rumination*. Middle-aged women characterized by being highly action oriented showed less of an increase in depressive symptoms over 3 years than women less instrumental, after controlling for potential confounders, in one longitudinal study.[31] Studies of midlife women have also suggested that trait anxiety/ neuroticism (a tendency to experience chronic negative emotions), rumination/ self-consciousness, and pessimism are significantly associated with the risk for MDD and/or depressive symptoms.[18,32,33] It is also the case that negative attitudes toward menopause and/or aging are conceptually related to neuroticism and pessimism and predict depressive, anxious, and negative mood in midlife women.[26,34–36]

Social factors

Similar to other times in life, the quality of one's social environment can impact the risk for depression and depressive symptoms during menopause.[26] Social risk factors include acute and chronic stressors, daily hassles, lack of environmental resources, and poor social relationships.[34,37–39] Midlife women with depression report a higher prevalence of interpersonal problems, major events happening to significant others, and financial difficulties compared with their nondepressed counterparts.[40] Stressful events have been associated with depressive symptoms in perimenopausal compared with premenopausal women.[21] Among perimenopausal women, there were a greater number of adverse events in the 6 months before clinical depression occurrence than in the same period of time in nondepressed women.[41] Although vasomotor symptom severity is often correlated with depressive symptoms, they are not predictive[42]; adverse life events are a more significant risk factor for MDD among perimenopausal women.[17] Hence, the fluctuating hormonal milieu of perimenopause may reduce the threshold for depression in the presence of adverse life events,[21,43–45] perhaps because of hormonal effects on neurotransmitters and brain regions implicated in the regulation of mood, cognition, and the stress response.[46–48]

Adequate social support can buffer the individual from the adverse effects of stressful life events and daily hassles. There are different types of support: instrumental (eg, help with chores), structural/social network (eg, number of close friends or relatives, organization memberships), and emotional (eg, someone to confide in or talk to). The most salient type of social support, is emotional support. Research has shown that an adequate number and quality of social relationships can protect perimenopausal women from depression and depressive symptoms. For example, the Melbourne Women's Health Study[35] found that the magnitude of negative mood reported across the MT was associated with the woman's negative feelings for her partner or lack of a partner entirely. Similarly, in the SWAN cohort, marital dissatisfaction having low social support, and few close family members and friends were significantly associated with high depressive symptoms and MDD even after adjusting for multiple confounders (stressful events and negative attitudes toward aging and menopause).[18,34]

Psychosocial stress and adversity

Child adversity includes, but is not limited to, abuse/neglect, family problems, and low childhood socioeconomic status, poverty, and unsafe environments. These stressors and other significantly early life stressors or traumatic events can have enduring effects on stress-sensitive biological systems as well as behaviors that are detrimental to mental and physical health.[44,49,50] Childhood adversity is associated with an increased lifetime risk for MDD as well as new-onset MDD and depressive symptoms during perimenopause.[45,51–53] Cumulative burden of depressive symptoms over 15 years has been shown to be greater for middle-aged women who grew up impoverished and had parents with low educational attainment versus those with parents of low educational attainment only.[51] Five adult factors (financial strain, lower education, low social support, low social function, and high bodily pain) jointly attenuated the association, suggesting a potential pathway between early adversity and midlife depressive symptom burden.[51]

Health-related factors

Depression and depressive symptoms are associated with suboptimal health behaviors, including smoking, inactivity, and sleep problems during midlife.[25,54,55] Prospective studies of middle-aged women indicate that physical activity and depression and depressive symptoms are inversely associated.[56–58] The SWAN[57] and the ASWH[58] reported that the dose of moderate-intensity physical activity that is consistent with public health guidelines is protective for depressed mood. Sleep difficulties are more frequently reported during perimenopause (50%) than premenopause (30%).[59] Although sleep disturbance is one of the cardinal symptoms of depression, the relationship between the two is bidirectional.[60] There is some evidence that sleep disturbance predicts subsequent depression[61] and a more severe depression course. In midlife women, those who reported sleep problems at study entry were 8 times more likely to experience a persistent or recurrent pattern of major depression over 13 years, independent of lifetime depression history and other covariates, than a single episode, minor depression, or no depression.[62] Additionally, in a clinical study, improvement in perceived sleep quality was associated with improvement in depressive symptoms among women with depression during the MT.[63]

Poor self-reported physical health and functioning are associated with depressive symptoms in midlife women.[18,64] Depression often is associated with medical illnesses and risk factors, including subclinical cardiovascular conditions, such as coronary and aortic calcification[65] and carotid atherosclerosis[66] as well as physical functioning.[67] Although it is difficult to disentangle the direction of the relationship between depression and decline in physical functioning, evidence supports a reciprocal relationship in older populations.[68] Depressive symptoms are also correlated with somatic symptoms in perimenopausal and postmenopausal women in numerous cross-sectional studies[69–71] including dizziness, headaches, tiredness, aches and stiff joints, and urinary incontinence. Although some studies find vasomotor symptoms (VMS) are correlated with depressive symptoms or disorder,[72] others do not[17] or they note that the onset of depressive symptoms precedes the onset of VMS when they co-occur.[42] As noted above, in SWAN, stressful life events were a stronger predictor of subsequent major depression than were VMS.[17]

BIOLOGICAL FACTORS

Similar to psychosocial and health related factors, the biological factors contributing to risk and resilience for depression during the MT are complex and inter-related. For example, genetic vulnerability may be observed solely in the context of having experienced childhood adversity or significant stressful events during adulthood.[73,74] Research focusing on this gene by environment (G × E) interaction has rarely considered the potential for sex differences, despite the female bias for affective disorders, sex differences in response to early life stress, and the potential for sex to modify risk associated with specific genetic polymorphisms.[44] Perhaps for some women, the risk associated with this G × E interaction is sufficient to result in an episode of MDD in the absence of hormonal flux/reproductive transitions. For others, the erratic fluctuations of gonadal steroids during perimenopause may be necessary to unmask the risk for MDD either alone or in concert with stress history and genetics for a G × E × sex hormone interaction.[45]

Genes, Environment, and Race/Ethnicity

The heritability of MDD is approximately 35% to 40%.[75,76] As with MDD occurring in the general population, there is some evidence that multiple hits, genetic risk, *and* environmental factors, such as childhood adversity and/or significant current stressors (environment), are required in order to unmask the risk for MDD during perimenopause. Not surprisingly, genetic targets for investigation related to perimenopause or midlife onset of depression are those related to estrogen receptors and steroid metabolizing enzymes in addition to estradiol's downstream targets, such as the serotonin (5-HT) transporter (5-HTT), postsynaptic 5-HT type 2 receptor density, and tryptophan hydroxylase (TH), monoamine oxidase A (MAO-A), and catechol O-methyltransferase (COMT) gene expression.[77,78] TH is the rate-limiting enzyme for the conversion of tryptophan to serotonin, whereas COMT and MAO-A are the primary enzymes responsible for synaptic amine degradation. Overall, estradiol seems to promote increased neurotransmitter synthesis and/or decrease degradation, essentially prolonging synaptic neurotransmitter levels.[46]

Although a recent review of the literature provides strong support for a G × E interaction with respect to depression in the general population and a functional polymorphism in the SCL6A4 gene,[74] the impact of sex and/or reproductive status (premenopause vs perimenopause vs postmenopause) on this genetic polymorphism, which modulates the transcription and efficiency of the 5-HTT, has not been fully explored. The one study that examined polymorphisms in this gene, as well as the gene encoding MAO-A, and the risk for depression among menopausal women failed to find an association between genotype and depression risk.[79] Whether the findings would have been similar had the investigators focused specifically on depression onset during the perimenopause is not known.

As the genomic activity of estradiol is mediated through ER-α and ER-β, polymorphisms in the ER1 and ER2 genes could have a significant impact on receptor transcription and binding efficacy. Moreover, the antidepressant effects of estradiol are thought to be mediated primarily through ER-β. Several polymorphisms in ER1 and ER2 (which encode ER-α and ER-β, respectively) have been studied in relation to the risk for late-life depression among 3525 women who would have been postmenopausal at the time of depression onset. The presence of the A allele for ER2 rs1256049 polymorphism was associated with the onset of late-life depression but only in women not currently using hormone therapy (HT), suggesting a protective effect of HT even in the face of a potential genetic risk factor.[80] Similarly, in a study of unmedicated reproductive-aged women (aged 18–39 years) and menopausal women (aged 40–60 years) experiencing their first episode of MDD and with a minimum score of 21 (at least moderate severity) on the Hamilton Depression Rating Scale (HAM-D), a genetic polymorphism in the gene encoding ER-β distinguished those with and without MDD regardless of reproductive stage. However, when lifetime adverse life event scores were considered, a G × E interaction was observed for both the ER2 polymorphisms studied (rs1256049 and rs4986938)[81] but only in the menopausal group. These data are interesting in light of additional findings from the POAS that childhood adversity was associated with a 2- to 3-fold increased risk for lifetime depression as well as *new-onset* depression during the MT.[82] Together these data support the need to consider a G × E × hormone interaction for depression during the MT.

Findings from the POAS and SWAN implicate not only genetic variations in steroid metabolizing enzymes in risk for perimenopausal depression but also highlight the potential modifying effect of race/ethnicity.[78,83] In the POAS, which included a community cohort of women (50% African American [AA], 50% European American [EA]) assessed yearly from premenopause to postmenopause over 14 years, interactions between the cytochrome p450 enzymes CYP1B1*3 and CYP1B1*4 and the menopause stage were observed for depressive symptoms among AA women only. CYP1B1s, which are highly expressed in estrogen target tissue, are responsible for the hydroxylation of estradiol. This process creates 4- hydroxyestradiol, which generates free radicals that could negatively affect target tissues.[84] Outside of altering local estradiol levels, the mechanism by which of CYP1B1s could impact depression during the perimenopause is unknown. In contrast, the sulfotransferase SULT1A1*3, which converts estradiol to the biologically inactive estradiol sulfate, was associated with a decreased risk for depressive symptoms, but increased risk of hot flashes among EA women. This disconnect between depressive symptoms and VMS is interesting, given that depressive symptoms are often (41% in the POAS cohort), but not always, comorbid with severe VMS.[42] No significant relationship between depression, menopause stage, and genes encoding COMT, CYP19, CYP1B1, CYP1A2, CYP1A1, or CYP3A4 were found for the entire group or by race.[78]

Similarly, a SWAN substudy demonstrated a relationship between estrogen-metabolizing enzymes and depression risk, which differed by race. Although the sample size was large (n = 1538), menopause status was not considered with respect to depression onset (ie, women may have also experienced MDD during the premenopause). In contrast to the POAS, SWAN found that EAs with the CYP1A1 rs2606345 CC and AC genotypes had 2-fold greater odds of having depressive symptoms than those homozygous for the A allele. This relationship between the CC genotype was even greater for AA women (10-fold). Among Japanese women, those homozygous for the T allele in the single nucleotide polymorphism (SNP) CYP19 rs936306 were nearly 5 times as likely to have depressive symptoms as those with the CC genotype. For Chinese women, the TT genotype at the SNP rs615942 for the 17 hydroxysteroid dehydrogenase gene was associated with a 7- to 11-fold increased risk.[83]

Finally, genetic analyses from the Seattle Midlife Women's Health Study focused on the estrogen synthesis pathway, specifically CYYP19 and 17-HSD, but this time in relationship to severity of symptom clusters identified through a latent class analysis of typical perimenopausal symptoms.[85] Although hot flash severity served as the basis for these clusters, depressed mood was included. Investigators found that a 17-beta hydroxysteroid dehydrogenase gene polymorphism was associated with the high-severity group, which included women with high-severity hot flashes and moderate sleep, mood, cognitive, and pain symptoms. Again, unlike the POAS, analyses conducted in the Seattle Midlife Women's Health Study did not consider the menopause stage with respect to depression onset in their analyses and clustering of symptoms limits interpretation of their findings with respect to the genetics of perimenopause depression.

Gonadal Steroid Levels and Fluctuations

The fact that the years leading up to the final menstrual period are characterized by an enhanced depression risk compared with subsequent years,[24] particularly among women with only perimenopausal onset of MDD, implicates dynamic hormonal changes in endogenous reproductive steroids versus absolute hypogonadism in this heightened risk. Given the robust impact of estradiol on brain neurochemistry, structure, and function,[46] it is not surprising that investigators have examined the timing of the onset of menopause, rapidity of progression through menopause, the degree of hormonal fluctuations, and absolute levels of gonadal steroids in the pathophysiology of perimenopause depression. Reproductive steroid (estradiol, progesterone, testosterone, and dehydroepiandrosterone sulfate) levels at discrete time points or across the MT are associated with depressive symptoms in some,[37,86–90] but not all, studies.[23,91] The directionality of this relationship also varies by study, hormone, and sample population. An increase in follicle-stimulating hormone and the variability of estradiol across the MT, particularly in relationship to women's own mean fluctuations, were significantly associated with a greater risk for incident perimenopausal depression after controlling for smoking status, body mass index, poor sleep, hot flashes, and history of premenstrual syndrome.[19] Likewise, postmenopausal women with a decline in estradiol levels over a 2-year follow-up period were 3 times as likely to experience depressive symptoms, suggesting that changes in estradiol levels even after the final menstrual period can impact the depression risk.[91] Finally, studies, including a recent meta-analysis, indicate that a longer reproductive period, defined as a later age at the time of the final menstrual period, or greater number of years between menarche and the onset of the MT was associated with a reduced risk for midlife depression.[92,93]

Clinical Studies of Estradiol Treatment

Two double-blind placebo-controlled studies indicate that conventional HT estradiol doses are more effective than placebo in reducing depressive symptoms among women who presented with perimenopausal MDD.[94,95] In a similar randomized clinical trial in postmenopausal women, estradiol did not differ in effectiveness from placebo.[96] Moreover, a recent study in which euthymic perimenopausal women randomized to receive estradiol (0.1 mg/d) plus intermittent progesterone (200 mg/d for 12 days every 3 months) versus those randomized to placebo were less likely to have potentially clinically significant depressive symptoms at any time during the 12-month assessment period.[97] On average, CES-D scores were higher in the placebo versus estradiol group across the study. When considering menopause stage, the positive effect of the hormone regimen on mood was limited to those in the early MT versus those in the late perimenopause or early postmenopause stages. These findings support the notion of a window of opportunity during which women are more likely to be responsive to the antidepressant effects of estradiol.[98]

CLINICAL IMPLICATIONS

This review highlights the importance of clinical screening for depression among middle-aged women, as the risk for MDD and depressive symptoms are increased during the MT even among those without a personal history of depression. Multiple factors contribute to the risk for depression. Social factors play a critical role in depression onset and persistence. As midlife women are often in transition with respect to interpersonal relationships, adequacy of social support, and current stressors, gynecologists treating menopausal women should periodically assess the current stressors as well as the quality of their patients' intimate relationships and friendships. The current stressors among midlife women often include caring for aging parents at the same time that women are managing their children's transitions to adulthood, stressful job changes, and conflict with their spouse/partner. Given the association of lifetime traumas or childhood adversity with depression, clinicians may want to screen for these as well.

There are numerous screening instruments for clinicians to use in the routine assessment of depression symptoms and their severity. Although self-rated scales are not diagnostic for MDD or minor depressive disorder, they can give the clinician an understanding of the range of symptoms and their individual severity. For example, the CES-D can be used to measure both key symptoms of MDD (anhedonia and low mood) as well as symptoms of anxiety and sleep disturbance, which can also impair quality of life. Women scoring 16 or greater on the CES-D should be evaluated by their clinician for potential treatment in the primary care setting and/or referral to specialty behavioral health.

Although genetic polymorphisms and reproductive hormone fluctuations play a role in the manifestation of risk for MDD during perimenopause, the measurement of these genetic differences is not yet recommended. Future research is needed to confirm the relationship between genotype and risk for depression during periods of dynamic hormonal flux, such as perimenopause.

Estradiol treatment was shown to be more effective than placebo for perimenopausal women meeting the criteria for MDD.[95] The impact of estradiol treatment on depression seemed to be independent of the hormone's effect on VMS and sleep.

For menopausal women who experienced premenopausal episodes of MDD requiring psychiatric treatment, moderate-severe symptoms for the first time during the perimenopause, or those with suicidal thinking, the standard of care would be treatment with antidepressants (assuming no history of bipolar disorder or current hypomania) and referral to a behavioral health specialist if one is available. Antidepressants may be started in the primary care setting in uncomplicated cases when the diagnosis is clear and there is no suicidal thinking. However, follow-up should occur within 1 to 2 weeks to assess for side effects and potential dose titration.

SUMMARY

Depressive symptoms and diagnosis are common during the MT and early postmenopause. Multiple psychosocial and biological factors are involved. Evaluation for depression and treatment may be conducted in the primary care practice and includes consideration of HT and antidepressants, alone or in combination, and cognitive behavioral therapy.

REFERENCES

1. Kessler RC, McGonagle KA, Zhao S, et al. Lifetime and 12-month prevalence of DSM-III-R psychiatric disorders in the United States. Arch Gen Psychiatry 1994; 51:8–19.
2. Hantsoo L, Epperson CN. Premenstrual dysphoric disorder: epidemiology and treatment. Curr Psychiatry Rep 2015;17:87.
3. Santoro N, Epperson CN, Mathews SB. Menopausal symptoms and their management. Endocrinol Metab Clin North Am 2015;44:497–515.
4. Freeman EW, Sammel MD, Liu L, et al. Hormones and menopausal status as predictors of depression in women in transition to menopause. Arch Gen Psychiatry 2004;61:62–70.
5. American Psychiatric Association. Diagnostic and statistical manual of mental disorders. 5th edition. Washington, DC: American Psychiatric Association; 2013.
6. Ayuso-Mateos JL, Nuevo R, Verdes E, et al. From depressive symptoms to depressive disorders: the relevance of thresholds. Br J Psychiatry 2010;196: 365–71.
7. Radloff LS. The CES-D scale: a self-report depression scale for research in the general population. Appl Psychol Meas 1977;1:385–401.
8. Beck AT, Beamesderfer A. Assessment of depression: the depression inventory. In: Pichot P, editor. Psychological measurements in psychopharmacology, vol. 7. Basel (Switzerland): Karger Press; 1974. p. 151–69.
9. Spitzer RL, Williams JB, Kroenke K, et al. Validity and utility of the PRIME-MD patient health questionnaire in assessment of 3000 obstetric-gynecologic patients: the PRIME-MD patient health questionnaire obstetrics-gynecology study. Am J Obstet Gynecol 2000;183:759–69.
10. Spitzer RL, Kroenke K, Williams JB. Validation and utility of a self-report version of PRIME-MD: the PHQ primary care study. Primary care evaluation of mental disorders. patient health questionnaire. JAMA 1999;282:1737–44.
11. Moriarty AS, Gilbody S, McMillan D, et al. Screening and case finding for major depressive disorder using the Patient Health Questionnaire (PHQ-9): a meta-analysis. Gen Hosp Psychiatry 2015;37:567–76.
12. Siu AL, Bibbins-Domingo K, Grossman DC, et al. Screening for depression in adults: US preventive services task force recommendation statement. JAMA 2016;315:380–7.

13. Hardeveld F, Spijker J, De GR, et al. Prevalence and predictors of recurrence of major depressive disorder in the adult population. Acta Psychiatr Scand 2010; 122:184–91.

14. Kessler RC. The effects of stressful life events on depression. Annu Rev Psychol 1997;48:191–214.

15. Rossler W, Ajdacic-Gross V, Riecher-Rossler A, et al. Does menopausal transition really influence mental health? Findings from the prospective long-term Zurich study. World Psychiatry 2016;15:146–54.

16. Vesco KK, Haney EM, Humphrey L, et al. Influence of menopause on mood: a systematic review of cohort studies. Climacteric 2007;10:448–65.

17. Bromberger JT, Kravitz HM, Chang YF, et al. Major depression during and after the menopausal transition: Study of Women's Health Across the Nation (SWAN). Psychol Med 2011;41:1879–88.

18. Bromberger JT, Schott L, Kravitz HM, et al. Risk factors for major depression during midlife among a community sample of women with and without prior major depression: are they the same or different? Psychol Med 2015;45:1653–64.

19. Freeman EW, Sammel MD, Lin H, et al. Associations of hormones and menopausal status with depressed mood in women with no history of depression. Arch Gen Psychiatry 2006;63:375–82.

20. Freeman EW. Associations of depression with the transition to menopause. Menopause 2010;17:823–7.

21. Cohen LS, Soares CN, Vitonis AF, et al. Risk for new onset of depression during the menopausal transition: the Harvard study of moods and cycles. Arch Gen Psychiatry 2006;63:385–90.

22. Hickey M, Schoenaker DA, Joffe H, et al. Depressive symptoms across the menopause transition: findings from a large population-based cohort study. Menopause 2016;23:1287–93.

23. Woods NF, Smith-Dijulio K, Percival DB, et al. Depressed mood during the menopausal transition and early postmenopause: observations from the Seattle Midlife Women's Health Study. Menopause 2008;15:223–32.

24. Freeman EW, Sammel MD, Boorman DW, et al. Longitudinal pattern of depressive symptoms around natural menopause. JAMA Psychiatry 2014;71:36–43.

25. Bromberger JT, Assmann SF, Avis NE, et al. Persistent mood symptoms in a multiethnic community cohort of pre- and perimenopausal women. Am J Epidemiol 2003;158:347–56.

26. Gibbs Z, Lee S, Kulkarni J. What factors determine whether a woman becomes depressed during the perimenopause? Arch Womens Ment Health 2012;15: 323–32.

27. Harlow BL, Cohen LS, Otto MW, et al. Prevalence and predictors of depressive symptoms in older premenopausal women: the Harvard Study of Moods and Cycles. Arch Gen Psychiatry 1999;56:418–24.

28. Bromberger JT, Harlow S, Avis N, et al. Racial/ethnic differences in the prevalence of depressive symptoms among middle-aged women: The Study of Women's Health Across the Nation (SWAN). Am J Public Health 2004;94: 1378–85.

29. Liang J, Xu X, Quinones AR, et al. Multiple trajectories of depressive symptoms in middle and late life: racial/ethnic variations. Psychol Aging 2011;26:761–77.

30. Spence NJ, Adkins DE, Dupre ME. Racial differences in depression trajectories among older women: socioeconomic, family, and health influences. J Health Soc Behav 2011;52:444–59.

31. Bromberger JT, Matthews KA. A "feminine" model of vulnerability to depressive symptoms: a longitudinal investigation of middle-aged women. J Pers Soc Psychol 1996;70:591–8.

32. Bromberger JT, Matthews KA. A longitudinal study of the effects of pessimism, trait anxiety, and life stress on depressive symptoms in middle-aged women. Psychol Aging 1996;11:207–13.

33. Kuh D, Hardy R, Rodgers B, et al. Lifetime risk factors for women's psychological distress in midlife. Soc Sci Med 2002;55:1957–73.

34. Bromberger JT, Matthews KA, Schott LL, et al. Depressive symptoms during the menopausal transition: the Study of Women's Health Across the Nation (SWAN). J Affect Disord 2007;103:267–72.

35. Dennerstein L, Lehert P, Burger H, et al. Mood and the menopausal transition. J Nerv Ment Dis 1999;187:685–91.

36. Ayers B, Forshaw M, Hunter MS. The impact of attitudes towards the menopause on women's symptom experience: a systematic review. Maturitas 2010;65:28–36.

37. Bromberger JT, Schott LL, Kravitz HM, et al. Longitudinal change in reproductive hormones and depressive symptoms across the menopausal transition: results from the Study of Women's Health Across the Nation (SWAN). Arch Gen Psychiatry 2010;67:598–607.

38. Pimenta F, Leal I, Maroco J, et al. Menopausal symptoms: do life events predict severity of symptoms in peri- and post-menopause? Maturitas 2012;72:324–31.

39. Woods NF, Mitchell ES. Pathways to depressed mood for midlife women: observations from the Seattle Midlife Women's Health Study. Res Nurs Health 1997;20:119–29.

40. Bromberger JT, Kravitz HM, Matthews K, et al. Predictors of first lifetime episodes of major depression in midlife women. Psychol Med 2009;39:55–64.

41. Schmidt PJ, Murphy JH, Haq N, et al. Stressful life events, personal losses, and perimenopause-related depression. Arch Womens Ment Health 2004;7:19–26.

42. Freeman EW, Sammel MD, Lin H. Temporal associations of hot flashes and depression in the transition to menopause. Menopause 2009;16:728–34.

43. Gordon JL, Rubinow DR, Eisenlohr-Moul TA, et al. Estradiol variability, stressful life events, and the emergence of depressive symptomatology during the menopausal transition. Menopause 2016;23:257–66.

44. Bale TL, Epperson CN. Sex differences and stress across the lifespan. Nat Neurosci 2015;18:1413–20.

45. Epperson CN, Sammel MD, Bale TL, et al. Adverse childhood experiences and risk for first-episode major depression during the menopause transition. J Clin Psychiatry 2017;78:e298–307.

46. Shanmugan S, Epperson CN. Estrogen and the prefrontal cortex: towards a new understanding of estrogen's effects on executive functions in the menopause transition. Hum Brain Mapp 2014;35:847–65.

47. Shanmugan S, Satterthwaite TD, Sammel MD, et al. Impact of early life adversity and tryptophan depletion on functional connectivity in menopausal women: a double-blind, placebo-controlled crossover study. Psychoneuroendocrinology 2017;84:197–205.

48. Shanmugan S, Loughead J, Cao W, et al. Impact of tryptophan depletion on executive system function during menopause is moderated by childhood adversity. Neuropsychopharmacology 2017;42:2398–406.

49. Anda RF, Croft JB, Felitti VJ, et al. Adverse childhood experiences and smoking during adolescence and adulthood. JAMA 1999;282:1652–8.

50. Anda RF, Felitti VJ, Bremner JD, et al. The enduring effects of abuse and related adverse experiences in childhood. A convergence of evidence from neurobiology and epidemiology. Eur Arch Psychiatry Clin Neurosci 2006;256:174–86.

51. Bromberger JT, Schott LL, Matthews KA, et al. Childhood socioeconomic circumstances and depressive symptom burden across 15 years of follow-up during midlife: Study of Women's Health Across the Nation (SWAN). Arch Womens Ment Health 2017;20:495–504.

52. Felitti VJ, Anda RF, Nordenberg D, et al. Relationship of childhood abuse and household dysfunction to many of the leading causes of death in adults. The Adverse Childhood Experiences (ACS) Study. Am J Prev Med 1998;14:245–58.

53. Heim C, Binder EB. Current research trends in early life stress and depression: review of human studies on sensitive periods, gene-environment interactions, and epigenetics. Exp Neurol 2012;233:102–11.

54. Freeman EW, Sammel MD, Lin H, et al. Symptoms in the menopausal transition: hormone and behavioral correlates. Obstet Gynecol 2008;111:127–36.

55. Gallicchio L, Schilling C, Miller SR, et al. Correlates of depressive symptoms among women undergoing the menopausal transition. J Psychosom Res 2007; 63:263–8.

56. Brown WJ, Ford JH, Burton NW, et al. Prospective study of physical activity and depressive symptoms in middle-aged women. Am J Prev Med 2005;29:265–72.

57. Dugan SA, Bromberger JT, Segawa E, et al. Association between physical activity and depressive symptoms: midlife women in SWAN. Med Sci Sports Exerc 2015; 47:335–42.

58. van Uffelen JG, van Gellecum YR, Burton NW, et al. Sitting-time, physical activity, and depressive symptoms in mid-aged women. Am J Prev Med 2013;45:276–81.

59. Polo-Kantola P. Sleep problems in midlife and beyond. Maturitas 2011;68:224–32.

60. Alvaro PK, Roberts RM, Harris JK. A systematic review assessing bidirectionality between sleep disturbances, anxiety, and depression. Sleep 2013;36:1059–68.

61. Breslau N, Roth T, Rosenthal L, et al. Sleep disturbance and psychiatric disorders: a longitudinal epidemiological study of young adults. Biol Psychiatry 1996;39:411–8.

62. Bromberger JT, Kravitz HM, Youk A, et al. Patterns of depressive disorders across 13 years and their determinants among midlife women: SWAN mental health study. J Affect Disord 2016;206:31–40.

63. Joffe H, Crawford SL, Freeman MP, et al. Independent contributions of nocturnal hot flashes and sleep disturbance to depression in estrogen-deprived women. J Clin Endocrinol Metab 2016;101:3847–55.

64. Bauld R, Brown RF. Stress, psychological distress, psychosocial factors, menopause symptoms and physical health in women. Maturitas 2009;62:160–5.

65. Agatisa PK, Matthews KA, Bromberger JT, et al. Coronary and aortic calcification in women with a history of major depression. Arch Intern Med 2005;165:1229–36.

66. Jones DJ, Bromberger JT, Sutton-Tyrrell K, et al. Lifetime history of depression and carotid atherosclerosis in middle-aged women. Arch Gen Psychiatry 2003; 60:153–60.

67. Tomey K, Sowers MR, Harlow S, et al. Physical functioning among mid-life women: associations with trajectory of depressive symptoms. Soc Sci Med 2010;71:1259–67.

68. Ormel J, Rijsdijk FV, Sullivan M, et al. Temporal and reciprocal relationship between IADL/ADL disability and depressive symptoms in late life. J Gerontol B Psychol Sci Soc Sci 2002;57:338–47.

69. Terauchi M, Hiramitsu S, Akiyoshi M, et al. Associations among depression, anxiety and somatic symptoms in peri- and postmenopausal women. J Obstet Gynaecol Res 2013;39:1007–13.

70. Wang HL, Booth-LaForce C, Tang SM, et al. Depressive symptoms in Taiwanese women during the peri- and post-menopause years: associations with demographic, health, and psychosocial characteristics. Maturitas 2013;75:355–60.

71. Waetjen LE, Liao S, Johnson WO, et al. Factors associated with prevalent and incident urinary incontinence in a cohort of midlife women: a longitudinal analysis of data: study of women's health across the nation. Am J Epidemiol 2007;165: 309–18.

72. Joffe H, Hall JE, Soares CN, et al. Vasomotor symptoms are associated with depression in perimenopausal women seeking primary care. Menopause 2002; 9:392–8.

73. Caspi A, Sugden K, Moffitt TE, et al. Influence of life stress on depression: moderation by a polymorphism in the 5-HTT gene. Science 2003;301:386–9.

74. Sharpley CF, Palanisamy SK, Glyde NS, et al. An update on the interaction between the serotonin transporter promoter variant (5-HTTLPR), stress and depression, plus an exploration of non-confirming findings. Behav Brain Res 2014;273: 89–105.

75. Otte C, Gold SM, Penninx BW, et al. Major depressive disorder. Nat Rev Dis Primers 2016;2:16065.

76. Sullivan PF, Neale MC, Kendler KS. Genetic epidemiology of major depression: review and meta-analysis. Am J Psychiatry 2000;157:1552–62.

77. Kugaya A, Epperson CN, Zoghbi S, et al. Increase in prefrontal cortex serotonin 2A receptors following estrogen treatment in postmenopausal women. Am J Psychiatry 2003;160:1522–4.

78. Rebbeck TR, Su HI, Sammel MD, et al. Effect of hormone metabolism genotypes on steroid hormone levels and menopausal symptoms in a prospective population-based cohort of women experiencing the menopausal transition. Menopause 2010;17:1026–34.

79. Grochans E, Jurczak A, Szkup M, et al. Evaluation of the relationship between 5-HTT and MAO gene polymorphisms, mood and level of anxiety among postmenopausal women. Int J Environ Res Public Health 2014;12:268–81.

80. Ryan J, Scali J, Carriere I, et al. Oestrogen receptor polymorphisms and late-life depression. Br J Psychiatry 2011;199:126–31.

81. Zhang J, Chen L, Ma J, et al. Interaction of estrogen receptor beta and negative life events in susceptibility to major depressive disorder in a Chinese Han female population. J Affect Disord 2017;208:628–33.

82. Epperson CN, Shanmugan S, Kim DR, et al. New onset executive function difficulties at menopause: a possible role for lisdexamfetamine. Psychopharmacology (Berl) 2015;232:3091–100.

83. Kravitz HM, Janssen I, Lotrich FE, et al. Sex steroid hormone gene polymorphisms and depressive symptoms in women at midlife. Am J Med 2006;119: S87–93.

84. Tsuchiya Y, Nakajima M, Yokoi T. Cytochrome P450-mediated metabolism of estrogens and its regulation in human. Cancer Lett 2005;227:115–24.

85. Woods NF, Cray LA, Mitchell ES, et al. Polymorphisms in estrogen synthesis genes and symptom clusters during the menopausal transition and early postmenopause: observations from the Seattle Midlife Women's Health Study. Biol Res Nurs 2018;20(2):153–60.

86. Colangelo LA, Ouyang P, Golden SH, et al. Do sex hormones or hormone therapy modify the relation of n-3 fatty acids with incident depressive symptoms in post-menopausal women? The MESA Study. Psychoneuroendocrinology 2017;75: 26–35.

87. Milman LW, Sammel MD, Barnhart KT, et al. Higher serum total testosterone levels correlate with increased risk of depressive symptoms in Caucasian women through the entire menopausal transition. Psychoneuroendocrinology 2015;62: 107–13.

88. Morrison MF, Ten HT, Freeman EW, et al. DHEA-S levels and depressive symptoms in a cohort of African American and Caucasian women in the late reproductive years. Biol Psychiatry 2001;50:705–11.

89. Santoro N, Torrens J, Crawford S, et al. Correlates of circulating androgens in mid-life women: the study of women's health across the nation. J Clin Endocrinol Metab 2005;90:4836–45.

90. Schmidt PJ, Murphy JH, Haq N, et al. Basal plasma hormone levels in depressed perimenopausal women. Psychoneuroendocrinology 2002;27:907–20.

91. Ryan J, Burger HG, Szoeke C, et al. A prospective study of the association between endogenous hormones and depressive symptoms in postmenopausal women. Menopause 2009;16:509–17.

92. Marsh WK, Bromberger JT, Crawford SL, et al. Lifelong estradiol exposure and risk of depressive symptoms during the transition to menopause and postmenopause. Menopause 2017;24:1351–9.

93. Georgakis MK, Thomopoulos TP, Diamantaras AA, et al. Association of age at menopause and duration of reproductive period with depression after menopause: a systematic review and meta-analysis. JAMA Psychiatry 2016;73: 139–49.

94. Schmidt PJ, Nieman L, Danaceau MA, et al. Estrogen replacement in perimenopause-related depression: a preliminary report. Am J Obstet Gynecol 2000;183:414–20.

95. Soares CN, Almeida OP, Joffe H, et al. Efficacy of estradiol for the treatment of depressive disorders in perimenopausal women: a double-blind, randomized, placebo-controlled trial. Arch Gen Psychiatry 2001;58:529–34.

96. Morrison MF, Kallan MJ, Ten HT, et al. Lack of efficacy of estradiol for depression in postmenopausal women: a randomized, controlled trial. Biol Psychiatry 2004; 55:406–12.

97. Gordon JL, Rubinow DR, Eisenlohr-Moul TA, et al. Efficacy of transdermal estradiol and micronized progesterone in the prevention of depressive symptoms in the menopause transition: a randomized clinical trial. JAMA Psychiatry 2018; 75:149–57.

98. Soares CN, Maki PM. Menopausal transition, mood, and cognition: an integrated view to close the gaps. Menopause 2010;17:812–4.

Sleep, Health, and Metabolism in Midlife Women and Menopause: Food for Thought

Howard M. Kravitz, DO, MPH[a,b,*], Rasa Kazlauskaite, MD, MSc[c], Hadine Joffe, MD, MSc[d]

KEYWORDS

- Sleep health • Metabolic health • Immunometabolism • Menopause
- Menopausal transition • Midlife

KEY POINTS

- Sleep health includes subjective sleep satisfaction, regularity, appropriate timing of sleep, adequate duration, sleep efficiency/continuity, and sustained alertness during waking hours.
- Metabolic health depends largely on lifestyle and extends to every human body system because energy metabolism is involved in every biological function.
- Circadian rhythms regulate many functions related to sleep and metabolism, including sleep propensity, hormonal rhythms, feeding behavior/appetite, and the glucose and lipid metabolism rhythmicity.

Continued

Disclosure Statement: Dr H.M. Kravitz and Dr R. Kazlauskaite report no relationship with a commercial company that has a direct financial interest in subject matter or materials discussed in this article or with a company making a competing product. Dr H. Joffe reports research grants from Merck and Pfizer, and consulting fees from Merck, KaNDy, and Sojournix.
The Study of Women's Health Across the Nation (SWAN) has grant support from the National Institutes of Health (NIH), DHHS, through the National Institute on Aging (NIA), the National Institute of Nursing Research (NINR), and the NIH Office of Research on Women's Health (ORWH) (Grants U01NR004061; U01AG012505, U01AG012535, U01AG012531, U01AG012539, U01AG012546, U01AG012553, U01AG012554, U01AG012495). Dr H. Joffe also has support from National Institute on Aging (R01AG053838).

[a] Department of Psychiatry, Rush University Medical Center, Rush West Campus, 2150 West Harrison Street, Room 278, Chicago, IL 60612, USA; [b] Department of Preventive Medicine, Rush University Medical Center, 1700 West Van Buren Street, Triangle Office Building, Suite 470, Chicago, IL, USA; [c] Department of Medicine, Division of Endocrinology and Metabolism, Rush University Medical Center, 1750 West Harrison Street, Suite 604w Jelke, Chicago, IL 60612, USA; [d] Department of Psychiatry and Connors Center for Women's Health, Brigham and Women's Hospital, Dana Farber Cancer Institute, Harvard Medical School, 75 Francis Street, Boston, MA 02115, USA
* Corresponding author. Department of Psychiatry, Rush University Medical Center, Rush West Campus, 2150 West Harrison Street, Room 278, Chicago, IL 60612.
E-mail address: hkravitz@rush.edu

Obstet Gynecol Clin N Am 45 (2018) 679–694
https://doi.org/10.1016/j.ogc.2018.07.008
0889-8545/18/© 2018 Elsevier Inc. All rights reserved.

Continued

- Changes in sleep patterns associated with menopause and aging may reflect voluntary lifestyle modifications and disturbances in sleep health may result in metabolic health consequences.
- Menopause-related sleep disturbance may affect eating behaviors and timing, directly affect immunometabolism, and interact with other triggers of immunometabolic dysfunction, particularly abdominal adiposity (adipose inflammation).

INTRODUCTION

"If sleep does not serve an absolutely vital function, then it is the biggest mistake the evolutionary process has ever made."[1] In the half-century since Allan Rechtschaffen's declaration, studies of sleep and sleep deprivation have demonstrated that as a universal behavior sleep serves a variety of physiologic functions. As a behavior essential for survival, and one in which humans engage in for nearly one-third of their life, sleep is as necessary as food and water.[2] Although the function(s) associated with the complex phenomenon of sleep, which involves many interacting regulatory mechanisms, remain to be fully elucidated, one of its key roles is metabolic homeostasis.[3] Moreover, the health of populations is increasingly defined by positive attributes such as wellness, performance, and adaptation, and not merely by the absence of disease,[4] as well as prolongation of healthspan, not just extension of lifespan.[5] In this article, the authors examine the concepts of sleep health and metabolic health, and their relationships to reproductive and chronologic aging in middle aged and older adult women.

SLEEP AND SLEEP HEALTH

The 2007 report of the Sleep in America poll brought national attention to the public health relevance of sleep, particularly for women.[6] Sleep disturbances are a common complaint during the menopausal transition (MT).[7,8] In their review of studies of perceived sleep quality, Shaver and Woods[7] described that more women in MT stages (ie, perimenopause) reported poor sleep than did women in late reproductive age to an extent that was beyond anticipated age effects. Closely inter-related psychological, social, and cultural factors associated with the transition to midlife shape a woman's experience of menopause and contribute to sleep disturbances.[9] Menopause-specific factors, aging, stress and other psychological factors, social realities/social transitions and their associated lifestyle changes, coexisting health conditions, and cultural factors can contribute to sleep problems and poor sleep health.

Much information has accrued about the impact of sleep and sleep disorders on women's health since the release of the Sleep in America report. Consistent findings have confirmed that women's sleep disturbances increase with age, more so than in men, and the prevalence of their sleep problems increase as they traverse the MT.[10] Both sex (biological and physiologic) and gender (environmental, social, and cultural influences on the biological factors) differences may help to explain why men and women sleep differently and may underlie their differential risk for sleep disorders.[11,12] However, because menopause is associated with changes in behavior and other biological functions such as mood swings, anxiety/depression, and stress, in addition to sleep disturbances, symptoms that are associated with reproductive aging may be difficult to differentiate from symptoms owing to chronologic aging. Vasomotor symptoms (VMS), hormonal changes, age-associated changes in sleep, comorbid conditions, and psychosocial factors all have been cited as factors that contribute to the increasing prevalence of disturbed sleep in midlife women as they transition to menopause.[13] Recent data from the Study of Women's Health Across the Nation (SWAN)[14] and the Penn Ovarian Aging Study,[15] which used the final menstrual period (FMP) rather than MT stages, suggest that premenopausal sleep complaints predict poor sleep around the FMP, consistent with a diagnosis of a menopause-related form of sleep disturbance. However, aside from a subgroup of approximately 15% of women whose sleep worsened in the years around the FMP, both the SWAN and the Penn Ovarian Aging Study found that, after the FMP, sleep complaints tended to be stable or increase slowly from pre-FMP to post-FMP from their premenopausal baseline.

In older adults, women as well as men, great variability in sleep characteristics are observed. Sleep is described as lighter, more easily disrupted, and associated with more frequent brief arousals and longer awakenings. It is shorter and less refreshing, and older adults are more likely to take daytime naps and/or adopt earlier bedtimes. In addition, older adults experience a greater burden of general health problems, and sleep problems, such as sleep apnea and restless legs, which become more prevalent, particularly in women during postmenopause. However, few studies have specifically examined the potential benefits of good sleep/sleep health in older adults.

Sleep Health

Good sleep health is important for successful aging.[16] Although sleep complaints are common in older adults, they are commonly associated with physical, environmental, and health factors. Foley and associates[17] found that respondents to the 2003 Sleep and Aging survey who were 65 years and older indicated an inverse association between self-perceived quality of sleep and the number of their comorbid conditions.

Buysse[4] defined sleep health as "a multidimensional pattern of sleep-wakefulness, adapted to individual, social, and environmental demands, that promotes physical and mental well-being." In developing this concept, he found that sleep health is a term that is mentioned infrequently in the literature and, when it is, it is typically not defined. A PubMed search for this exact term produced 150 results, and Google Scholar more than 3000, but the majority include a comma between the words "sleep" and "health," indicating 2 items in a list of related concepts. Moreover, sleep health consisted of a number of different sleep parameters, including sleep duration, sleep times, awakenings, sleepiness, and specific sleep disorder symptoms. We conducted a more recent Ovid Medline search (December 18, 2017) and obtained 370 documents, of which 302 (82%) were published between 2010 and the search date.

To assess sleep health, characteristics of sleep and sleep problems can be measured on a range of key quantifiable dimensions, including subjective sleep satisfaction, appropriate timing of sleep, adequate duration, sleep efficiency or continuity, sustained alertness/sleepiness during waking hours, and sleep regularity.[4,18] This definition does not pertain to any specific sleep disorder and can be used to characterize sleep multidimensionally across all persons. Buysse's[4] conceptual model of sleep health recognizes that relationships between sleep–wake function and molecular, cellular, systems, and organism-level outcomes are reciprocal; just as sleep affects function and health, so too function and health influence sleep–wake function.

Healthy People 2020, a US government-sponsored public health initiative, includes a section on sleep health that is designed to increase public awareness about the potential adverse consequences associated with sleep loss and sleep disorders.[19] Perturbations in various dimensions of sleep health may be manifested as metabolic health consequences[20] and psychological health consequences.[18]

METABOLIC HEALTH

Metabolic health is typically approached from the perspective of the metabolic syndrome (MetS), which is clinically defined using diagnostic thresholds (**Table 1**).[21] Most women with type 2 diabetes meet criteria for MetS and the majority with MetS are obese or overweight. Moreover, metabolic health extends to every human body system and relates to many chronic degenerative diseases and disability, because energy metabolism is involved in every biological function (**Fig. 1**). Thus, metabolism is an essential component of health.

Historically viewed as a product of insulin resistance, MetS has been recognized as a manifestation of immunometabolic dysfunction (nutrient–energy stress induced chronic low-grade inflammation, causing loss of metabolic control).[22] It is generally accepted that energy metabolism is in constant dynamic balance between catabolic processes to generate energy for physical and mental productivity (at the cellular and global levels), and anabolic processes to generate biomass (such as glucose, fatty acids, amino acids, etc) for repair, maintenance, detoxification, and storage.[23,24] This dynamic coupling of catabolic and anabolic processes is regulated by circadian,[25] neurologic, and hormonal systems,[26] and tightly intertwined with innate and adaptive immunity (thus referred to as immunometabolism).[22] The dynamic balance interval of energy metabolism (immunometabolic flexibility) narrows with age and other factors, increasing susceptibility to chronic disease and physical and neuropsychological frailty (for a conceptual model, see **Fig. 1**).[23]

In midlife women, accelerated reproductive aging is intertwined with chronologic aging. Changes in the reproductive hormone milieu lead to transformation of body and self-image, change in psychological and physical functioning, and adaptation

Table 1
Diagnostic criteria for metabolic syndrome

Criteria	Thresholds
Central obesity	Waist circumference[a] • Men: ≥102 cm (90 cm in Asians/Hispanics) • Women: ≥88 cm (80 cm in Asians/Hispanics)
Hypertension	≥130/85 mm Hg or hypertension treatment
Fasting blood glucose	≥100 mg/dL
High-density lipoprotein cholesterol	• Men: <40 mg/dL • Women: <50 mg/dL
Triglyceridemia	≥150 mg/dL

Diagnosis requires meeting threshold for at least 3 of the 5 criteria.

[a] Note that Asian and Hispanic men and women have different waist circumference thresholds than whites and non-Hispanic blacks (this is partially related to body size; they tend to be shorter on average).

Data from Alberti KG, Eckel RH, Grundy SM, et al. Harmonizing the metabolic syndrome: a joint interim statement of the International Diabetes Federation Task Force on Epidemiology and Prevention; National Heart, Lung, and Blood Institute; American Heart Association; World Heart Federation; International Atherosclerosis Society; and International Association for the Study of Obesity. Circulation 2009;120(16):1642.

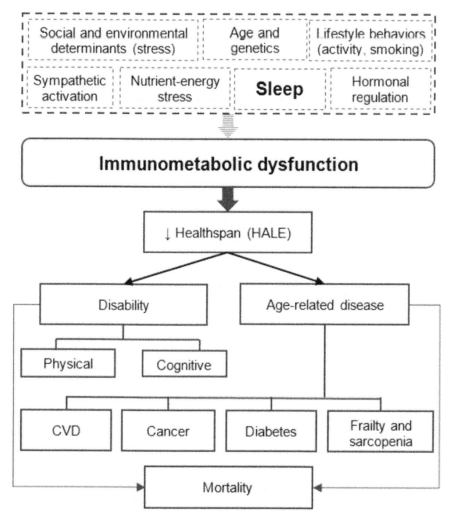

Fig. 1. Sleep with other triggers of immunometabolic dysfunction and relation to health-span, disease, and disability in midlife women. Sleep can affect immunometabolism directly and through interactions with other triggers. Hormonal regulation: reproductive hormones, adipokines, and other hormones. CVD, cardiovascular disease; HALE, healthy life expectancy. (*Data from* World Health Organization. WHO methods for life expectancy and healthy life expectancy. In: Global Health Estimates Technical Paper WHO/HIS/HSI/GHE/2014.5. 2014. Available at: http://www.who.int/healthinfo/statistics/LT_method_1990_2012.pdf. Accessed January 18, 2018; and *Courtesy of* R. Kazlauskaite, MD, MSc, FACE, Chicago, IL.)

(or maladaptation) of lifestyle behaviors. Moreover, immunometabolic changes during the MT relate to adipose tissue redistribution, often without changes in the overall body mass[27] with abdominal adiposity (adipose inflammation) being central to immunometabolic dysfunction and MetS.[28]

Metabolic health largely depends on individual's lifestyle. Among all lifestyle factors, nutrition (nutrient–energy stress) undisputedly has the most impact on metabolic abnormalities.[29] Yet food intake is affected by other lifestyle factors, with a substantial effect of sleep because nearly one-third of human life is spent sleeping.[30]

SLEEP HEALTH AND METABOLIC HEALTH: PATHOBIOLOGY OF ASSOCIATIONS

Sleep can affect immunometabolism directly and through interactions with the other triggers of immunometabolic dysfunction (see **Fig. 1**). Menopause-related sleep disturbance may affect eating behaviors and timing. Sleep disturbance is interconnected with mood, regulation of hunger and impulse control, thermoregulatory sensitivity, and other factors related to metabolic flexibility in response to nutrient–energy stress.[31–34] The relationship between sleep and energy metabolism seems to be bidirectional.[35–37]

Vasomotor Symptoms and Thermoregulation

VMS are associated with more sleep complaints and impaired sleep efficiency and continuity, with VMS primarily interrupting sleep but not shortening total sleep duration.[14,15,38] A narrow temperature sensitivity interval and core body temperature oscillations during the MT may explain the transitional nature of VMS, and in late postmenopause when women have lower body temperature, on average, compared with premenopausal women, these symptoms (hot flashes/flushes, night sweats) may subside.[39] A lower thermoregulatory threshold relative to an elevated core body temperature may plausibly prolong the duration of night sweats (and VMS), which in turn may be associated with extended exposure to an increased amount of wake after sleep onset time.

During sleep, changes in the respiratory quotient, reflecting energy metabolism, seem to follow the time course of core body temperature (decreases during the first one-half of sleep and increases during the second one-half), because energy metabolism and thermoregulation are closely associated.[40,41] Specifically, the respiratory quotient and glucose oxidation decrease during the first one-half of the nighttime sleep cycle, particularly the last hour of this interval. As such, MT-related sleep changes produce respiratory quotient shifts negatively affecting glucose and lipid use and storage, characteristic of the MetS.

Circadian Timing and Insulin Resistance

Circadian timing influences the regulation of many body functions, including sleep propensity, appetite/feeding, hormonal rhythms, and the rhythmicity of glucose and lipid metabolism.[42] Age-related changes in sleep and circadian rhythms may contribute to and interact with changes in nutrient intake, energy expenditure, resting metabolic rate, physical activity (exercise, nonexercise, sedentary time), and ultimately sarcopenia and greater body adiposity.[43] Misalignment of the sleep–wake cycle and melatonin rhythm may promote insulin resistance through regulation of the endocrine system, of peripheral clock genes, and of mitochondrial respiratory function. Sleep disturbances, including insufficient total sleep time, poor sleep quality and insomnia, and obstructive sleep apnea, are independent risk factors for the development and exacerbation of insulin resistance.[44] Dietary intake may modulate the effect of sleep loss on insulin resistance,[45] whereas exercise may potentially mitigate some of the metabolic damage and may improve sleep quality.[46] Thus, if older adults continue to work and engage in shiftwork, the incidence of metabolic disease may increase.[47]

In a sample of midlife women participating in SWAN, circadian misalignment beyond shift work (ie, greater variability in bedtime advance and delay) in non–shift-working midlife women was associated with adverse metabolic health.[48] Sex differences in age-related sleep and circadian rhythm disturbances and age-related changes in sex hormones also may contribute to metabolic disease in older adults, and the relationships between metabolic disease and sleep and circadian rhythm disturbance may be bidirectional.[49]

Metabolic Flexibility (the Capacity for the Organism to Adapt Fuel Oxidation to Fuel Availability, Maintaining Normal Metabolic Function)

Sleep typically represents a state of a relative quiescence from external environmental stressors (as sleep-related fasting), a state that allows for cell maintenance, repair, detoxification, cellular downscaling, and memory consolidation, which are required for daily maintenance of metabolic flexibility.[50] Evidence suggests that chronic exposure to environmental factors can shape the metabolic pathways directed by specific transcriptional programs that tightly regulate the enzymes involved in cell metabolism and dictate cell fate, contributing to metabolic flexibility.[51] The studies of transcriptome indicate that sleep loss affects metabolic adaptation and flexibility from the neurocognitive perspective,[52] and from the peripheral circadian regulation perspective.[53] Likewise, sleep may affect immunologic adaptation.[54,55] These restorative processes prevent the organism from disintegration (the entropy of the living systems tends to a maximum and repair requires time and additional energy). As such, sleep is a fundamental biological necessity.

In experimental settings, sleep-related fasting is modeled as time-restricted feeding, which is contrasted with random around-the-clock feeding time, representing a disrupted sleep–wake cycle. Time-restricted feeding exerts a profound effect on hepatic gene expression and metabolites, particularly related to glucose and lipid metabolism,[56] including cyclic adenosine monophosphate response element binding protein, mechanistic target of rapamycin, and adenosine monophosphate-activated protein kinase nutrient sensing pathways.[42] In addition, compared with random around-the-clock feeding times, restricted feeding results in smaller adipocyte size, less macrophage infiltration of adipose, lower inflammatory cytokine production, and more mitochondria. As such, time-restricted feeding may be associated with better adipose tissue function and immunometabolism.

Appetite, Mood, and Nutrient–energy Stress

Sleep restriction does not significantly affect 24-hour energy expenditure.[33,40] In contrast, sleep disturbance relates to positive energy balance owing to increased food intake, suggesting an additional indirect mechanism for sleep's effect on metabolic health.[35,40,57]

In experimental settings with a controlled eucaloric diet, sleep restriction results in significantly decreased concentrations of leptin, fasting peptide YY levels, glucagon-like peptide 1, and fullness, with significantly increased ghrelin, hunger, and appetite.[40,57–59] Experimental sleep restriction studies paired with ad libitum eating opportunities further demonstrate that sleep restriction increases food intake, especially in the evening, and in excess of that required for energy balance, resulting in weight gain despite changes in hunger and satiety hormones signaling excess energy stores. Relative to men, women maintain weight during adequate sleep, but increase food consumption and experience weight gain during insufficient sleep.[60] Thus, excess energy intake secondary to sleep restriction is driven by both adverse changes in orexigenic and anorexigenic hormones and food consumption.[31,61,62] However, only a small number of women have been included in experimental sleep restriction studies, so less is known about the role of adipokines in women's metabolic health. In addition, it is not known whether sleep fragmentation concurrent with normal sleep duration, the most common type of sleep problem linked with menopause and VMS, has the same metabolic and eating behavior consequences as observed in sleep restriction.

Menopause-related sleep disturbance is associated with negative changes in mood.[32,63,64] Moreover, negative memory bias exacerbates this association.[65] The proposed mechanisms to explain the association between sleep, mood, and excessive ad libitum food intake include sensitivity to food reward, disinhibited eating and psychological distress.[66] The relation of emotions and sleep is bidirectional: emotional processing can affect sleep, and sleep disturbance can be associated with stress reactivity and maladaptive coping including excessive food intake, alcohol consumption, and reduced physical activity, all factors that directly affect metabolism.

Menopausal Hormonal Milieu

The association of sleep with immunometabolic changes is stronger in midlife women than in men. Specifically, actigraphy-assessed sleep latency in women was associated with insulin resistance and partially explained by the indirect effect of inflammatory cytokines.[67] Loss of ovarian estradiol (E2) leads to much lower E2 concentrations in postmenopausal women than in midlife men of the same age,[68] partially explaining sex disparities in sleep and immunometabolism. Evidence suggests that there may be a significant bidirectional relationship in which sleep–wake cycles influence ovarian steroids and gonadotropins, and ovarian steroids and gonadotropin hormones influence sleep–wake cycles.[69–72] Marked fluctuations and changes in ovarian steroids and gonadotropins during the MT may contribute to the risks for and mechanism(s) involved in the development of menopause-related sleep disturbances and disorders.[73,74]

The estrogen action on immunometabolism has been extensively reviewed.[75] Because estrogens decrease food intake and upturn energy expenditure, menopausal loss of ovarian estrogen narrows the interval of metabolic flexibility, increasing susceptibility to metabolic abnormalities when exposed to sleep disturbances and nutrient–energy stress.[76] Menopausal hormone therapy seems to restore sleep health[69] and facilitates metabolic health.[77] E2 in the physiologic range mitigates immunometabolic dysfunction in adipose, cardiovascular, and neural in vitro systems,[78,79] partially explaining the pleiotropic effects of menopausal E2 loss on chronic degenerative conditions.

SLEEP APNEA, METABOLIC HEALTH, AND MENOPAUSE

The direct relationship between sleep health and immunometabolism is well-established,[80] with chronic hypoxia affecting oxidative metabolism and apnea-induced sleep fragmentation affecting appetite regulation, neurohormonal regulation, adipose tissue distribution, epigenetic phenomena, and immunometabolism overall. Multiple mechanisms link obstructive sleep apnea with abnormal immunometabolism.[81] Menopause is associated with an increased risk of sleep apnea.[82] Specifically, at the perimenopause, each additional year in the MT was associated with a 4% greater apnea–hypopnea index.[83] Moreover, metabolic markers improve with treatment of obstructive sleep apnea[84] and treatment of MetS using lifestyle modifications or bariatric surgery improve sleep apnea indices.[85,86]

METABOLIC OUTCOMES

Associations between sleep and metabolic outcomes have been explored in cross-sectional and longitudinal studies.[37] The prototypical metabolic outcomes pertaining to midlife women include obesity, diabetes, and MetS.

Obesity

A metaanalysis of 14 adult longitudinal studies reported overall 25% higher odds of obesity with short (≤5–6 hours) sleep duration but not with long (≥7–9 hours) sleep duration.[87] The metaanalysis of cross-sectional studies reported a negative relationship between sleep duration and abdominal adiposity.[88] These metaanalyses were not specific to midlife women, nor do they address the specific menopause- and VMS-related sleep problem of sleep interruption paired with normal sleep duration.

It is becoming increasingly recognized that sleep and nutrition are related, although the studies of these associations in clinical and community samples generally have been cross-sectional and have not involved midlife or older adults. Among 310 midlife women (mean age, 49.7 years; standard deviation, 2.0 years) who participated in the SWAN Sleep Study, cross-sectional associations between sleep duration and current body mass index (BMI) were independent of sleep-disordered breathing, but longitudinal associations between sleep duration and annual BMI change were not prospectively associated over approximately 4.6 years of follow-up in unadjusted and adjusted models.[89] Shortened sleep and sleep disturbances seem to be related to the accumulation of visceral adipose tissue in a study that included midlife women.[90] Although longitudinal studies, which are limited by reliance on self-reported sleep duration and generally do not account for potential confounding by sleep-disordered breathing, demonstrate no consistent association between sleep and BMI in midlife women, the evidence suggests a potential relationship between sleep and adipose tissue redistribution (visceral adiposity, increase in total body fat, and decrease in muscle), which is characteristic of the MetS.[27] These limitations highlight the need for a longitudinal investigation of sleep and adipose tissue distribution (with or without changes in total body fat) during the MT.

Diabetes Mellitus

A metaanalysis of 15 studies suggests a parabolic dose–response relationship in persons with diabetes between sleep duration and hemoglobin A1c, and a direct association between poor sleep quality and hemoglobin A1c.[91] Metaanalysis of 10 prospective studies with a follow-up of at least 3 years revealed an unambiguous and consistent parabolic relationship between sleep duration (both short, ie, <6 hours, or long, ie, >8 hours) or difficulties maintaining sleep and the risk of incident type 2 diabetes.[92] Moreover, a metaanalysis of 36 studies revealed that sleep disturbances, including difficulty initiating and maintaining sleep and obstructive sleep apnea, were associated with a risk of incident diabetes, with the effect sizes comparable to having a family history of diabetes or being overweight and exceeding the effect size of sedentary lifestyle on diabetes risk.[30] The magnitude of the sleep effect highlights the importance of sleep in diabetes risk.

The recently published results from 3 studies including midlife women—the Nurses' Health Study,[93] the Whitehall II study,[94] and the West of Scotland study[95]—suggest parabolic associations between sleep duration or quality and incident diabetes, with confounding effects of obesity and behavioral factors. The majority of studies involving individuals without diabetes, which are not limited to midlife or menopausal women, have reported independent associations between obstructive sleep apnea and insulin resistance or sensitivity and/or other measures of glycemic health, with a dose-dependent effect of obstructive sleep apnea on such measures of metabolic impairment, although some studies were confounded by obesity.[96]

Although the steepest increase in diabetes prevalence occurs at midlife, the relationship between reproductive aging and incident diabetes proved to be difficult to ascertain. Neither natural nor surgical menopause per se has been reported to have strong associations with diabetes risk.[77,97] Likewise, the evidence linking menopausal reproductive hormone changes with increased diabetes risk is weak, although rapid changes as observed with oophorectomy may increase risk, and menopausal hormone therapy seems to decrease the risk of diabetes. Moreover, diabetes may increase the risk of ovarian failure, although this relationship has been studied less extensively.[77] The effects of reproductive aging may be difficult to disentangle from the effects of chronologic aging in relation to incident diabetes owing to the insidious nature (leading to imprecise timing of diagnosis) and heterogeneity of diabetes. Moreover, results of longitudinal studies may be confounded by methodologic constraints, related to limited glycemic outcomes across the glycemic spectrum. Also, instead of long-term glycemic markers (eg, hemoglobin A1c or glycated albumin), most studies use short-term glycemic markers such as fasting glucose, which tend to have relatively poor reproducibility. The definitions of menopausal staging may also affect the associations between MT, metabolic outcomes, and sleep factors.

The Metabolic Syndrome

The MetS (see **Table 1**) is more prevalent in midlife women than in men[98] and adversely affects women more than men.[99] Women typically transition from prediabetes to diabetes with a worse cardiovascular risk profile and a higher BMI than men. The steepest progression of MetS to diabetes occurs at midlife.

The increased risk for the MetS during the MT[28] may be linked to dimensions of sleep affected by the MT, including subjective sleep complaints such as difficulty initiating or maintaining sleep,[100] and sleep-disordered breathing.[101,102] A metaanalysis of 3 longitudinal and 12 cross-sectional studies reported a higher odds of MetS with short ($\leq$5–6 hours), and long ($\geq$8–10 hours) sleep duration,[103] and the associations of short sleep duration with MetS are stronger in women than in men.[104] The SWAN investigators examined cross-sectional associations of subjective and objective measures of sleep with the MetS in a multiethnic sample of midlife women and found that objective indices of sleep continuity, depth, and sleep-disordered breathing were significant correlates of the MetS independent of race/ethnicity, menopausal status, and other factors that might otherwise account for these relationships, and these relationships did not differ by race/ethnicity.[20]

SUMMARY

Sleep is a biological necessity, a complex phenomenon that involves many interacting regulatory mechanisms, and one of its key roles is metabolic homeostasis. Sleep problems are common complaints of midlife women, particularly as they traverse the MT. Menopause-specific factors, aging, general health, psychosocial factors, and lifestyle changes are typical contributors to sleep problems and suboptimal sleep health. Sleep health, as defined and conceptualized by Buysse, is a multidimensional pattern of sleep–wakefulness, adapted to individual, social, and environmental demands, that promotes physical and mental well-being. Consisting of a number of different parameters, including sleep duration, sleep times, awakenings, and sleepiness, sleep health can be used to characterize sleep multidimensionally. The conceptual model recognizes that relationships between sleep–wake function and molecular, cellular, systems and organism-level outcomes are reciprocal—sleep affects function and health, and function and health influence sleep–wake function.

Metabolism, too, is an essential component of health, extending as it does to every human body system, because energy metabolism is involved in every biological function. Whereas metabolic health depends largely on individual's lifestyle, disturbances in dimensions of sleep health may be manifested as metabolic health consequences. Aging in women, both chronologic and reproductive, are associated with the onset and progression of chronic degenerative diseases and disability, because accelerated reproductive aging is intertwined with chronologic aging. The dynamic balance interval of energy metabolism, termed "immunometabolic flexibility" narrows with age and other factors, increasing the susceptibility to chronic disease and physical and neuropsychological frailty. Both sleep and metabolism are influenced by circadian timing, and age-related changes in sleep and circadian rhythms may contribute to and interact with changes in orexigenic and anorexigenic hormones, nutrient intake, energy expenditure, resting metabolic rate, physical activity (exercise, nonexercise, sedentary time), and ultimately lead to greater body adiposity.

To examine the associations between sleep and metabolism, we have reviewed hot flashes and sleep apnea as important causes of sleep disruption during the menopause transition together with common metabolic health conditions relevant to midlife women—obesity, diabetes, and the MetS. By addressing women's health care needs for these conditions, and encouraging healthy lifestyle behaviors and activities, clinicians will be assisting them to achieve sleep and metabolic health as well as help them on the path to successful aging beyond midlife.

ACKNOWLEDGMENTS

The content of this article is solely the responsibility of the authors and does not necessarily represent the official views of the NIA, NINR, ORWH, or the NIH.

REFERENCES

1. Rechtschaffen A. The control of sleep. Proceedings of the Symposium on Human Behavior and its Control. Meeting of the American Association for the Advancement of Science, Chicago, III, December, 1970. [cited in Aldrich MS. Normal human sleep. In: Sleep medicine. New York: Oxford University Press; 1999. p. 3-26 (p.20)].

2. Ross JJ. Neurological findings after prolonged sleep deprivation. Arch Neurol 1965;12:399–403.

3. Upender RP. Sleep medicine, public policy, and public health. In: Kryger M, Roth T, Dement WC, editors. Principles and practice of sleep medicine. 6th edition. Philadelphia: Elsevier, Inc.; 2017. p. 638–45.

4. Buysse DJ. Sleep health: can we define it? Does it matter? Sleep 2014;37:9–17.

5. World Health Organization. WHO methods for life expectancy and healthy life expectancy. In: Global health estimates technical paper WHO/HIS/HSI/GHE/2014.5. 2014. Available at: http://www.who.int/healthinfo/statistics/LT_method_1990_2012.pdf. Accessed January 18, 2018.

6. 2007 women and sleep. Sleep in America polls. National Sleep Foundation Web site. Available at: http://www.sleepfoundation.org/article/sleep-america-polls/2007-women-and-sleep. Accessed August 11, 2017.

7. Shaver JL, Woods NF. Sleep and menopause: a narrative review. Menopause 2015;22:899–915.

8. Xu Q, Lang CP, Rooney N. A systematic review of the longitudinal relationships between subjective sleep disturbance and menopausal stage. Maturitas 2014; 79:401–12.

9. Stotland NL. The contexts of midlife in women. In: Stewart DE, editor. Menopause: a mental health practitioner's guide. Washington, DC: American Psychiatric Press, Inc; 2005. p. 1–14.

10. Jehan S, Masters-Isarilov A, Salifu I, et al. Sleep disorders in postmenopausal women. J Sleep Disord Ther 2015;4:1000212.

11. Krishnan V, Collop NA. Gender differences in sleep disorders. Curr Opin Pulm Med 2006;12:383–9.

12. Mallampalli MP, Carter CL. Exploring sex and gender differences in sleep health: a Society for Women's Health Research Report. J Womens Health 2014;23:553–62.

13. Joffe H, Massler A, Sharkey KM. Evaluation and management of sleep disturbance during the menopause transition. Semin Reprod Med 2010;28:404–21.

14. Kravitz HM, Janssen I, Bromberger JT, et al. Sleep trajectories before and after the final menstrual period in the Study of Women's Health Across the Nation (SWAN). Curr Sleep Med Rep 2017;3:235–50.

15. Freeman EW, Sammel MD, Gross SA, et al. Poor sleep in relation to natural menopause: a population-based 14-year follow-up of midlife women. Menopause 2015;22:719–26.

16. Society for Women's Health Research Interdisciplinary Network on Sleep. Women & sleep. A guide for better health. Washington, DC: Society for Women's Health Research; 2017.

17. Foley D, Ancoli-Israel S, Britz P, et al. Sleep disturbances and chronic disease in older adults: results of the 2003 National Sleep Foundation Sleep in America Survey. J Psychosom Res 2004;56:497–502.

18. Furihata R, Hall MH, Stone KL, et al. An aggregate measure of sleep health is associated with prevalent and incident clinically significant depression symptoms among community-dwelling older women. Sleep 2017;40:zsw075.

19. HealthyPeople.gov.Sleep health. Available at: http://www.healthypeople.gov/2020/topicsobjectives2020/overview.aspx?topicid=38. Accessed December 25, 2017.

20. Hall M, Okun ML, Sowers M, et al. Sleep is associated with the metabolic syndrome in a multi-ethnic cohort of midlife women: the SWAN Sleep Study. Sleep 2012;35:783–90.

21. Alberti K, Eckel R, Grundy S, et al. Harmonizing the metabolic syndrome: a joint interim statement of the International Diabetes Federation Task Force on Epidemiology and Prevention; National Heart, Lung, and Blood Institute; American Heart Association; World Heart Federation; International Atherosclerosis Society; and International Association for the Study of Obesity. Circulation 2009; 120:1640–5.

22. Hotamisligil GS. Foundations of immunometabolism and implications for metabolic health and disease. Immunity 2017;47:406–20.

23. Feng Z, Hanson RW, Berger NA, et al. Reprogramming of energy metabolism as a driver of aging. Oncotarget 2016;7:15410–20.

24. Vander Heiden MG, Cantley LC, Thompson CB. Understanding the Warburg effect: the metabolic requirements of cell proliferation. Science 2009;324:1029–33.

25. Asher G, Sassone-Corsi P. Time for food: the intimate interplay between nutrition, metabolism, and the circadian clock. Cell 2015;161:84–92.

26. Samuel VT, Shulman GI. The pathogenesis of insulin resistance: integrating signaling pathways and substrate flux. J Clin Invest 2016;126:12–22.

27. Janssen I, Powell LH, Kazlauskaite R, et al. Testosterone and visceral fat in midlife women: the Study of Women's Health Across the Nation (SWAN) fat patterning study. Obesity (Silver Spring) 2010;18:604–10.

28. Janssen I, Powell LH, Crawford S, et al. Menopause and the metabolic syndrome: the Study of Women's Health Across the Nation. Arch Intern Med 2008;168:1568–75.

29. Hall KD, Heymsfield SB, Kemnitz JW, et al. Energy balance and its components: implications for body weight regulation. Am J Clin Nutr 2012;95:989–94.

30. Anothaisintawee T, Reutrakul S, Van Cauter E, et al. Sleep disturbances compared to traditional risk factors for diabetes development: systematic review and meta-analysis. Sleep Med Rev 2016;30:11–24.

31. Chaput J-P, St-Onge M-P. Increased food intake by insufficient sleep in humans: are we jumping the gun on the hormonal explanation? Front Endocrinol (Lausanne) 2014;5:116.

32. Kahn M, Sheppes G, Sadeh A. Sleep and emotions: bidirectional links and underlying mechanisms. Int J Psychophysiol 2013;89:218–28.

33. Klingenberg L, Sjodin A, Holmback U, et al. Short sleep duration and its association with energy metabolism. Obes Rev 2012;13:565–77.

34. Wilckens KA, Woo SG, Kirk AR, et al. Role of sleep continuity and total sleep time in executive function across the adult lifespan. Psychol Aging 2014;29:658–65.

35. Chapman CD, Benedict C, Brooks SJ, et al. Lifestyle determinants of the drive to eat: a meta-analysis. Am J Clin Nutr 2012;96:492–7.

36. Depner CM, Stothard ER, Wright KP. Metabolic consequences of sleep and circadian disorders. Curr Diab Rep 2014;14:507.

37. Schmid SM, Hallschmid M, Schultes B. The metabolic burden of sleep loss. Lancet Diabetes Endocrinol 2015;3:52–62.

38. Joffe H, Crawford S, Economou N, et al. A gonadotropin-releasing hormone agonist model demonstrates that nocturnal hot flashes interrupt objective sleep. Sleep 2013;36:1977–85.

39. Neff LM, Hoffmann ME, Zeiss DM, et al. Core body temperature is lower in postmenopausal women than premenopausal women: potential implications for energy metabolism and midlife weight gain. Cardiovasc Endocrinol 2016;5:151–4.

40. Hibi M, Kubota C, Mizuno T, et al. Effect of shortened sleep on energy expenditure, core body temperature, and appetite: a human randomised crossover trial. Sci Rep 2017;7:39640.

41. Park I, Kayaba M, Iwayama K, et al. Relationship between metabolic rate and core body temperature during sleep in human [Abstract]. Sleep Med 2015;16(Supplement 1):S186–7.

42. Manoogian ENC, Panda S. Circadian rhythms, time-restricted feeding, and healthy aging. Ageing Res Rev 2017;39:59–67.

43. Fung CH, Vitiello MV, Alessi CA, et al. Report and research agenda of the American Geriatrics Society and National Institute on Aging bedside-to-bench conference on sleep, circadian rhythms, and aging: new avenues for improving brain health, physical health, and functioning. J Am Geriatr Soc 2016;64:e238–47.

44. Van Cauter E. Sleep disturbances and insulin resistance. Diabet Med 2011;28:1455–62.

45. Nedeltcheva AV, Imperial JG, Penev PD. Effects of sleep restriction on glucose control and insulin secretion during diet-induced weight loss. Obesity (Silver Spring) 2012;20:1379–86.

46. Saner NJ, Bishop DJ, Bartlett JD. Is exercise a viable therapeutic intervention to mitigate mitochondrial dysfunction and insulin resistance induced by sleep loss? Sleep Med Rev 2018;37:60–8.

47. Tucker P, Marquie JC, Folkard S, et al. Shiftwork and metabolic dysfunction. Chronobiol Int 2012;29:549–55.

48. Taylor BJ, Matthews KA, Hasler BP, et al. Bedtime variability and metabolic health in midlife women: the SWAN Sleep Study. Sleep 2016;39:457–65.

49. Aurora RN, Punjabi NM. Obstructive sleep apnoea and type 2 diabetes mellitus: a bidirectional association. Lancet Respir Med 2013;1:329–38.

50. Cronise RJ, Sinclair DA, Bremer AA. Oxidative priority, meal frequency, and the energy economy of food and activity: implications for longevity, obesity, and cardiometabolic disease. Metab Syndr Relat Disord 2017;15:6–17.

51. Gluckman PD, Hanson MA, Buklijas T, et al. Epigenetic mechanisms that underpin metabolic and cardiovascular diseases. Nat Rev Endocrinol 2009;5:401–8.

52. Lane JM, Liang J, Vlasac I, et al. Genome-wide association analyses of sleep disturbance traits identify new loci and highlight shared genetics with neuropsychiatric and metabolic traits. Nat Genet 2017;49:274–81.

53. Archer SN, Oster H. How sleep and wakefulness influence circadian rhythmicity: effects of insufficient and mistimed sleep on the animal and human transcriptome. J Sleep Res 2015;24:476–93.

54. Westermann J, Lange T, Textor J, et al. System consolidation during sleep – A common principle underlying psychological and immunological memory formation. Trends Neurosci 2015;38:585–97.

55. O'Neill LAJ, Kishton RJ, Rathmell J. A guide to immunometabolism for immunologists. Nat Rev Immunol 2016;169:553–65.

56. Robinson SL, Hattersley J, Frost GS, et al. Maximal fat oxidation during exercise is positively associated with 24-hour fat oxidation and insulin sensitivity in young, healthy men. J Appl Physiol (1985) 2015;118:1415–22.

57. St-Onge M-P. Impact of sleep duration on food intake regulation: different mechanisms by sex? [Commentary]. Obesity (Silver Spring) 2016;24:11.

58. Spiegel K, Leproult R, L'hermite-Balériaux M, et al. Leptin levels are dependent on sleep duration: relationships with sympathovagal balance, carbohydrate regulation, cortisol, and thyrotropin. J Clin Endocrinol Metab 2004;89:5762–71.

59. Spiegel K, Tasali E, Penev P, et al. Brief communication: sleep curtailment in healthy young men is associated with decreased leptin levels, elevated ghrelin levels, and increased hunger and appetite. Ann Intern Med 2004;141:846–50.

60. Markwald RR, Melanson EL, Smith MR, et al. Impact of insufficient sleep on total daily energy expenditure, food intake, and weight gain. Proc Natl Acad Sci U S A 2013;110:5695–700.

61. Capers PL, Fobian AD, Kaiser KA, et al. A systemic review and meta-analysis of randomized controlled trials of the impact of sleep duration on adiposity and components of energy balance. Obes Rev 2015;16:771–82.

62. Nedeltcheva AV, Kilkus JM, Imperial J, et al. Sleep curtailment is accompanied by increased intake of calories from snacks. Am J Clin Nutr 2009;89:126–33.

63. Joffe H, Crawford SL, Freeman MP, et al. Independent contributions of nocturnal hot flashes and sleep disturbance to depression in estrogen-deprived women. J Clin Endocrinol Metab 2016;101:3847–55.

64. Prairie BA, Wisniewski SR, Luther J, et al. Symptoms of depressed mood, disturbed sleep, and sexual problems in midlife women: cross-sectional data from the Study of Women's Health Across the Nation. J Womens Health 2015; 24:119–26.

65. Hussain D, Shams W, Brake W. Estrogen and memory system bias in females across the lifespan. Transl Neurosci 2014;5:35.

66. Chaput J-P. Sleep patterns, diet quality and energy balance. Physiol Behav 2014;134:86–91.

67. Kim TH, Carroll JE, An SK, et al. Associations between actigraphy-assessed sleep, inflammatory markers, and insulin resistance in the Midlife Development in the United States (MIDUS) study. Sleep Med 2016;27-28:72–9.

68. Vandenput L, Ohlsson C. Estrogens as regulators of bone health in men. Nat Rev Endocrinol 2009;5:437–43.

69. Mong JA, Baker FC, Mahoney MM, et al. Sleep, rhythms, and the endocrine brain: influence of sex and gonadal hormones. J Neurosci 2011;31:16107–16.

70. Shaw ND, Gill S, Lavoie HB, et al. Persistence of sleep-associated decrease in GnRH pulse frequency in the absence of gonadal steroids. J Clin Endocrinol Metab 2011;96:2590–5.

71. Kravitz HM, Janssen I, Santoro N, et al. Relationship of day-to-day reproductive hormone levels to sleep in midlife women. Arch Intern Med 2005;165:2370–6.

72. Sowers MF, Zheng H, Kravitz HM, et al. Sex steroid hormone profiles are related to sleep measures from polysomnography and the Pittsburgh Sleep Quality Index. Sleep 2008;31:1339–49.

73. Polo-Kantolo P. Sleep problems in midlife and beyond. Maturitas 2011;68: 224–32.

74. Paul KN, Turek FW, Kryger MH. Influence of sex on sleep regulatory mechanisms. J Womens Health 2008;17:1201–8.

75. Monteiro R, Teixeira D, Calhau C. Estrogen signaling in metabolic inflammation. Mediators Inflamm 2014;2014:615917.

76. Jones MEE, Thorburn AW, Britt KL, et al. Aromatase-deficient (ArKO) mice have a phenotype of increased adiposity. Proc Natl Acad Sci U S A 2000;97: 12735–40.

77. Karvonen-Gutierrez CA, Park SK, Kim C. Diabetes and menopause. Curr Diab Rep 2016;16:20.

78. Ghisletti S, Meda C, Maggi A, et al. 17beta-estradiol inhibits inflammatory gene expression by controlling NF-kappaB intracellular localization. Mol Cell Biol 2005;25:2957–68.

79. Turgeon JL, Carr MC, Maki PM, et al. Complex actions of sex steroids in adipose tissue, the cardiovascular system, and brain: insights from basic science and clinical studies. Endocr Rev 2006;27:575–605.

80. Gileles-Hillel A, Kheirandish-Gozal L, Gozal D. Biological plausibility linking sleep apnoea and metabolic dysfunction. Nat Rev Endocrinol 2016;12:290–8.

81. Farr OM, Mantzoros CS. Sleep apnea in relation to metabolism: an urgent need to study underlying mechanisms and to develop novel treatments for this unmet clinical need. Metabolism 2017;69:207–10.

82. Tufik S, Santos-Silva R, Taddei JA, et al. Obstructive sleep apnea syndrome in the Sao Paulo Epidemiologic Sleep Study. Sleep Med 2010;11:441–6.

83. Mirer AG, Young T, Palta M, et al. Sleep-disordered breathing and the menopausal transition among participants in the Sleep in Midlife Women Study. Menopause 2017;24:157–62.

84. Jullian-Desayes I, Joyeux-Faure M, Tamisier R, et al. Impact of obstructive sleep apnea treatment by continuous positive airway pressure on cardiometabolic biomarkers: a systematic review from sham CPAP randomized controlled trials. Sleep Med Rev 2015;21:23–38.

85. Anandam A, Akinnusi M, Kufel T, et al. Effects of dietary weight loss on obstructive sleep apnea: a meta-analysis. Sleep Breath 2013;17:227–34.
86. Greenburg DL, Lettieri CJ, Eliasson AH. Effects of surgical weight loss on measures of obstructive sleep apnea: a meta-analysis. Am J Med 2009;122:535–42.
87. Wu Y, Zhai L, Zhang D. Sleep duration and obesity among adults: a meta-analysis of prospective studies. Sleep Med 2014;15:1456–62.
88. Sperry SD, Scully ID, Gramzow RH, et al. Sleep duration and waist circumference in adults: a meta-analysis. Sleep 2015;38:1269–76.
89. Appelhans BM, Janssen I, Cursio JF, et al. Sleep duration and weight change in midlife women: the SWAN Sleep Study. Obesity (Silver Spring) 2013;21:77–84.
90. Chaput J-P, Bouchard C, Tremblay A. Change in sleep duration and visceral fat accumulation over 6 years in adults. Obesity (Silver Spring) 2014;22:E9–12.
91. Lee SWH, Ng KY, Chin WK. The impact of sleep amount and sleep quality on glycemic control in type 2 diabetes: a systematic review and meta-analysis. Sleep Med Rev 2017;31:91–101.
92. Cappuccio FP, D'Elia L, Strazzullo P, et al. Quantity and quality of sleep and incidence of type 2 diabetes: a systematic review and meta-analysis. Diabetes Care 2010;33:414–20.
93. Cespedes EM, Bhupathiraju SN, Li Y, et al. Long-term changes in sleep duration, energy balance and risk of type 2 diabetes. Diabetologia 2016;59:101–9.
94. Ferrie JE, Kivimäki M, Akbaraly TN, et al. Change in sleep duration and type 2 diabetes: the Whitehall II Study. Diabetes Care 2015;38:1467–72.
95. Green MJ, Espie CA, Popham F, et al. Insomnia symptoms as a cause of type 2 diabetes incidence: a 20 year cohort study. BMC Psychiatry 2017;17:94.
96. Lui MM, Ip MS. Disorders of glucose metabolism in sleep-disordered breathing. Clin Chest Med 2010;31:271–85.
97. Kim C. Does menopause increase diabetes risk? Strategies for diabetes prevention in midlife women. Womens Health (Lond) 2012;8:155–67.
98. Beigh SH, Jain S. Prevalence of metabolic syndrome and gender differences. Bioinformation 2012;8(13):613–6.
99. Rossi MC, Cristofaro MR, Gentile S, et al. Sex disparities in the quality of diabetes care: biological and cultural factors may play a different role for different outcomes: a cross-sectional observational study from the AMD Annals initiative. Diabetes Care 2013;36:3162–8.
100. Akbaraly TN, Jaussent I, Besset A, et al. Sleep complaints and metabolic syndrome in an elderly population: the Three-City Study. Am J Geriatr Psychiatry 2015;23:818–28.
101. Resta O, Bonfitto P, Sabato R, et al. Prevalence of obstructive sleep apnoea in a sample of obese women: effect of menopause. Diabetes Nutr Metab 2004;17:296–303.
102. Young T, Finn L, Austin D, et al. Menopausal status and sleep-disordered breathing in the Wisconsin Sleep Cohort Study. Am J Respir Crit Care Med 2003;167:1181–5.
103. Ju SY, Choi WS. Sleep duration and metabolic syndrome in adult populations: a meta-analysis of observational studies. Nutr Diabetes 2013;3:e65.
104. Xi B, He D, Zhang M, et al. Short sleep duration predicts risk of metabolic syndrome: a systematic review and meta-analysis. Sleep Med Rev 2014;18:293–7.

Bone Health During the Menopause Transition and Beyond

Arun S. Karlamangla, PhD, MD[a],*,
Sherri-Ann M. Burnett-Bowie, MD, MPH[b],
Carolyn J. Crandall, MD, MS[c]

KEYWORDS

- Perimenopause • Bone strength • Bone turnover markers
- Transmenopausal bone loss • Race/ethnicity differences • Bone loss trajectories
- Osteoporosis • Fracture

KEY POINTS

- The substantial differences in fracture risk between race/ethnicity groups are not explained by between-group differences in bone mineral density.
- Composite indices of femoral neck strength capture the combined impact of bone density, bone size, and body size on fracture risk and explain observed racial/ethnic differences in fracture risk.
- Bone resorption begins increasing 2 years before the final menstrual period (FMP), peaks approximately 1.5 years after the FMP and then plateaus.
- In concert with increases in bone resorption, there is a rapid phase of bone loss during the menopause transition, in a 3-year period around the FMP.
- Metabolic factors during the menopause transition, such as insulin resistance, inflammation, and obesity, are associated with lower bone strength and increased fracture risk.

SWAN has grant support from the National Institutes of Health (NIH), Department of Health and Human Services, through the National Institute on Aging (NIA), the National Institute of Nursing Research (NINR), and the NIH Office of Research on Women's Health (ORWH) (grants U01NR004061, U01AG012505, U01AG012535, U01AG012531, U01AG012539, U01AG012546, U01AG012553, U01AG012554, and U01AG012495). The content of this review article is solely the responsibility of the authors and does not necessarily represent the official views of the NIA, NINR, ORWH, or the NIH.
[a] Division of Geriatrics, David Geffen School of Medicine at UCLA, 10945 Le Conte Avenue #2339, Los Angeles, CA 90095, USA; [b] Endocrinology Division, Massachusetts General Hospital, Harvard Medical School, 55 Fruit Street, Boston, MA 02114, USA; [c] Division of General Internal Medicine and Health Services Research, David Geffen School of Medicine at UCLA, 911 Broxton Avenue, 1st floor, Los Angeles, CA 90024, USA
* Corresponding author.
E-mail address: AKarlamangla@mednet.ucla.edu

Obstet Gynecol Clin N Am 45 (2018) 695–708
https://doi.org/10.1016/j.ogc.2018.07.012
0889-8545/18/© 2018 Elsevier Inc. All rights reserved.

INTRODUCTION

The Study of Women's Health Across the Nation (SWAN) has significantly added to understanding of changes in women's bone health over the menopause transition (MT), advancing the knowledge base regarding a critical period that has major impact on osteoporosis risk in older ages. SWAN is one of a few, large, race/ethnically diverse cohorts with comprehensive longitudinal measures of bone health over the MT and serves as a primary source for this review. Conducted in a large multiethnic population of more than 2000 women followed for more than 20 years across 5 clinical centers in the United States, the SWAN bone study has also contributed greatly to understanding race/ethnicity differences in both premenopausal and postmenopausal bone health. This review begins with recent findings on bone health over the MT, with a discussion of racial/ethnic differences in various aspects of bone health, and then provides a broad overview of changes in bone metabolism and strength during the MT, briefly summarizing new data on factors that influence fracture risk in the perimenopause and postmenopause.

RACIAL/ETHNIC DIFFERENCES

The incidence of low-trauma fracture varies substantially across race/ethnicity groups, both nationally and worldwide. Low-trauma fractures of the hip for instance, which are a major cause of morbidity, physical disability, and early mortality in older Americans,[1] are considerably more common in white women than in Asian women, black women, and Hispanic women in the United States.[2–4] Although low bone mineral density (BMD) by dual-energy x-ray absorptiometry (DXA) is the most reliable predictor of hip fracture risk within race/ethnicity groups,[5–8] BMD does not account for the differences in fracture risk between race/ethnicity groups. Japanese women for example, who have lower risk of hip fracture than white women, also have lower BMD on average than white women.[9,10] On the other hand, black women have fewer fractures than white women, even after controlling for differences in BMD.[6]

At the SWAN baseline, BMD in the femoral neck, which is considered the best bone site at which to measure BMD for hip fracture prediction,[11] was significantly higher in black women than in white women and lower still in Chinese women and Japanese women, with mean differences of 14% to 24% between black women and the other groups.[12,13] Although some of these differences in BMD can be explained by body weight, the discrepancy between BMD and fracture rate differences by race/ethnicity is not completely explained by body weight differences between the groups.

Racial/Ethnic Differences in Bone Size and Geometry

Differences by race/ethnicity in bone size and geometry might add explanatory power. Hip structural analysis showed that although black women have greater BMD in the femoral neck (the site of 45% of osteoporotic hip fractures) than white women in SWAN, the width (or outer diameter) of the femoral neck is smaller in black women.[14] At a given BMD, a smaller femoral neck width (FNW) means there is less bone mineral content in a cross-section and thus less strength to resist fracture forces.[15] It seems that the BMD advantage in black women may be offset by their smaller FNW. In contrast, Japanese women had lower BMD in the femoral neck than white women, but this relative disadvantage was offset by their larger FNW, demonstrating the importance of not examining BMD in isolation.

In addition to the amount of bone mineral in a cross-section of the femoral neck, which is determined by both BMD and FNW, the ability of the femoral neck to resist fracture is also affected by how the bone mineral content is distributed in the cross-section. If it is mostly confined to a thin cortical shell, it increases the likelihood of buckling like a thin straw. The buckling ratio, the ratio of outer diameter to width of the cortical shell, is a measure of susceptibility to fracture from buckling.[16] Compared with white women in SWAN, the buckling ratio in the femoral neck was higher on average in black women and Japanese women and lower in Chinese women.[14]

Racial/Ethnic Differences in Composite Indices of Femoral Neck Strength

Other than the bone's ability to resist fracture forces, risk of fracture also depends on the magnitude of the forces on bone during a fall. These forces increase with both body weight and body height, which implies that a level of BMD and bone size/geometry that is adequate to prevent fractures in a lighter or shorter individual may not be adequate in a taller or heavier one.[17] Composite indices of femoral neck strength integrate these major determinants of fracture risk (namely, BMD and FNW obtained from routinely obtained DXA scans and body height and weight) to capture bone strength relative to the load that bone would be exposed to in a fall from standing height. They have been shown to be inversely associated with hip fracture risk in community-dwelling older adults.[18] In SWAN, at the baseline visit, when all women were either premenopausal or in early perimenopause, despite having lower BMD in the femoral neck, both Japanese women and Chinese women had higher average values of femoral neck composite strength indices than white women, consistent with the lower risk for fracture in Asian women.[13]

Not only do the racial/ethnic differences in femoral neck strength indices explain the paradox of lower fracture risk in Asian women despite their lower BMD, they also reduce the importance of race/ethnicity as a determinant of fracture risk. Each SD increment in the composite strength indices measured at the SWAN baseline visit was associated with a 34% to 41% decrement in fracture hazard over 9 years of follow-up. In addition, whereas race/ethnicity predicted incident fractures independent of BMD, it did not add independent prediction or discrimination ability over that provided by the femoral neck composite strength indices.[19]

Racial/Ethnic Differences in Trabecular Microstructure

In addition to macrostructural aspects of bone, bone microarchitecture also contributes to bone strength. Thinned trabecula and diminished connectivity are seen in the bones of postmenopausal women, which lead to reduction in load-bearing capacity of older bones.[20] Femoral neck composite strength indices may capture aspects of cortical bone strength relative to load, but, like BMD, they ignore the contribution of trabecular microarchitectural integrity to bone strength, which is especially important in vertebral bodies in the spine, which are the site of compression deformities, also a significant source of morbidity in older men and women. Not surprisingly, trabecular bone score (TBS), an index of trabecular thickness and connectivity obtained from DXA images of the lumbar spine,[21] predicts incident fracture risk independent of BMD.[22,23]

Several studies have documented racial/ethnic differences in trabecular microarchitecture. One study found TBS is lower in Japanese women than in age-matched white women and that the difference increases with age.[24] *National Health and Nutrition Examination Survey* data from 2005 to 2008 show that non-Hispanic whites have higher TBS than non-Hispanic Blacks or Mexican Americans in all age groups.[25] These TBS comparisons need to be considered in light of body mass index (BMI) differences between race/ethnicity groups, because TBS, as currently measured, is underestimated in individuals with more soft tissue around the lumbar spine.[26]

There are also differences by race/ethnicity in the shape and structure of individual trabeculae, with postmenopausal black women in SWAN having more platelike trabeculae and white women having more rodlike trabeculae, in high-resolution peripheral quantitative CT (HR-pQCT) images.[27]

BONE LOSS DURING THE MENOPAUSE TRANSITION

The MT is a critical period of change in bone strength in women, which sets the stage for development of osteoporosis and fracture susceptibility in older ages.[28] It has been suggested that the MT represents a time-limited window of opportunity to intervene to prevent rapid bone loss and microarchitectural damage to stave off osteoporosis in later years.[29] Data from SWAN have provided substantial new knowledge and insights about these changes during the MT.

Changes in Bone Mineral Density Over the Menopause Transition

Several prospective cohorts have documented declines in BMD over the MT,[30,31] and SWAN established that there is a rapid phase of bone loss in a 3-year period around final menstrual period (FMP); BMD begins to decline at approximately 1 year prior to the FMP and continues to decrease in early postmenopause, with a slight reduction in loss rate around 2 years after the FMP[32] (**Fig. 1**). This pattern of initial acceleration of change before the FMP and a deceleration after the FMP is seen in a variety of hormonal, metabolic, and other indicators of health, which has led researchers to refer to this interval as the transmenopause. This interval includes both perimenopause and early postmenopause but is best defined using the date of the FMP and not menstrual bleeding patterns, because of the large between-women variability in the length

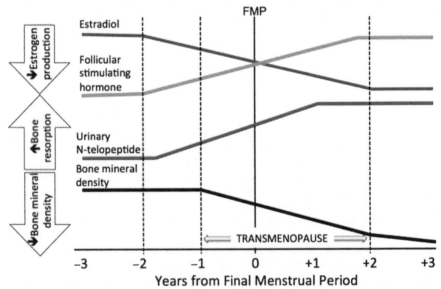

Fig. 1. Schematic depiction of the trajectories of sex steroid hormones (estradiol [*blue*] and FSH [*green*]), bone resorption marker U-NTX (*red*), and BMD (*black*) over the MT. Rapid bone loss occurs during transmenopause, a period that lasts from 1 year before to 2 years after the FMP. Changes in hormone levels and in U-NTX start approximately 1 year before the transmenopause. (*Courtesy of* A. Shieh, MD, Los Angeles, CA.)

of the different menstrually defined MT stages. Even in the year after the FMP, 30% of women would be classified as early perimenopausal based on bleeding patterns.[32]

During the 3-year-long rapid bone loss phase in the transmenopause, the average rate of decline in BMD in white women was 2.5% per year in the lumbar spine and 1.8% per year in the femoral neck.[32] Prior to the transmenopause, there was no appreciable change in BMD at either bone site. Adjusted for BMI, black women had smaller percentage losses at both bone sites (2.2% per year in the spine and 1.4% in the femoral neck) and Japanese women and Chinese women had larger losses at the femoral neck (2.1% and 2.2% per year, respectively).[32]

Not surprisingly, changes in estradiol and follicle-stimulating hormone (FSH) levels during the MT seem to be driving these changes in bone mass. The pattern of hormonal changes mirror those in BMD, with the most rapid increases in FSH and decreases in estradiol occurring in the years around the FMP (see **Fig. 1**). Every doubling of FSH level during the transmenopause was associated with an additional 0.3% decline per year in BMD at both the femoral neck and lumbar spine.[33] Consistent with a causal role for estrogen is the finding from at least 2 studies that women with vasomotor symptoms (hot flashes and night sweats), which have been etiologically linked to declining estradiol levels, have lower BMD.[34,35] Also consistent with a causal role for hormones, women in SWAN who initiated sex steroid hormone therapy during the MT had 0.4% per year less decline in BMD.[36]

Analysis of initiation of other medications in SWAN also suggests that the women who use thiazide diuretics may lose less bone mass at the femoral neck than women who use angiotensin-converting enzyme inhibitors or who do not use antihypertensive medications.[37] Similar analysis of initiation of proton pump inhibitors, H_2 receptor antagonists, and antidepressants by participants did not reveal any links between these medications and the rate of bone loss over the MT.[36]

Changes in Composite Strength Indices Over the Menopause Transition

Declines in cortical bone mass during the transmenopause result from endosteal resorption by osteoclasts, which leads to compensatory bone formation at the outer periosteal surface. This results in increases in the outer diameter of long bones, such as the radius and the femoral neck.[38,39] The width of the femoral neck increases on average by 0.4% per year during the MT, but it is not adequate to compensate for the decline in BMD, so the composite indices of femoral neck strength decline on average by 0.7% per year.[40] The compensatory increase in external bone size (the outer diameter) of cortical long bones during the MT comes at a cost; it increases the susceptibility of long bones to failure by buckling.[16] In SWAN, the buckling ratio—a measure of this susceptibility—increased during the transmenopause by 2% each year.[40]

The composite indices reflect bone strength relative to load borne, and load is proportional to body weight; thus, changes in the composite indices are also affected by changes in body weight. Body weight generally increases in midlife; the average increase in white women in SWAN was 0.4% per year. There were racial/ethnic differences in the rate of change in both bone size (FNW) and body weight. Both Japanese women and Chinese women had smaller increases in body weight than white women, but the increase in FNW was also smaller in Japanese women. The combined effect was that the composite strength indices declined at the slowest rate in Chinese women and the fastest in Japanese women. Despite these differences in decline rate, the strength indices remained consistently lower in white women than in black, Chinese, and Japanese women throughout the study.[40]

Because the external bone size of cortical bones reflects cortical bone remodeling, correlations have been observed between FNW and both cortical thickness and intra-cortical porosity.[41] This has led to the hypothesis that women who start with a wider femoral neck at baseline experience greater bone loss during and after the MT. An analysis of longitudinal SWAN data from the Pittsburgh study site did show that bone lost over 14 years of follow-up was greater in women who had wider femoral necks,[42] pointing to the importance of measuring bone size in addition to BMD in assessing a woman's risk for osteoporosis and fractures.

Changes in Bone Turnover Markers Over the Menopause Transition

The pattern of bone loss over the MT parallels changes in markers of bone turnover: Markers of both bone resorption and formation increase over the MT.[31] Urinary N-terminal telopeptide of type I collagen (U-NTX), a marker of type I collagen break-down, starts increasing 2 years before the FMP, peaks approximately 1.5 years after the FMP, and plateaus thereafter[43] (see **Fig. 1**). Decreases in levels of circulating estra-diol and increases in FSH occur on nearly the same time frame, whereas decreases in BMD lag by approximately 6 months, consistent with a causal pathway from hormones to bone resorption to bone mass (see **Fig. 1**). Further support comes from the obser-vation that women who report frequent vasomotor symptoms (6 or more days in 2 weeks), which may indicate either larger declines in circulating estradiol levels or heightened sensitivity to the decline, have significantly higher levels of U-NTX.[44]

After restricting the comparisons to women with BMI under 29 kg/m^2, Japanese women had the highest level and black women the lowest level of peak (postmeno-pausal) U-NTX,[43] consistent, with the rate of BMD decline being greatest in Japanese women and smallest in black women.[32]

If the increase in bone resorption during the MT is causally related to transmeno-pausal bone loss, then measurement of U-NTX during the MT might be useful in esti-mating the magnitude of bone loss in the rapid phase. SWAN longitudinal data show that U-NTX measured both in early postmenopause (when U-NTX has peaked and plateaued) and in late perimenopause (when U-NTX has risen considerably but not yet peaked) does strongly predict the rate of bone loss in transmenopause in the femoral neck and lumbar spine. U-NTX measured when women were still premeno-pausal or in early perimenopause, however, did not predict the rate of transmeno-pausal bone loss.[45]

Because bone formation and resorption are coupled, markers of both formation and resorption increase when there is bone turnover, regardless of whether there is net bone gain (as after initiating an exercise regimen) or bone loss. Therefore, in younger women, some of whom may not yet have entered the rapid phase of MT-related bone loss, bone resorption markers, such as U-NTX, may not be able to predict who is losing bone and how much. SWAN measured serum levels of bone formation marker, osteocalcin, from fasting morning blood. The in-balance relationship between osteo-calcin and U-NTX was estimated from measurements of the 2 turnover markers in 685 women who were more than 5 years before their FMP at the time and presumably in a state of balance between bone formation and resorption. This estimated in-balance relationship was used to create, for every woman in the cohort, a bone balance index (BBI) that reflects her level of bone formation that is in excess of bone resorption. Not only was the BBI smaller (less favorable) in women who were closer to the FMP (0.3 SD smaller for every year closer to the FMP; $P = .007$) but also BBI predicted the rate of BMD decline in the lumbar spine over the next 3 years to 4 years. Each SD decrement in BBI was associated with 38% higher odds of faster-than-average loss of BMD in the lumbar spine ($P = .008$, C statistic 0.76).[46]

FRACTURE RISK DURING AND AFTER THE MENOPAUSAL TRANSITION

Fractures during the MT are not uncommon, although women are still in midlife and few meet criteria for osteoporosis. Between the ages of 42 years and 58 years, which included a median of 6 years after the FMP, 1 in 6 women in SWAN had 1 or more fractures, at a rate of 11 first fractures per 1000 person-years. A majority (59%) of these fractures were not minimum-trauma fractures attributable solely to osteoporosis. Yet low BMD, low indices of femoral neck composite strength, and high levels of U-NTX did strongly predict the risk of fracture in this midlife period.[19,47] In addition, 3.2% of women had a vertebral compression deformity by the eighth to tenth follow-up visits, when mean age was 54 years, and, as expected, low BMD at the SWAN baseline visit was a major risk factor, with the odds increasing by 61% per SD decrement in BMD in the lumbar spine. Over the next 7 years (until the thirteenth follow-up visit), the observed incidence of new vertebral deformities was 2 per 1000 person-years.[48]

In addition to low BMD, several other factors increase the risk of fracture over the MT. Among indicators of socioeconomic status (SES), low education, but not low income, was associated with greater incidence of fracture in nonwhite women.[49] That this association was seen only in nonwhite women may be partly explained by the increased prevalence of risk factors for low bone accrual in childhood and young adulthood (such as inadequate vitamin D intake, smoking, and depression) in under-privileged minority communities in the United States; the combination of low SES and minority race/ethnicity status may be synergistically deleterious to bone health. Increased parity is often seen in low SES and minority women, and both parity and lactation have been linked to poor bone health. In SWAN, lifetime parity was associated positively with composite indices of femoral neck strength, whereas accumulated duration of lactation was associated negatively with BMD in the lumbar spine; yet there were no associations between either lifetime parity or accumulated duration of lactation with fracture hazard after age 42.[50] Both low SES and minority race/ethnicity status are also associated with obesity and increased prevalence of chronic inflammation and diabetes, all of which have been linked to increased fracture risk.

Metabolic Risk Factors and Fracture Risk

Several observational studies have noted that diabetics have more fractures despite having higher BMD than matched nondiabetics. Women with diabetes at the baseline SWAN visit had higher BMD at both the hip and spine than nondiabetics, yet they had twice as many fractures over the first 8 years of follow-up. This can be only partly explained by the observed faster rate of decline in hip BMD in diabetic women but is inconsistent with their slower rate of decline in spine BMD.[51] Consistent with their higher fracture risk, diabetic women in SWAN did have lower levels of femoral neck composite strength indices (0.2 SD lower) at the baseline visit than nondiabetic women. In those without diabetes, there was a graded inverse relationship between insulin resistance and femoral neck strength indices, such that each doubling of homeostasis model assessment–insulin resistance was associated with 2.4% decline in the strength indices.[52] There are also differences in bone microarchitecture in diabetic women that are not captured by either BMD or the strength indices. In postmenopausal SWAN women, although there were no differences in BMD at the radius by diabetes status, diabetic women had 26% greater cortical porosity, as measured by HR-pQCT, than women without diabetes.[53]

Chronic inflammation is also a risk factor for osteoporosis and fractures, but in the absence of inflammatory conditions, like rheumatoid arthritis and inflammatory bowel disease, associations have not been consistently found between subclinical chronic inflammation and low BMD. In SWAN, in the general population of women going through the MT, fracture hazard increased monotonically with serum levels of inflammatory biomarker, C-reactive protein (CRP), above a threshold level of 3 mg/L, yet there was no association between CRP level and BMD at the baseline visit. CRP level was inversely associated, however, with femoral neck composite strength indices (0.04 SD decrement per doubling of CRP level), and the association explained the link between high CRP and increased fracture hazard.[54] Increased plasma levels of triglycerides, another component of the metabolic syndrome, is also an independent risk factor for fracture in midlife. Women with triglycerides level at the SWAN baseline visit higher than 300 mg/dL had a 2.5-fold greater hazard for nontraumatic fractures than women with baseline triglycerides lower than 150 mg/dL.[55]

Pleiotropic Effects of Obesity on Fracture Risk

Obesity has multiple effects on bone health, some positive and others negative. Greater body weight in an obese individual can stimulate bone formation and lead to greater BMD, and the increased tissue padding at potential sites of impact in a fall (such as over the greater trochanter) can also protect against fractures, but other aspects of an obese body habitus increase fracture risk, for example, by increasing impact forces in a fall from standing height. In SWAN, greater BMI was associated with greater BMD but smaller composite indices of femoral neck strength, suggesting that although BMD increases with greater skeletal loading in heavier individuals, the increase may not be sufficient to compensate for the increase in fall impact forces. After controlling for BMD, greater BMI was associated with increased fracture risk, consistent with the greater impact forces in a heavier individual. With controls for the femoral neck composite strength indices (which also account for greater impact force in heavier individuals), greater BMI was associated with reduced fracture risk (5% reduction in fracture hazard per unit increment in BMI), consistent with a protective role for soft tissue padding in obese women. This protective association was eliminated when control for hip circumference, a surrogate marker for soft tissue padding over the hip, was added to the model, confirming the multiple ways by which obesity influences fracture risk in women.[56]

SUMMARY AND CLINICAL IMPLICATIONS

In summary, the prospective assessment of bone health in a large, multiethnic cohort of women through and after the MT has confirmed previously seen differences by race/ethnicity in older women, pointed out the importance of looking beyond traditional BMD measurement to include macrostructural and microstructural aspects of bone in the context of body size, and documented the trajectories of change in various aspects of bone health across the MT. It has also highlighted the role of SES and metabolic risk factors in bone health during this critical period and illuminated the pleiotropic effects of obesity on fracture risk in women.

These findings point to the importance of early intervention, including but not necessarily limited to, lifestyle modification, to ward off osteoporosis and fractures in later years. To this end, data from SWAN show that greater physical activity in midlife in each of the domains of home, work, active living (daily routine), and sports, is associated with larger femoral neck composite strength indices.[57] The importance of a healthy diet cannot be ignored, especially the need to maintain an adequate calcium and vitamin D intake. In longitudinal follow-up of the Aberdeen Prospective

Osteoporosis Screening Study, greater dietary intake of calcium was associated with smaller loss of BMD in the femoral neck during the MT.[58] In SWAN women, levels of serum 25-hydroxyvitamin D below 20 ng/mL at the third follow-up visit (when mean age was 48.5 years) were associated with 85% higher hazard for incident nontraumatic fractures.[59] Greater intake of isoflavones (such as from soy products) was also associated with greater BMD at the baseline visit.[60,61] More of a good thing, however, is not always better. Just as excessive exercise may have deleterious effects on health,[62] excessive calcium and vitamin D supplementation can also be harmful: excess calcium intake can lead to nephrolithiasis,[63] and high-dose vitamin D supplementation in older ages can increase falls[64,65] and raise the risk of fractures.[66]

Screening and Treatment

Current guidelines (from the US Preventive Services Task Force) for osteoporosis screening in midlife (between the ages of 50 years and 64 years) recommend using the Fracture Risk Assessment Tool (FRAX) (https://www.sheffield.ac.uk/FRAX/) to estimate the 10-year risk for osteoporotic fracture as a first step and to proceed only if the estimated 10-year risk exceeds 9.3%. In those 50 years old to 64 years old, however, only approximately one-third of the women who would meet treatment criteria by BMD (T score ≤ -2.5) and only one-quarter of the women who experience a fracture over the next 10 years would meet the FRAX-based threshold for screening.[67,68] As a result, the current clinically used strategy for screening does not identify the majority of women who could benefit from treatment. Unfortunately, data on treatment options in midlife are also limited. Currently available drugs for treating osteoporosis have significant adverse effects that increase with duration of treatment. Data on the benefits versus harms of pharmacotherapy beginning in the 50s and continued for multiple decades are not available. Use of drug treatment in younger ages may also leave women with fewer options for pharmacotherapy in their 70s, when their risk for hip fracture begins to increase.[69]

FUTURE WORK

Because bone mass declines rapidly during the transmenopause and it is accompanied by deleterious changes in trabecular and cortical microarchitecture (including decreased trabecular number, increased trabecular spacing, conversion of trabecular plates to rods, and increased cortical thinning and porosity),[70,71] which may be irreversible, the start of the transmenopause may be the optimal, but time-limited, window for early interventions to prevent osteoporosis and reduce the risk of debilitating fractures in older ages. To develop and test such a strategy, we need to be able to determine before substantial bone loss has occurred, whether transmenopausal bone loss is imminent (to be able to time the intervention optimally) and which women will lose the most bone during the transmenopausal rapid loss phase (to select the women who will gain the most from early intervention). The rapid bone loss phase of transmenopause begins 1 year before the FMP, but the FMP date is not knowable until 1 year after it has passed, by which time 2 of the 3 years of the rapid bone loss phase will have passed. Sex steroid hormones, bone turnover markers, and antimüllerian hormone measurements are all potential indicators of the onset of the transmenopause, and future work will examine their ability to jointly do so. The same biomarkers, in combination with metabolic risk factors, may be of use in identifying the women who are likely to lose the most bone mass over the MT.

ACKNOWLEDGMENTS

The authors would like to thank Gail A. Greendale, MD (David Geffen School of Medicine at UCLA), for her expert review and suggestions for improvement of this article.

REFERENCES

1. Quah C, Boulton C, Moran C. The influence of socioeconomic status on the incidence, outcome and mortality of fractures of the hip. J Bone Joint Surg Br 2011; 93(6):801–5.
2. Ross PD, Norimatsu H, Davis JW, et al. A comparison of hip fracture incidence among native Japanese, Japanese Americans, and American Caucasians. Am J Epidemiol 1991;133(8):801–9.
3. Lauderdale DS, Jacobsen SJ, Furner SE, et al. Hip fracture incidence among elderly Asian-American populations. Am J Epidemiol 1997;146(6):502–9.
4. Robbins J, Aragaki AK, Kooperberg C, et al. Factors associated with 5-year risk of hip fracture in postmenopausal women. JAMA 2007;298(20):2389–98.
5. Johnell O, Kanis JA, Oden A, et al. Predictive value of BMD for hip and other fractures. J Bone Miner Res 2005;20(7):1185–94.
6. Barrett-Connor E, Siris ES, Wehren LE, et al. Osteoporosis and fracture risk in women of different ethnic groups. J Bone Miner Res 2005;20(2):185–94.
7. Mackey DC, Eby JG, Harris F, et al. Prediction of clinical non-spine fractures in older black and white men and women with volumetric BMD of the spine and areal BMD of the hip: the health, aging, and body composition study. J Bone Miner Res 2007;22(12):1862–8.
8. Fujiwara S, Kasagi F, Masunari N, et al. Fracture prediction from bone mineral density in Japanese men and women. J Bone Miner Res 2003;18(8):1547–53.
9. Yano K, Wasnich RD, Vogel JM, et al. Bone mineral measurements among middle-aged and elderly Japanese residents in Hawaii. Am J Epidemiol 1984; 119(5):751–64.
10. Norimatsu H, Mori S, Uesato T, et al. Bone mineral density of the spine and proximal femur in normal and osteoporotic subjects in Japan. Bone Miner 1989;5(2): 213–22.
11. Cummings SR, Black DM, Nevitt MC, et al. Bone density at various sites for prediction of hip fractures. The Study of Osteoporotic Fractures Research Group. Lancet 1992;341(8837):72–5.
12. Finkelstein JS, Lee ML, Sowers M, et al. Ethnic variation in bone density in premenopausal and early perimenopausal women: effects of anthropometric and lifestyle factors. J Clin Endocrinol Metab 2002;87(7):3057–67.
13. Ishii S, Cauley JA, Greendale GA, et al. Ethnic differences in composite indices of femoral neck strength. Osteoporos Int 2011;23:1381–90.
14. Danielson ME, Beck TJ, Lian Y, et al. Ethnic variability in bone geometry as assessed by hip structure analysis: findings from the hip strength across the menopausal transition study. J Bone Miner Res 2013;28(4):771–9.
15. Cheng XG, Lowet G, Boonen S, et al. Assessment of the strength of proximal femur in vitro: relationship to femoral bone mineral density and femoral geometry. Bone 1997;20:213–8.
16. Young WC. Elastic stability formulas for stress and strain. In: Young WC, editor. Roark's formulas for stress and strain. 6th edition. New York: McGraw-Hill; 1989. p. 688.
17. Allolio B. Risk factors for hip fracture not related to bone mass and their therapeutic implications. Osteoporos Int 1999;9(Suppl 2):S9–16.

18. Karlamangla AS, Barrett-Connor E, Young J, et al. Hip fracture risk assessment using composite indices of femoral neck strength: the Rancho Bernardo study. Osteoporos Int 2004;15(1):62–70.

19. Ishii S, Greendale G, Cauley J, et al. Fracture risk assessment without race/ethnicity information. J Clin Endocrinol Metab 2012;97(10):3593–602.

20. Fields AJ, Keaveny TM. Trabecular architecture and vertebral fragility in osteoporosis. Curr Osteoporos Rep 2012;10(2):132–40.

21. Silva BC, Leslie WD, Resch H, et al. Trabecular bone score: a noninvasive analytical method based upon the DXA image. J Bone Miner Res 2014;29(3):518–30.

22. Iki M, Tamaki J, Kadowaki E, et al. Trabecular bone score (TBS) predicts vertebral fractures in japanese women over 10 years independently of bone density and prevalent vertebral deformity: The Japanese Population-Based Osteoporosis (JPOS) Cohort Study. J Bone Miner Res 2014;29(2):399–407.

23. Krueger D, Fidler E, Libber J, et al. Spine trabecular bone score subsequent to bone mineral density improves fracture discrimination in women. J Clin Densitom 2014;17(1):60–5.

24. Iki M, Tamaki J, Sato Y, et al. Age-related normative values of trabecular bone score (TBS) for Japanese women: the Japanese Population-based Osteoporosis (JPOS) study. Osteoporos Int 2015;26(1):245–52.

25. Looker AC, Safrazi Isfahani N, Fan B, et al. Trabecular bone scores and lumbar spine bone mineral density of US adults: Comparison of relationships with demographic and body size variables. Osteoporos Int 2016;27(8):2467–75.

26. Amnuaywattakorn S, Sritara C, Utamukul C, et al. Simulated increased soft tissue thickness artefactually decreases trabecular bone score: a phantom study. BMC Musculoskelet Disord 2016;17:17.

27. Putnam MS, Yu EW, Lin D, et al. Differences in trabecular microstructure between black and white women assessed by individual trabecular segmentation analysis of HR-pQCT images. J Bone Miner Res 2017;32(5):1100–8.

28. Riis BJ, Hansen MA, Jensen AM, et al. Low bone mass and fast rate of bone loss at menopause: equal risk factors for future fracture: a 15-year follow-up study. Bone 1996;19:9–12.

29. Zaidi M, Turner C, Canalis E, et al. Bone loss or lost bone: rationale and recommendations for the diagnosis and treatment of early postmenopausal bone loss. Curr Osteoporos Rep 2009;7(4):118–26.

30. Guthrie JR, Dennerstein L, Taffe JR, et al. The menopausal transition: a 9-year prospective population-based study. The Melbourne Women's Midlife Health Project. Climacteric 2004;7:375–89.

31. Seifert-Klauss V, Fillenberg S, Schneider H, et al. Bone loss in premenopausal, perimenopausal and postmenopausal women: results of a prospective observational study over 9 years. Climacteric 2012;15(5):433–40.

32. Greendale GA, Sowers MF, Han WJ, et al. Bone mineral density loss in relation to the final menstrual period in a multi-ethnic cohort: results from the Study of Women's Health Across the Nation (SWAN). J Bone Miner Res 2012;27(1):111–8.

33. Crandall CJ, Tseng C-H, Karlamangla AS, et al. Serum sex steroid levels and longitudinal changes in bone density in relation to the final menstrual period. J Clin Endocrinol Metab 2013;98(4):E654–63.

34. Gast GM, Grobbee DE, Pop VJM, et al. Vasomotor symptoms are associated with a lower bone mineral density. Menopause 2009;16(2):231–8.

35. Crandall CJ, Zheng Y, Crawford SL, et al. Presence of vasomotor symptoms is associated with lower bone mineral density. A longitudinal analysis. Menopause 2009;16(2):239–46.

36. Solomon DH, Diem SJ, Ruppert K, et al. Bone mineral density changes among women initiating proton pump inhibitors or H2 receptor antagonists: a SWAN cohort study. J Bone Miner Res 2015;30(2):232–9.

37. Solomon DH, Ruppert K, Zhao Z, et al. Bone mineral density changes among women initiating blood pressure lowering drugs: a SWAN cohort study. Osteoporos Int 2016;27(3):1181–9.

38. Heaney RP, Barger-Lux MJ, Davies KM, et al. Bone dimensional change with age: interactions of genetic, hormonal, and body size variables. Osteoporos Int 1997; 7:426–31.

39. Ahlborg HG, Johnell O, Turner CH, et al. Bone loss and bone size after menopause. N Engl J Med 2003;349:327–34.

40. Ishii S, Cauley JA, Greendale GA, et al. Trajectories of femoral neck strength in relation to the final menstrual period in a multi-ethnic cohort. Osteoporos Int 2013;24(9):2471–81.

41. Zebaze RM, Ghasem-Zadeh A, Bohte A, et al. Intracortical remodelling and porosity in the distal radius and post-mortem femurs of women: a cross-sectional study. Lancet 2010;375(9727):1729–36.

42. Jepsen KJ, Kozminski A, Bigelow EMR, et al. Femoral neck external size but not aBMD predicts structural and mass changes for women transitioning through menopause. J Bone Miner Res 2017;32(6):1218–28.

43. Sowers MR, Zheng H, Greendale GA, et al. Changes in bone resorption across the menopause transition: Effects of reproductive hormones, body size, and ethnicity. J Clin Endocrinol Metab 2013;98(7):2854–63.

44. Crandall CJ, Tseng C-H, Crawford SL, et al. Association of menopausal vasomotor symptoms with increased bone turnover during the menopausal transition. J Bone Miner Res 2011;26(4):840–9.

45. Shieh A, Ishii S, Greendale GA, et al. Urinary N-telopeptide, and rate of bone loss over the menopause transition and early postmenopause. J Bone Miner Res 2016;31(11):2057–64.

46. Shieh A, Han WJ, Ishii S, et al. Quantifying the balance between bone formation and resorption: an index of net bone formation. J Clin Endocrinol Metab 2016; 101(7):2802–9.

47. Cauley JA, Danielson ME, Greendale GA, et al. Bone resorption and fracture across the menopausal transition: The Study of Women's Health Across the Nation. Menopause 2012;19(11):1200–7.

48. Greendale G, LeClair H, Huang MH, et al. Prevalent and incident vertebral deformities in midlife women: results from the Study of Women's Health Across the Nation (SWAN). PLoS One 2016;11(9):e0162664.

49. Crandall CJ, Han W-J, Greendale GA, et al. Socioeconomic status in relation to incident fracture risk in the Study of Women's Health Across the Nation. Osteoporos Int 2014;25:1379–88.

50. Mori T, Ishii S, Greendale GA, et al. Parity, lactation, bone strength, and 12-year fracture risk in adult women: Findings from the Study of Women's Health Across the Nation. Bone 2015;73:160–6.

51. Khalil N, Sutton-Tyrell K, Strotmeyer ES, et al. Menopausal bone changes and incident fractures in diabetic women: a cohort study. Osteoporos Int 2011;22: 1367–76.

52. Ishii S, Cauley J, Crandall C, et al. Diabetes and femoral neck strength: findings from the hip strength across the menopausal transition study. J Clin Endocrinol Metab 2012;97(1):190–7.

53. Yu EW, Putman MS, Derrico N, et al. Defects in cortical microarchitecture among African-American women with type 2 diabetes. Osteoporos Int 2015;26(2):673–9.
54. Ishii S, Cauley JA, Greendale GA, et al. C-reactive protein, femoral neck strength, and 9-year fracture risk. Data from The Study of Women's Health Across the Nation. J Bone Miner Res 2013;28(7):1688–98.
55. Chang P-Y, Gold EB, Cauley Jane A, et al. Triglyceride levels and fracture risk in midlife women: Study of Women's Health Across the Nation (SWAN). J Clin Endocrinol Metab 2016;101(9):3297–305.
56. Ishii S, Cauley J, Greendale G, et al. Pleiotropic effects of obesity on fracture risk: The Study of Women's Health Across the Nation. J Bone Miner Res 2014;29(12): 2561–70.
57. Mori T, Ishii S, Greendale GA, et al. Physical activity as determinant of femoral neck strength in adult women. Findings from the hip strength across the menopausal transition study. Osteoporos Int 2014;25:265–72.
58. Macdonald HM, New HA, Golden MHN, et al. Nutritional associations with bone loss during the menopausal transition: evidence of a beneficial effect of calcium, alcohol, and fruit and vegetable nutrients and of a detrimental effect of fatty acids. Am J Clin Nutr 2004;79(1):155–65.
59. Cauley JA, Greendale GA, Ruppert K, et al. Serum 25 Hydroxyvitamin D, bone mineral density and fracture risk across the menopause. J Clin Endocrinol Metab 2015;100(5):2046–54.
60. Greendale GA, FitzGerald G, Huang M-H, et al. Dietary soy isoflavones and bone mineral density: results from the Study of Women's Health Across the Nation. Am J Epidemiol 2002;155:746–54.
61. Greendale GA, Tseng C-H, Han W, et al. Dietary isoflavones and bone mineral density during midlife and the menopausal transition: cross-sectional and longitudinal results from the Study of Women's Health Across the Nation Phytoestrogen Study. Menopause 2015;22(3):279–88.
62. Eijsvogels TMH, Molossi S, Lee D, et al. Exercise at the extremes. The amount of exercise to reduce cardiovascular events. J Am Coll Cardiol 2016;67:316–29.
63. Institute of Medicine. Dietary reference intakes for calcium and Vitamin D. Washington, DC: National Academies Press; 2011.
64. Bischoff-Ferrari HA, Dawson-Hughes B, Orav J, et al. Monthly high-dose vitamin D treatment for the prevention of functional decline: a randomized clinical trial. JAMA Intern Med 2016;176(2):175–83.
65. Ginde AA, Blatchford P, Breese K, et al. High-dose monthly vitamin D for prevention of acute respiratory infection in older long-term care residents: a randomized clinical trial. J Am Geriatr Soc 2017;65(3):496–503.
66. Sanders KM, Stuart AI, Williamson EJ, et al. Annual high-dose oral vitamin D and falls and fractures in older women. A randomized controlled trial. JAMA 2010; 303(18):1815–22.
67. Crandall CJ, Larson J, Gourlay ML, et al. Osteoporosis screening in postmenopausal women 50 to 64 years old: comparison of US Preventive Services Task Force strategy and two traditional strategies in the Women's Health Initiative. J Bone Miner Res 2014;29(7):1661–6.
68. Crandall CJ, Larson JB, Watts NB, et al. Comparison of fracture risk prediction by the US Preventive Services Task Force strategy and two alternative strategies in women 50–64 years old in the Women's Health Initiative. J Clin Endocrinol Metab 2014;99(12):4514–22.
69. Ensrud KE, Crandall CJ. Osteoporosis. Ann Intern Med 2017;167(3):ITC17–32.

70. Akhter M, Lappe J, Davies K, et al. Transmenopausal changes in the trabecular bone structure. Bone 2007;41(1):111–6.
71. Cooper D, Thomas C, Clement J, et al. Age-dependent change in the 3D structure of cortical porosity at the human femoral midshaft. Bone 2007; 40(4):957–65.

Female Sexual Function at Midlife and Beyond

Holly N. Thomas, MD, MS[a],*, Genevieve S. Neal-Perry, MD, PhD[b], Rachel Hess, MD, MS[c,d]

KEYWORDS

- Sexual function • Menopause • Perimenopause • Sexual dysfunction

KEY POINTS

- A sizable minority of women report sexual dysfunction during the perimenopause and menopausal years; about 15% endorse personal distress as a result.
- Genitourinary syndrome of menopause, vulvovaginal atrophy, and pelvic organ prolapse can cause vaginal and sexual pain and remain underrecognized and undertreated.
- Relationship and social factors, as well as sexual trauma, are important predictors of midlife sexual function.
- A variety of pharmacologic treatments are available with varying efficacy; more information is needed to help clinicians target treatments effectively.

INTRODUCTION

Sexual function is an important aspect of life for many women, regardless of age. Sexual function is closely correlated with overall well-being and relationship satisfaction.[1–3] Most women continue to consider sexual function important as they age.[4–6] However, 45% of midlife women have sexual problems,[2,7] and 15% have a sexual problem that causes significant personal distress.[7] Female sexual dysfunction remains underrecognized and undertreated by health care providers. In this article, the authors review the definition of female sexual dysfunction, examine how sexual function changes during the midlife transition, define factors

Disclosure Statement: Dr R. Hess reports no disclosures; Dr G.S. Neal-Perry is a member of the Scientific Advisory Board for Astellas and a past Data and Safety Monitoring Board member for Ferring Pharmaceuticals. Dr H.N. Thomas is funded by a grant from the National Institute of Health's National Institute on Aging; grant number K23AG052628.
^a Department of Medicine, Center for Women's Health Research and Innovation (CWHRI), University of Pittsburgh, 230 McKee Place, Suite 600, Pittsburgh, PA 15213, USA; ^b Department of Obstetrics and Gynecology, University of Washington, 4245 Roosevelt Way NE, 4th Floor, Seattle, WA 98105, USA; ^c Department of Population Health Sciences, University of Utah, 295 Chipeta Way 1N492, Salt Lake City, UT 84108, USA; ^d Department of Internal Medicine, University of Utah, 295 Chipeta Way 1N492, Salt Lake City, UT 84108, USA
* Corresponding author.
E-mail address: thomashn@upmc.edu

Obstet Gynecol Clin N Am 45 (2018) 709–722
https://doi.org/10.1016/j.ogc.2018.07.013
0889-8545/18/© 2018 Elsevier Inc. All rights reserved.

obgyn.theclinics.com

that are associated with sexual dysfunction at midlife, and discuss new and emerging treatments.

DEFINITIONS

Sexual dysfunction, as defined in the *Diagnostic and Statistical Manual of Mental Disorders (DSM-5)*, is a heterogeneous group of disorders characterized by clinically significant disturbances in sexual response or the experience of sexual pleasure.[8] A key element of the *DSM-5* definition is *significant personal distress*. Revision of the *DSM* between versions 4 and 5 included substantive changes to female sexual dysfunction terminology (**Fig. 1**). Notably, Hypoactive Sexual Desire Disorder and Female Sexual Arousal Disorder were combined into a single diagnosis, Female Sexual Interest and Arousal Disorder,[8] because there is considerable overlap between the disorders, and the concepts of desire and arousal are virtually indistinguishable for many women.[9,10] These changes were controversial,[11-13] and some experts still favor the older terminology. It is also essential to consider overall sexual satisfaction. For many women, the end goal of sex is not "functional" sex, where all the parts are working well, but emotional and physical satisfaction and increased intimacy with one's partner.

CHANGES IN SEXUAL FUNCTION DURING MIDLIFE

Sexual function declines during midlife. The Study of Women's Health Across the Nation and others found that this decline corresponds with the menopausal transition, including in women who have hysterectomies.[14,15] Although symptoms such as vaginal dryness increase over the same period, changes in sexual function are

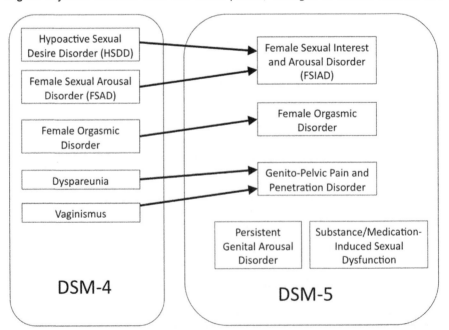

Fig. 1. Female sexual dysfunction terminology. (*Data from* American Psychiatric Association. Diagnostic and statistical manual of mental disorders. 4th edition. Washington, DC: American Psychiatric Publishing; 2000; and American Psychiatric Association. Diagnostic and statistical manual of mental disorders, 5th edition. Washington, DC: American Psychiatric Publishing; 2013.)

independent of other symptoms associated with the menopausal transition. Declines in sexual activity during midlife are multifactorial (discussed later). One prominent reason that women do not engage in sexual activity is lack of a partner.[16]

Women who are sexually active before menopause appear to continue to engage in sexual activities during midlife, despite poor "functional sex."[5] Lifestyle factors, including sufficient sleep and physical activity, contribute to more positive sexual functioning during midlife.[16] Alternative models of sexual function may provide more insight into the impact of these changes during menopause. In contrast to the traditional linear model posited by Masters and Johnson,[17] Basson[18] suggests that the sexual response, particularly in women, is more circular and dependent on emotional connection and fulfillment. This model offers an explanation for the dichotomy of decline in sexual function, with endurance of sexual activities as a means to express and maintain connected partnerships.

FACTORS THAT AFFECT FEMALE SEXUAL FUNCTION AT MIDLIFE
Biologic Factors: Hormones, Menopausal Symptoms

Menopause is characterized by ovarian follicular exhaustion and hypogonadism. Reduced ovarian steroidogenesis leads to the development of genitourinary syndrome of menopause (GSM),[19] which adversely affects the genital system and lower urinary tract in menopausal women and significantly contributes to sexual dysfunction.[20] More than half of menopausal women experience GSM, which is responsive to local estradiol. Unlike vasomotor symptoms, which often decrease over time, GSM does not resolve and recurs after discontinuation of estrogen.[21,22]

Vulvovaginal atrophy (VVA), also known as vulvovaginitis, is a key component of GSM and can result in postcoital vaginal bleeding, vaginal burning, irritation, and pain and discomfort with sex. Symptomatic GSM is often accompanied by diminished secretions from vulvar sebaceous glands and reduced vaginal lubrication during sexual stimulation. Hypoestrogenic menopausal women often experience a shift of the vaginal microbiome from lactic acid–producing lactobacilli to gram- negative and -positive bacteria.[23] This shift in the vaginal microbiome results in increased vaginal pH, local immune changes, and increased cytokine synthesis, which worsens symptoms of vaginal dryness and burning[23] and contributes to sexual dysfunction. These external genital changes are covered in detail in Caroline M. Mitchell and L. Elaine Waetjen's article, "Genitourinary Changes with Aging," in this issue.

Pelvic organ prolapse (POP) involves descent of one or more female genital organs (anterior and/or posterior vaginal wall, the uterus or the apex of the vagina). The incidence of pelvic floor relaxation increases with aging and is hypothesized to result from a combination of connective tissue degradation, pelvic denervation, and devascularization, all of which predispose to prolapse.[24] Dyspareunia, chronic pelvic pain, and reduced self-image are associated with POP. Any one of these adverse anatomic changes can devastate sexual interest and function.[25] Estrogen treatment may reduce the risk for POP, especially in postmenopausal women who have undergone hysterectomy and require transvaginal reconstructive surgery.[26]

Medical Problems and Medications

Multiple medical problems, including diabetes, hypertension, and breast cancer, have been associated with female sexual dysfunction (**Box 1**). These conditions become more common as women move through midlife.

Both type 1 and 2 diabetes are associated with a 2 to 3 times higher rate of female sexual dysfunction.[27] Biologically, diabetes imparts chronic microvascular damage

---

Box 1
Medical and psychiatric conditions that are associated with female sexual dysfunction

Cardiovascular disease[108]

Diabetes mellitus[109]

Neurologic disease (stroke, multiple sclerosis, spinal cord injury)[110]

Hypertension[28]

Substance use disorders[111]

Genitourinary syndrome of menopause[57,112]

Breast, ovarian, uterine, and cervical cancer[113–115]

History of gynecologic surgery[116,117]

Chronic renal failure[118,119]

Urinary incontinence[120,121]

---

that could affect small nerves and blood vessels in the clitoris and associated structures, leading to impaired arousal and lubrication. Through similar mechanisms, hypertension has a 3-fold higher risk of sexual dysfunction in women,[28] with the strongest effects on the domain of lubrication.[29] Although early studies suggested that certain antihypertensives, especially beta-blockers, may negatively affect sexual function in women,[30] newer studies have found no association between antihypertensives and female sexual dysfunction.[31–33] In fact, antihypertensive medications that work on the renin-angiotensin system may be associated with *better* sexual function.[31,34]

Breast cancer can negatively affect sexual function in both the short and long term.[35–37] Around 50% of women with a history of breast cancer report sexual problems,[37] and the prevalence increases to 70% among women with invasive cancer.[38] The causes are multifactorial. Receipt of chemotherapy is one of the strongest risk factors,[39] particularly if it results in premature menopause.[40] Aromatase inhibitors are associated with vaginal dryness and sexual pain,[38,41] whereas tamoxifen does not have strong effects on sexual function.[38] Mastectomy can negatively affect body image[39] and in turn sexual function.[37–39,42] Among women with diabetes, hypertension, or breast cancer, depression is highly correlated with sexual dysfunction.[35,37,43,44] These findings highlight the importance of screening for and treating mood disorders in these populations.

Other medications have been associated with female sexual dysfunction (**Box 2**). Among the most common offenders are antidepressants, including

---

Box 2
Medications that are associated with female sexual dysfunction

Antidepressants (selective serotonin reuptake inhibitors, serotonin norepinephrine reuptake inhibitors, tricyclic antidepressants)[46,47,122,123]

Opiates[111]

Cancer therapies, especially for breast and gynecologic cancer[113,124–126]

Antihypertensives (mixed evidence), particularly beta-blockers[30,127]

Antiepileptics[128,129]

Benzodiazepines[130,131]

---

selective-serotonin reuptake inhibitors, serotonin-norepinephrine reuptake inhibitors, and tricyclic antidepressants.[45] Although depression itself is associated with sexual dysfunction, odds of sexual dysfunction are 4 to 6 times higher for women taking a medication.[46] Sexual side effects are less common with bupropion[46,47] and mirtazapine.[47,48] Providers should counsel women about the potential for sexual side effects when starting these medications. Small studies have shown sildenafil and bupropion to be effective antidotes for antidepressant-associated sexual dysfunction.[49,50]

Psychosocial

Several of the following psychosocial factors that are common during midlife are associated with sexual dysfunction:

- Mood symptoms, such as depression and anxiety
- Life stressors, such as career and family demands
- A history of trauma, particularly sexual trauma

The development of depression and anxiety symptoms during the menopausal transition is common.[51-53] Mood disorders and sexual dysfunction are highly comorbid,[54] with 25% to 75% of depressed women reporting sexual problems[55] even when controlling for other factors.[56-58] It is important for providers to screen women with sexual complaints for depression and anxiety symptoms and recognize that not all women with sexual dysfunction have a mood disorder. Everyday life stressors also have a negative impact.[59-61] Midlife women may be caring for children of their own, may have adult children return home, and/or be caring for aging parents.[59] Job-related stress and financial concerns are also common.[59] Providers should be attuned to the effects of life stressors and work with women to develop stress reduction strategies, such as mindfulness meditation.

Women who are victims of violence are at increased risk for sexual dysfunction,[62] with those who have experienced sexual trauma, up to 44% of women over their lifetime,[63] at particularly high risk.[64] The relationship between trauma history and sexual dysfunction is not entirely explained by mental health disorders, such as depression, anxiety, and posttraumatic stress disorder. It is important to use evidence-based, trauma-informed care techniques to screen for these events when providing care for women with sexual dysfunction.[65,66]

Interpersonal Factors

Most midlife women are sexually active with a partner,[5] and partner-associated issues can affect the woman's sexual function, as follows:

- Positive relationship aspects: higher relationship satisfaction and intimacy are associated with better sexual function,[67,68] and the ability to openly communicate with one's partner is of key importance.[59]
- Loss or gain of a partner: Many women experience the loss of a partner (to death, divorce, or separation) at midlife, and some gain a new partner, both of which can affect sexual function.[57,69] Gain of a new partner is associated with increased desire, arousal, and emotional satisfaction with sex.[57]
- Issues affecting aging partners: Partners may develop medical problems, medications, or sexual dysfunction that can affect the woman's sexual function. In particular, erectile dysfunction in male partners is associated with decreased sexual function and satisfaction in female partners.[59,70]

NEW AND EMERGING TREATMENTS
Female Sexual Interest and Arousal Disorder

There is only one Food and Drug Administration (FDA) -approved medication for the treatment of hypoactive sexual desire disorder: flibanserin. Although only approved for use in premenopausal women, it is efficacious in postmenopausal women.[71] Flibanserin increases satisfying sexual events by about 0.5 per month compared with placebo, with statistically significant improvements in desire, overall sexual function, and sexually related distress.[72–75] Some have questioned whether these improvements are clinically significant.[75] Providers should be aware of the following:

- Common adverse effects include somnolence, dizziness, and nausea[73,75]
- Flibanserin interacts with some common medications (macrolide antibiotics, azole antifungals, and calcium channel blockers)
- Women cannot drink alcohol while using flibanserin
- Health care providers must be certified to prescribe flibanserin

Testosterone has been studied for the treatment of hypoactive sexual desire disorder, but is not FDA approved for this purpose. Most testosterone studies were conducted among surgically menopausal women,[76–78] although a few studies included naturally menopausal women.[79,80] All but 2 studies[79,81] paired testosterone with estrogen therapy. Consistent positive effects were seen on sexual desire, overall sexual function, and sexual distress.[76–80,82–84] Common adverse effects were acne and hirsutism, occurring in 5% to 20% of women.[76–82] Negative effects on lipid parameters were not observed.[77,84] However, randomized trial data beyond 24 weeks are sparse, and a recent analysis suggests only women who achieve supraphysiologic testosterone levels have a significant response.[85] Observational studies have suggested there may be an increased risk of cardiovascular disease[86] and invasive breast cancer[81,87] when testosterone is added to traditional hormone therapy, but findings are inconsistent.[88,89]

Behavioral interventions, most notably mindfulness-based therapies, have shown positive effects on sexual desire, sexual distress, and overall sexual function.[90–92] These methods may improve sexual function by increasing bodily awareness[93] and improving concordance between physiologic and psychological arousal.[94] However, these studies are relatively small, limited by use of wait-list controls or no control group, and lack comparison to pharmaceutical interventions.

Genitourinary Syndrome of Menopause and Sexual Pain

Many women have been dissatisfied with prior treatment of GSM and sexual pain.[95,96] These symptoms remain underrecognized and undertreated by health care providers.[95,97,98] Newer options include ospemifene, prasterone, estradiol softgels, and carbon dioxide laser therapy.

Ospemifene is an FDA-approved selective estrogen receptor modifier that results in significant improvements in vaginal symptoms and dyspareunia.[99,100] Adverse effects include hot flashes (7%–10%)[101,102] and endometrial proliferation (2%–12%), although no cases of hyperplasia or endometrial cancer were reported.[101] Prasterone, intravaginal dehydroepiandrosterone, was recently approved for the treatment of dyspareunia due to GSM, with the only adverse effect being vaginal discharge (6%).[103] A new formulation of vaginal estradiol, a softgel tablet, has shown promising results in early trials.[104,105] Finally, carbon dioxide laser use is emerging as another potential treatment[106,107]; however, trials have lacked adequate control groups, and further research is necessary. Data beyond 52 weeks are not available for any of these newer treatments, and it is unclear how they compare to older treatments in terms of efficacy or safety.

FUTURE DIRECTIONS

Much progress has been made in the field of women's sexual function. However, much work remains. Sexual health education for providers in training needs to be better developed and tested. Easy-to-use, efficient screening methods for sexual problems in primary care settings are needed. Research should seek to define protective factors, ways that women adapt to the changes that occur with the midlife transition, and how they are able to maintain sexual function and satisfaction. Data on how sexual function changes with aging are needed among sexual minority groups. Research should explore how the traditional and newer treatment options for GSM compare with one another, not just placebo, and define which treatments are safest and most effective for specific patient groups. Treatments for desire and arousal difficulties remain lacking; behavioral interventions hold promise, and ongoing research should explore which aspects of these interventions are most powerful, and how they can be scaled up to reach the women in need. Helping women preserve healthy sexual function with aging is an essential component of maintaining quality of life into older adulthood.

REFERENCES

1. Leiblum SR, Koochaki PE, Rodenberg CA, et al. Hypoactive sexual desire disorder in postmenopausal women: US results from the Women's International Study of Health and Sexuality (WISHeS). Menopause 2006;13(1):46–56.
2. Laumann EO, Paik A, Rosen RC. Sexual dysfunction in the United States: prevalence and predictors. JAMA 1999;281(6):537–44.
3. Lindau ST, Gavrilova N. Sex, health, and years of sexually active life gained due to good health: evidence from two US population based cross sectional surveys of ageing. BMJ 2010;340:c810.
4. Cain VS, Johannes CB, Avis NE, et al. Sexual functioning and practices in a multi-ethnic study of midlife women: baseline results from SWAN. J Sex Res 2003;40(3):266–76.
5. Thomas HN, Chang CC, Dillon S, et al. Sexual activity in midlife women: importance of sex matters. JAMA Intern Med 2014;174(4):631–3.
6. Flynn KE, Lin L, Bruner DW, et al. Sexual satisfaction and the importance of sexual health to quality of life throughout the life course of U.S. adults. J Sex Med 2016;13(11):1642–50.
7. Shifren JL, Monz BU, Russo PA, et al. Sexual problems and distress in United States women: prevalence and correlates. Obstet Gynecol 2008;112(5):970–8.
8. American Psychiatric Association. DSM-5 task force. Diagnostic and statistical manual of mental disorders: DSM-5. 5th edition. Washington, DC: American Psychiatric Association; 2013.
9. Brotto LA. The DSM diagnostic criteria for hypoactive sexual desire disorder in women. Arch Sex Behav 2010;39(2):221–39.
10. Binik YM, Brotto LA, Graham CA, et al. Response of the DSM-V sexual dysfunctions subworkgroup to commentaries published in JSM. J Sex Med 2010;7(7):2382–7.
11. DeRogatis LR, Clayton AH, Rosen RC, et al. Should sexual desire and arousal disorders in women be merged? Arch Sex Behav 2011;40(2):217–9 [author reply: 221–5].

12. Balon R, Clayton AH. Female sexual interest/arousal disorder: a diagnosis out of thin air. Arch Sex Behav 2014;43(7):1227–9.

13. McCabe MP, Sharlip ID, Atalla E, et al. Definitions of sexual dysfunctions in women and men: a consensus statement from the Fourth International Consultation on Sexual Medicine 2015. J Sex Med 2016;13(2):135–43.

14. Dennerstein L, Dudley E, Burger H. Are changes in sexual functioning during midlife due to aging or menopause? Fertil Steril 2001;76(3):456–60.

15. Avis NE, Colvin A, Karlamangla AS, et al. Change in sexual functioning over the menopausal transition: results from the Study of Women's Health Across the Nation. Menopause 2017;24(4):379–90.

16. Hess R, Conroy MB, Ness R, et al. Association of lifestyle and relationship factors with sexual functioning of women during midlife. J Sex Med 2009;6(5):1350–60.

17. Masters WH, Johnson VE. Human sexual response. Boston: Little, Brown & Co; 1966.

18. Basson R. The female sexual response: a different model. J Sex Marital Ther 2000;26(1):51–65.

19. Portman DJ, Gass ML. Genitourinary syndrome of menopause: new terminology for vulvovaginal atrophy from the International Society for the Study of Women's Sexual Health and the North American Menopause Society. J Sex Med 2014;11(12):2865–72.

20. Cuerva MJ, Gonzalez D, Canals M, et al. The sexual health approach in postmenopause: the five-minutes study. Maturitas 2018;108:31–6.

21. Kroll R, Archer DF, Lin Y, et al. A randomized, multicenter, double-blind study to evaluate the safety and efficacy of estradiol vaginal cream 0.003% in postmenopausal women with dyspareunia as the most bothersome symptom. Menopause 2018;25(2):133–8.

22. Archer DF, Labrie F, Montesino M, et al. Comparison of intravaginal 6.5mg (0.50%) prasterone, 0.3mg conjugated estrogens and 10mug estradiol on symptoms of vulvovaginal atrophy. J Steroid Biochem Mol Biol 2017;174:1–8.

23. Hummelen R, Macklaim JM, Bisanz JE, et al. Vaginal microbiome and epithelial gene array in post-menopausal women with moderate to severe dryness. PLoS One 2011;6(11):e26602.

24. Mannella P, Palla G, Bellini M, et al. The female pelvic floor through midlife and aging. Maturitas 2013;76(3):230–4.

25. Shatkin-Margolis A, Pauls RN. Sexual function after prolapse repair. Curr Opin Obstet Gynecol 2017;29(5):343–8.

26. Rahn DD, Carberry C, Sanses TV, et al. Vaginal estrogen for genitourinary syndrome of menopause: a systematic review. Obstet Gynecol 2014;124(6):1147–56.

27. Pontiroli AE, Cortelazzi D, Morabito A. Female sexual dysfunction and diabetes: a systematic review and meta-analysis. J Sex Med 2013;10(4):1044–51.

28. Doumas M, Tsiodras S, Tsakiris A, et al. Female sexual dysfunction in essential hypertension: a common problem being uncovered. J Hypertens 2006;24(12):2387–92.

29. Duncan LE, Lewis C, Jenkins P, et al. Does hypertension and its pharmacotherapy affect the quality of sexual function in women? Am J Hypertens 2000;13(6 Pt 1):640–7.

30. A randomized trial of propranolol in patients with acute myocardial infarction. I. Mortality results. JAMA 1982;247(12):1707–14.

31. Thomas HN, Evans GW, Berlowitz DR, et al. Antihypertensive medications and sexual function in women: baseline data from the SBP intervention trial (SPRINT). J Hypertens 2016;34(6):1224–31.

32. Grimm RH Jr, Grandits GA, Prineas RJ, et al. Long-term effects on sexual function of five antihypertensive drugs and nutritional hygienic treatment in hypertensive men and women. Treatment of Mild Hypertension Study (TOMHS). Hypertension 1997;29(1 Pt 1):8–14.

33. Wassertheil-Smoller S, Blaufox MD, Oberman A, et al. Effect of antihypertensives on sexual function and quality of life: the TAIM Study. Ann Intern Med 1991;114(8):613–20.

34. Ma R, Yu J, Xu D, et al. Effect of felodipine with irbesartan or metoprolol on sexual function and oxidative stress in women with essential hypertension. J Hypertens 2012;30(1):210–6.

35. Speer JJ, Hillenberg B, Sugrue DP, et al. Study of sexual functioning determinants in breast cancer survivors. Breast J 2005;11(6):440–7.

36. Broeckel JA, Thors CL, Jacobsen PB, et al. Sexual functioning in long-term breast cancer survivors treated with adjuvant chemotherapy. Breast Cancer Res Treat 2002;75(3):241–8.

37. Fobair P, Stewart SL, Chang S, et al. Body image and sexual problems in young women with breast cancer. Psychooncology 2006;15(7):579–94.

38. Panjari M, Bell RJ, Davis SR. Sexual function after breast cancer. J Sex Med 2011;8(1):294–302.

39. Avis NE, Crawford S, Manuel J. Psychosocial problems among younger women with breast cancer. Psychooncology 2004;13(5):295–308.

40. Ganz PA, Rowland JH, Desmond K, et al. Life after breast cancer: understanding women's health-related quality of life and sexual functioning. J Clin Oncol 1998;16(2):501–14.

41. Avis NE, Crawford S, Manuel J. Quality of life among younger women with breast cancer. J Clin Oncol 2005;23(15):3322–30.

42. Greendale GA, Petersen L, Zibecchi L, et al. Factors related to sexual function in postmenopausal women with a history of breast cancer. Menopause 2001;8(2): 111–9.

43. Nascimento ER, Maia AC, Nardi AE, et al. Sexual dysfunction in arterial hypertension women: the role of depression and anxiety. J Affect Disord 2015;181: 96–100.

44. Foy CG, Newman JC, Berlowitz DR, et al. Blood pressure, sexual activity, and dysfunction in women with hypertension: baseline findings from the Systolic Blood Pressure Intervention Trial (SPRINT). J Sex Med 2016;13(9):1333–46.

45. Montgomery SA, Baldwin DS, Riley A. Antidepressant medications: a review of the evidence for drug-induced sexual dysfunction. J Affect Disord 2002;69(1–3): 119–40.

46. Clayton AH, Pradko JF, Croft HA, et al. Prevalence of sexual dysfunction among newer antidepressants. J Clin Psychiatry 2002;63(4):357–66.

47. Serretti A, Chiesa A. Treatment-emergent sexual dysfunction related to antidepressants: a meta-analysis. J Clin Psychopharmacol 2009;29(3):259–66.

48. Gelenberg AJ, McGahuey C, Laukes C, et al. Mirtazapine substitution in SSRI-induced sexual dysfunction. J Clin Psychiatry 2000;61(5):356–60.

49. Nurnberg HG, Hensley PL, Heiman JR, et al. Sildenafil treatment of women with antidepressant-associated sexual dysfunction: a randomized controlled trial. JAMA 2008;300(4):395–404.

50. Labbate LA, Grimes JB, Hines A, et al. Bupropion treatment of serotonin reuptake antidepressant-associated sexual dysfunction. Ann Clin Psychiatry 1997; 9(4):241–5.

51. Cohen LS, Soares CN, Vitonis AF, et al. Risk for new onset of depression during the menopausal transition: the Harvard study of moods and cycles. Arch Gen Psychiatry 2006;63(4):385–90.

52. Bromberger JT, Kravitz HM, Chang YF, et al. Major depression during and after the menopausal transition: Study of Women's Health Across the Nation (SWAN). Psychol Med 2011;41(9):1879–88.

53. Bromberger JT, Matthews KA, Schott LL, et al. Depressive symptoms during the menopausal transition: the Study of Women's Health Across the Nation (SWAN). J Affect Disord 2007;103(1–3):267–72.

54. Lonnee-Hoffmann RA, Dennerstein L, Lehert P, et al. Sexual function in the late postmenopause: a decade of follow-up in a population-based cohort of Australian women. J Sex Med 2014;11(8):2029–38.

55. Williams K, Reynolds MF. Sexual dysfunction in major depression. CNS Spectr 2006;11(8 Suppl 9):19–23.

56. Dennerstein L, Guthrie JR, Hayes RD, et al. Sexual function, dysfunction, and sexual distress in a prospective, population-based sample of mid-aged, Australian-born women. J Sex Med 2008;5(10):2291–9.

57. Avis NE, Brockwell S, Randolph JF Jr, et al. Longitudinal changes in sexual functioning as women transition through menopause: results from the Study of Women's Health Across the Nation. Menopause 2009;16(3):442–52.

58. Cyranowski JM, Bromberger J, Youk A, et al. Lifetime depression history and sexual function in women at midlife. Arch Sex Behav 2004;33(6):539–48.

59. Thomas HN, Hamm M, Hess R, et al. Changes in sexual function among midlife women: "I'm older… and I'm wiser". Menopause 2018;25(3):286–92.

60. Hamilton LD, Julian AM. The relationship between daily hassles and sexual function in men and women. J Sex Marital Ther 2014;40(5):379–95.

61. Bodenmann G, Atkins DC, Schar M, et al. The association between daily stress and sexual activity. J Fam Psychol 2010;24(3):271–9.

62. Golding JM. Sexual assault history and women's reproductive and sexual health. Psychol Women Q 1996;20:101–21.

63. Breiding MJ, Smith SG, Basile KC, et al. Prevalence and characteristics of sexual violence, stalking, and intimate partner violence victimization–national intimate partner and sexual violence survey, United States, 2011. MMWR Surveill Summ 2014;63(8):1–18.

64. Rellini A, Meston C. Sexual function and satisfaction in adults based on the definition of child sexual abuse. J Sex Med 2007;4(5):1312–21.

65. Ghandour RM, Campbell JC, Lloyd J. Screening and counseling for intimate partner violence: a vision for the future. J Womens Health (Larchmt) 2015; 24(1):57–61.

66. Harris M, Fallot RD. Using trauma theory to design service systems: new directions for mental health services. San Francisco (CA): Jossey-Bass; 2001.

67. Sprecher S. Sexual satisfaction in premarital relationships: associations with satisfaction, love, commitment, and stability. J Sex Res 2002;39(3):190–6.

68. Byers ES. Relationship satisfaction and sexual satisfaction: a longitudinal study of individuals in long-term relationships. J Sex Res 2005;42(2):113–8.

69. Gunst A, Ventus D, Karna A, et al. Female sexual function varies over time and is dependent on partner-specific factors: a population-based longitudinal analysis of six sexual function domains. Psychol Med 2017;47(2):341–52.

70. Fisher WA, Rosen RC, Eardley I, et al. Sexual experience of female partners of men with erectile dysfunction: the female experience of men's attitudes to life events and sexuality (FEMALES) study. J Sex Med 2005;2(5):675–84.

71. Portman DJ, Brown L, Yuan J, et al. Flibanserin in postmenopausal women with hypoactive sexual desire disorder: results of the PLUMERIA study. J Sex Med 2017;14(6):834–42.

72. Derogatis LR, Komer L, Katz M, et al. Treatment of hypoactive sexual desire disorder in premenopausal women: efficacy of flibanserin in the VIOLET Study. J Sex Med 2012;9(4):1074–85.

73. Katz M, DeRogatis LR, Ackerman R, et al. Efficacy of flibanserin in women with hypoactive sexual desire disorder: results from the BEGONIA trial. J Sex Med 2013;10(7):1807–15.

74. Goldfischer ER, Breaux J, Katz M, et al. Continued efficacy and safety of flibanserin in premenopausal women with Hypoactive Sexual Desire Disorder (HSDD): results from a randomized withdrawal trial. J Sex Med 2011;8(11): 3160–72.

75. Jaspers L, Feys F, Bramer WM, et al. Efficacy and safety of Flibanserin for the treatment of hypoactive sexual desire disorder in women: a systematic review and meta-analysis. JAMA Intern Med 2016;176(4):453–62.

76. Shifren JL, Braunstein GD, Simon JA, et al. Transdermal testosterone treatment in women with impaired sexual function after oophorectomy. N Engl J Med 2000; 343(10):682–8.

77. Buster JE, Kingsberg SA, Aguirre O, et al. Testosterone patch for low sexual desire in surgically menopausal women: a randomized trial. Obstet Gynecol 2005;105(5 Pt 1):944–52.

78. Braunstein GD, Sundwall DA, Katz M, et al. Safety and efficacy of a testosterone patch for the treatment of hypoactive sexual desire disorder in surgically menopausal women: a randomized, placebo-controlled trial. Arch Intern Med 2005; 165(14):1582–9.

79. Panay N, Al-Azzawi F, Bouchard C, et al. Testosterone treatment of HSDD in naturally menopausal women: the ADORE study. Climacteric 2010;13(2): 121–31.

80. Shifren JL, Davis SR, Moreau M, et al. Testosterone patch for the treatment of hypoactive sexual desire disorder in naturally menopausal women: results from the INTIMATE NM1 Study. Menopause 2006;13(5):770–9.

81. Davis SR, Moreau M, Kroll R, et al. Testosterone for low libido in postmenopausal women not taking estrogen. N Engl J Med 2008;359(19):2005–17.

82. Achilli C, Pundir J, Ramanathan P, et al. Efficacy and safety of transdermal testosterone in postmenopausal women with hypoactive sexual desire disorder: a systematic review and meta-analysis. Fertil Steril 2017;107(2):475–82.e5.

83. Elraiyah T, Sonbol MB, Wang Z, et al. Clinical review: the benefits and harms of systemic testosterone therapy in postmenopausal women with normal adrenal function: a systematic review and meta-analysis. J Clin Endocrinol Metab 2014;99(10):3543–50.

84. El-Hage G, Eden JA, Manga RZ. A double-blind, randomized, placebo-controlled trial of the effect of testosterone cream on the sexual motivation of menopausal hysterectomized women with hypoactive sexual desire disorder. Climacteric 2007;10(4):335–43.

85. Huang G, Basaria S, Travison TG, et al. Testosterone dose-response relationships in hysterectomized women with or without oophorectomy: effects on

sexual function, body composition, muscle performance and physical function in a randomized trial. Menopause 2014;21(6):612–23.

86. Rahman HA, Malik A, Rahman A, et al. Risk of stroke in women with use of testosterone-containing hormone replacement therapy. Stroke 2017;48(S1):197.

87. Hall SA, Araujo AB, Kupelian V, et al. Testosterone and breast cancer. J Sex Med 2010;7(2 Pt 2):1035–6 [author reply: 1036–7].

88. Dimitrakakis C, Jones RA, Liu A, et al. Breast cancer incidence in postmenopausal women using testosterone in addition to usual hormone therapy. Menopause 2004;11(5):531–5.

89. Davis SR, Wolfe R, Farrugia H, et al. The incidence of invasive breast cancer among women prescribed testosterone for low libido. J Sex Med 2009;6(7):1850–6.

90. Brotto LA, Basson R, Luria M. A mindfulness-based group psychoeducational intervention targeting sexual arousal disorder in women. J Sex Med 2008;5(7):1646–59.

91. Brotto LA, Basson R. Group mindfulness-based therapy significantly improves sexual desire in women. Behav Res Ther 2014;57:43–54.

92. Hucker A, McCabe MP. An online, mindfulness-based, cognitive-behavioral therapy for female sexual difficulties: impact on relationship functioning. J Sex Marital Ther 2014;40(6):561–76.

93. Silverstein RG, Brown AC, Roth HD, et al. Effects of mindfulness training on body awareness to sexual stimuli: implications for female sexual dysfunction. Psychosom Med 2011;73(9):817–25.

94. Brotto LA, Chivers ML, Millman RD, et al. Mindfulness-based sex therapy improves genital-subjective arousal concordance in women with sexual desire/arousal difficulties. Arch Sex Behav 2016;45(8):1907–21.

95. Nappi RE, Palacios S, Panay N, et al. Vulvar and vaginal atrophy in four European countries: evidence from the European REVIVE Survey. Climacteric 2016;19(2):188–97.

96. Palma F, Volpe A, Villa P, et al. Vaginal atrophy of women in postmenopause. Results from a multicentric observational study: the AGATA study. Maturitas 2016;83:40–4.

97. Kingsberg SA, Krychman M, Graham S, et al. The women's EMPOWER survey: identifying women's perceptions on vulvar and vaginal atrophy and its treatment. J Sex Med 2017;14(3):413–24.

98. Kingsberg SA, Wysocki S, Magnus L, et al. Vulvar and vaginal atrophy in postmenopausal women: findings from the REVIVE (REal Women's VIews of Treatment Options for Menopausal Vaginal ChangEs) survey. J Sex Med 2013;10(7):1790–9.

99. Constantine G, Graham S, Portman DJ, et al. Female sexual function improved with ospemifene in postmenopausal women with vulvar and vaginal atrophy: results of a randomized, placebo-controlled trial. Climacteric 2015;18(2):226–32.

100. Portman D, Palacios S, Nappi RE, et al. Ospemifene, a non-oestrogen selective oestrogen receptor modulator for the treatment of vaginal dryness associated with postmenopausal vulvar and vaginal atrophy: a randomised, placebo-controlled, phase III trial. Maturitas 2014;78(2):91–8.

101. Simon JA, Lin VH, Radovich C, et al. One-year long-term safety extension study of ospemifene for the treatment of vulvar and vaginal atrophy in postmenopausal women with a uterus. Menopause 2013;20(4):418–27.

102. Simon J, Portman D, Mabey RG Jr. Long-term safety of ospemifene (52-week extension) in the treatment of vulvar and vaginal atrophy in hysterectomized postmenopausal women. Maturitas 2014;77(3):274–81.
103. Labrie F, Archer DF, Koltun W, et al. Efficacy of intravaginal dehydroepiandrosterone (DHEA) on moderate to severe dyspareunia and vaginal dryness, symptoms of vulvovaginal atrophy, and of the genitourinary syndrome of menopause. Menopause 2016;23(3):243–56.
104. Kingsberg SA, Kroll R, Goldstein I, et al. Patient acceptability and satisfaction with a low-dose solubilized vaginal estradiol softgel capsule, TX-004HR. Menopause 2017;24(8):894–9.
105. Kingsberg SA, Derogatis L, Simon JA, et al. TX-004HR improves sexual function as measured by the female sexual function index in postmenopausal women with vulvar and vaginal atrophy: the REJOICE trial. J Sex Med 2016;13(12): 1930–7.
106. Perino A, Calligaro A, Forlani F, et al. Vulvo-vaginal atrophy: a new treatment modality using thermo-ablative fractional CO2 laser. Maturitas 2015;80(3):296–301.
107. Salvatore S, Nappi RE, Parma M, et al. Sexual function after fractional microablative CO(2) laser in women with vulvovaginal atrophy. Climacteric 2015; 18(2):219–25.
108. Lewis RW, Fugl-Meyer KS, Bosch R, et al. Epidemiology/risk factors of sexual dysfunction. J Sex Med 2004;1(1):35–9.
109. Enzlin P, Mathieu C, Van den Bruel A, et al. Sexual dysfunction in women with type 1 diabetes: a controlled study. Diabetes Care 2002;25(4):672–7.
110. Rees PM, Fowler CJ, Maas CP. Sexual function in men and women with neurological disorders. Lancet 2007;369(9560):512–25.
111. Peugh J, Belenko S. Alcohol, drugs and sexual function: a review. J Psychoactive Drugs 2001;33(3):223–32.
112. Mishra G, Kuh D. Sexual functioning throughout menopause: the perceptions of women in a British cohort. Menopause 2006;13(6):880–90.
113. Falk SJ, Dizon DS. Sexual dysfunction in women with cancer. Fertil Steril 2013; 100(4):916–21.
114. Gilbert E, Ussher JM, Perz J. Sexuality after breast cancer: a review. Maturitas 2010;66(4):397–407.
115. Jensen PT, Groenvold M, Klee MC, et al. Longitudinal study of sexual function and vaginal changes after radiotherapy for cervical cancer. Int J Radiat Oncol Biol Phys 2003;56(4):937–49.
116. Thakar R, Manyonda I, Stanton SL, et al. Bladder, bowel and sexual function after hysterectomy for benign conditions. Br J Obstet Gynaecol 1997;104(9): 983–7.
117. Carlson KJ. Outcomes of hysterectomy. Clin Obstet Gynecol 1997;40(4): 939–46.
118. Strippoli GF, Vecchio M, Palmer S, et al. Sexual dysfunction in women with ESRD requiring hemodialysis. Clin J Am Soc Nephrol 2012;7(6):974–81.
119. Palmer BF. Sexual dysfunction in men and women with chronic kidney disease and end-stage kidney disease. Adv Ren Replace Ther 2003;10(1):48–60.
120. Salonia A, Zanni G, Nappi RE, et al. Sexual dysfunction is common in women with lower urinary tract symptoms and urinary incontinence: results of a cross-sectional study. Eur Urol 2004;45(5):642–8 [discussion: 648].
121. Handa VL, Harvey L, Cundiff GW, et al. Sexual function among women with urinary incontinence and pelvic organ prolapse. Am J Obstet Gynecol 2004; 191(3):751–6.

122. Kennedy SH, Eisfeld BS, Dickens SE, et al. Antidepressant-induced sexual dysfunction during treatment with moclobemide, paroxetine, sertraline, and venlafaxine. J Clin Psychiatry 2000;61(4):276–81.

123. Coleman CC, King BR, Bolden-Watson C, et al. A placebo-controlled comparison of the effects on sexual functioning of bupropion sustained release and fluoxetine. Clin Ther 2001;23(7):1040–58.

124. Baumgart J, Nilsson K, Evers AS, et al. Sexual dysfunction in women on adjuvant endocrine therapy after breast cancer. Menopause 2013;20(2):162–8.

125. Mok K, Juraskova I, Friedlander M. The impact of aromatase inhibitors on sexual functioning: current knowledge and future research directions. Breast 2008; 17(5):436–40.

126. Gershenson DM, Miller AM, Champion VL, et al. Reproductive and sexual function after platinum-based chemotherapy in long-term ovarian germ cell tumor survivors: a Gynecologic Oncology Group Study. J Clin Oncol 2007;25(19): 2792–7.

127. Fogari R, Preti P, Zoppi A, et al. Effect of valsartan and atenolol on sexual behavior in hypertensive postmenopausal women. Am J Hypertens 2004; 17(1):77–81.

128. Newman LC, Broner SW, Lay CL. Reversible anorgasmia with topiramate therapy for migraine. Neurology 2005;65(8):1333–4.

129. Morrell MJ, Flynn KL, Done S, et al. Sexual dysfunction, sex steroid hormone abnormalities, and depression in women with epilepsy treated with antiepileptic drugs. Epilepsy Behav 2005;6(3):360–5.

130. Lydiard RB, Howell EF, Laraia MT, et al. Sexual side effects of alprazolam. Am J Psychiatry 1987;144(2):254–5.

131. Ghadirian AM, Annable L, Belanger MC. Lithium, benzodiazepines, and sexual function in bipolar patients. Am J Psychiatry 1992;149(6):801–5.

Physical Activity and Physical Function

Moving and Aging

Sheila A. Dugan, MD[a,b,*], Kelley Pettee Gabriel, MS, PhD[c,d],
Brittney S. Lange-Maia, MPH, PhD[b,e],
Carrie Karvonen-Gutierrez, MPH, PhD[f]

KEYWORDS

- Physical activity • Physical functioning • Midlife women • Aging

KEY POINTS

- Midlife women do not meet guidelines for physical activity participation for a variety of reasons, missing out on the proven physical and mental health benefits.
- Evidence suggests that the disablement process begins in midlife when women have multiple decades to live.
- Recent studies link physical activity to reduced declines in physical functioning in midlife women.

Continued

Disclosure Statement: The authors have no commercial or financial conflicts of interest to disclose.

Funding: The Study of Women's Health Across the Nation (SWAN) has grant support from the National Institutes of Health (NIH), DHHS, through the National Institute on Aging (NIA), the National Institute of Nursing Research (NINR), and the NIH Office of Research on Women's Health (ORWH) (Grants U01NR004061, U01AG012505, U01AG012535, U01AG012531, U01AG012539, U01AG012546, U01AG012553, U01AG012554, U01AG012495). The content of this article is solely the responsibility of the authors and does not necessarily represent the official views of the NIA, NINR, ORWH or the NIH.

[a] Department of Physical Medicine and Rehabilitation, Rush University Medical Center, 1725 W. Harrison Street, Suite 885, Chicago, IL 60612, USA; [b] Department of Preventive Medicine, Rush University Medical Center, 1700 W. Van Buren, Suite 470, Chicago, IL 60612, USA; [c] Department of Epidemiology, Human Genetics, and Environmental Sciences, University of Texas Health Science Center at Houston, School of Public Health, Austin Campus, Michael and Susan Dell Center for Healthy Living, 1616 Guadalupe Street, Suite 6.300, Austin, TX 78701, USA; [d] Department of Women's Health, The University of Texas at Austin, Dell Medical School, Medical Park Tower, 1301 W. 38th Street, Suite 705, Austin, TX 78705, USA; [e] Rush University Medical Center, Center for Community Health Equity, 600 S. Paulina Street, Suite 480, AAC, Chicago, IL 60612, USA; [f] Department of Epidemiology, University of Michigan, School of Public Health, 1415 Washington Heights, Room 6618, Ann Arbor, MI 48109-2029, USA
* Corresponding author. Rush University Medical Center, 1725 W. Harrison Street, Suite 855, Chicago, IL 60612.
E-mail address: Sheila_dugan@rush.edu

Obstet Gynecol Clin N Am 45 (2018) 723–736
https://doi.org/10.1016/j.ogc.2018.07.009
0889-8545/18/© 2018 Elsevier Inc. All rights reserved.

Continued

- Providing messages about the benefits of moving may shift the needle on participation, changing the trajectory not only for disablement but also for chronic disease.
- Future work should expand on exploring the role of reproductive aging beyond solely chronologic aging in midlife.

INTRODUCTION

Regular participation in physical activity (PA) has many health benefits, perhaps none more important to midlife women than combating the decline in physical functioning (PF) accompanying aging. This article reviews the existing literature relevant to PA and PF, including definitions, measurement approaches, and descriptive and intervention studies, drawing on findings from the Study of Women's Health Across the Nation (SWAN) and other relevant studies. Evidence supports the conclusion that the physical disablement process starts earlier than previously thought, with many limitations beginning in midlife rather than old age, when women still have many years to live. Understanding that restrictions in PF begin in the midlife for women is a strong argument for changing one's behavior to include regular PA.

PHYSICAL ACTIVITY

PA is defined as a behavior that involves human movement, resulting in physiologic attributes including increased energy expenditure and improved physical fitness.[1] Evidence gleaned from several decades of exercise training and public health studies has demonstrated the benefit of PA on a wide range of health outcomes in adults.[2] Nevertheless, despite the well-established benefits, most midlife women (defined as ages 45–64 years) are not sufficiently physically active to meet *2008 Physical Activity Guidelines for Americans* (henceforth *Guidelines*).[2] Current aerobic *Guidelines* encourage adults to engage in at least 150 minutes per week of moderate intensity (activity types between 3 and 6 metabolic equivalent of task [METs], such as a brisk walk), or at least 75 minutes per week of vigorous intensity (activity types $\geq$6 METs, such as jogging), or an equivalent combination of moderate to vigorous intensity PA. In addition, all adults should incorporate moderate- or high-intensity muscle strengthening activities that involve all major muscle groups on 2 or more days of the week. The *Guidelines* also encourage adults to avoid inactivity and directly state that some PA is better than none. Finally, *Guideline* targets for aerobic and muscle strengthening activities have no specific requirements for the following:

1. Activity mode or type,
2. Minimum duration per session, or
3. Frequency of sessions per week.

This flexibility in the behavioral targets included in the *Guidelines* may particularly resonate with women who aspire to become more physically active.

Public health surveillance data are particularly useful for monitoring trends in PA behaviors, including examining differences in prevalence estimates by various population subgroups. The prevalence estimates can provide important information on which groups of US adults are in greatest need of targeted health promotion efforts. Based on 2015 Behavioral Risk Factor Surveillance System (BRFSS) data,[3] 31.1% (standard error [SE] $\pm$ 0.47) of women aged 45 to 54 years met aerobic *Guidelines* only, 7.0%

(SE ± 0.25) met muscle strengthening *Guidelines* only, and just 17.4% (SE ± 0.37) met both aerobic and muscle strengthening *Guidelines.* Strikingly, 44.4% (SE ± 0.50) of women aged 45 to 54 years did not meet *Guidelines* for either aerobic or muscle strengthening, which is a higher proportion than similarly aged men (41.2% [SE ± 0.55]). Among older midlife women (ages 55–64 years), the prevalence estimates for meeting *Guidelines* were similar. More specifically, 33.8% (SE ± 0.44), 6.4% (SE ± 0.22), and 15.9% (SE ± 0.31) met aerobic guidelines only, muscle-strengthening guidelines only, or met both guidelines, respectively. The prevalence of women aged 55 to 64 years that did not meet *Guidelines* for either the aerobic or muscle strengthening was slightly lower than women aged 45 to 54 years (43.8% [SE ± 0.46]). Nevertheless, similar to younger midlife women, this was a slightly higher proportion compared with similarly aged men (41.3% [SE ± 0.51]) (**Fig. 1**).

In the National Health and Nutrition Examination Survey (NHANES), PA levels of a US representative sample were also directly measured via accelerometers.[4] Because behavioral targets included in the *Guidelines* were established with a body of literature that primarily used participant reported measures, there is some controversy among PA experts about operationalizing accelerometer-derived data using the same intensity-based dose thresholds. Nonetheless, prevalence estimates for meeting *Guidelines* are strikingly lower with accelerometers, compared with those based on self-report. Using the most current, publically available accelerometer data from the NHANES 2003 to 2006, 26.7% (SE ± 2.4) and 18.0% (SE ± 2.6) of midlife women, aged 45 to 54 and 55 to 64 years, respectively, met aerobic *Guidelines* (see **Fig. 1**).

Nevertheless, data from surveillance systems only provide a snapshot view or point prevalence estimates reflecting meeting or not meeting *Guidelines*. Furthermore, estimates generalize the entire subpopulation, with no acknowledgment that there may be different levels of PA within a defined population, and individual-level change in PA with trigger points that correspond to certain life

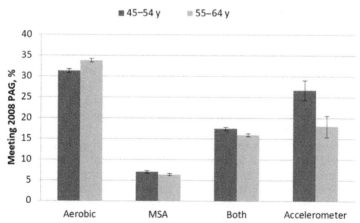

Fig. 1. Prevalence of meeting 2008 Physical Activity Guidelines (PAG) for midlife American women (aged 45–54 years and 55–64 years) based on self-reported data from the 2015 Behavioral Risk Factor Surveillance System (ie, aerobic guidelines, muscle strengthening [MSA] guidelines, and both aerobic and muscle strengthening guidelines) and accelerometer data from 2003 to 2006 NHANES. (*Data from* Centers for Disease Control and Prevention (CDC). 2015 Behavioral risk factor surveillance system. Available at: https://www.cdc.gov/brfss/annual_data/annual_2015.html. Accessed November 10, 2017; and Centers for Disease Control and Prevention (CDC). National Health and Nutrition Examination Survey. Available at: https://wwwn.cdc.gov/nchs/nhanes/Default.aspx. Accessed November 10, 2017.)

events that characterize various adult life-course transitions. In women, major life events that coincide with midlife that could potentially increase PA levels include change in employment status or family structure.[5,6] Nevertheless, these events may not always lead to increased PA. A woman may opt to engage in more sedentary pursuits to fill the added discretionary hours of the day due to retirement or may have reduced PA due to changes in health status. However, for some, a recent diagnosis may serve as a prompt for behavioral modification (eg, joining a fitness club) to manage symptoms or progression of disease or disability. Finally, other life events that are not necessarily rooted in midlife may also result in positive or negative changes to PA behaviors. These events include changes in relationship status or changes in residence.

The availability of longitudinal data from cohort studies provides the necessary evidence to characterize patterns of PA change during a period of life, rather than during a single point in time. Although the availability of prospective cohort studies focused on midlife women's health is limited, the Australian Longitudinal Study on Women's Health (ALSWH) and the US-based SWAN are 2 examples of studies that are poised to make significant contributions to improve the understanding of the patterns of PA change across the life course.

The ALSWH is an ongoing longitudinal survey of more than 58,000 women recruited in 1996 and enrolled as part of 3 age cohorts, including 18 to 23, 45 to 50, or 70 to 75 years, using a mail-based survey once every 3 years to assess physical and mental health.[7] In a 2009 study by Brown and colleagues,[8] the associations between life events and PA change were examined. Based on reported walking and moderate- and vigorous-intensity PA during leisure (or discretionary) time, 33.4% of the midlife cohort were classified as "active," 15.6% as "low active," and 7.0% as "none," consistently more than 3 years of follow-up, whereas 17.6% moved into a lower PA category (decreasing) and 26.5% moved into a higher category (increasing). Life events associated with higher odds of "increasing" PA in midlife women, after adjustment for area of residence and potential confounders, included retirement, changing conditions at work, major personal achievement, death of a spouse or partner, and decreased income (all $P<.05$). Nevertheless, birth of a grandchild had lower odds of membership in the "increasing" PA group. Conversely, after full adjustment, life events associated with higher odds of "decreasing" PA in midlife women (17.6%) included being pushed, grabbed, or shoved and having a family member being arrested or jailed (both $P<.05$). Women reporting infidelity of their spouse/partner or a major personal achievement had lower odds of being classified in the "decreasing" PA group (both $P<.05$).

Established at a similar time as the ALSWH, the SWAN study included 3302 midlife women aged 42 to 52 years who were recruited and enrolled between 1996 and 1997 into one of 7 clinical sites across the United States.[9] The primary objective of SWAN is to evaluate the impact of reproductive aging on the health outcomes of women during midlife. In SWAN, reported PA data (ie, moderate- and vigorous-intensity activity during leisure time) were collected from baseline through the most recent visit in 2015/16. Using latent class growth modeling[10] to examine patterns of PA change, 5 major patterns of PA emerged from SWAN data, including maintain low (26.2%), increasing (13.4%), decreasing (22.4%), maintain middle or moderate (23.9%), and maintain high (14.1%) PA.[11] Hispanic and black women were more likely to be in the maintain low PA group, and white women were least likely. Other characteristics associated with the maintain low PA group include income <$35,000, single/never married, fair/poor overall health status, obesity, current cigarette smoker, severe/very severe bodily pain, reported physical difficulties, and osteoarthritis (all $P<.01$).

Adherence to Physical Activity Guidelines in Midlife

Because midlife women are not adhering to recommended PA guidelines, there is room for improvement when it comes to health promotion messaging. One strategy is to link more immediate health benefits when one establishes a new PA routine, including favorable relationships to body composition, sleep, pain, and PF. More distal outcomes like chronic disease reduction and changing the trajectory of physical and cognitive functioning decline may also be more relevant when viewed through the lens of midlife but may be perceived as an insufficient or delayed consequence given midlife women's lack of discretionary hours.

Vasomotor Symptoms and Physical Activity

Although PA is recommended to address vasomotor symptoms of menopause, the impact on menopausal symptoms is not conclusive. A review by Pettee Gabriel and colleagues[12] presents the evidence on the relationship between PA and vasomotor symptoms of menopause, primarily hot flashes and night sweats. Although evidence from several cross-sectional studies reported a significant association between PA (measured by self-report and accelerometry) and self-reported vasomotor symptoms, more recent prospective cohort studies showed variable results.[13–15] Randomized controlled trials, including MsFlash, show no association between PA, including both yoga and aerobic exercise, and vasomotor symptoms.[16,17] Daley and colleagues[18] in the 2014 Cochrane Report conclude there was insufficient evidence to demonstrate that PA is effective in managing vasomotor symptoms. The review noted variability among the observational studies with smaller studies reporting negative or no associations and larger studies reporting positive associations.

Sleep and Physical Activity

Given the prevalence of sleep disturbance in midlife,[19] informing menopausal women about the conclusive evidence linking PA to improved sleep quality may be an effective behavior change message. The Dose-response to Exercise in postmenopausal Women Study found significant improvements in sleep quality in women randomized to all 3 exercise groups compared with the control group with a dose-response effect.[20] In the MsFlash trial, exercise group participants had greater subjective sleep quality and reduced insomnia, but differences were small and no longer statistically significant in adjusted analyses.[17]

Body Composition and Physical Activity

More positively, multiple studies support an inverse association between PA and weight gain. In the Biobehavioral Health in Diverse Midlife Women Study, women in the *increase in PA* group had significantly less weight and waist circumference gain than those in the *decrease PA* group.[21] An increase in leisure time PA, including walking and cycling over 6 years, was inversely associated with weight gain in the Nurses' Health Study II.[22] In the Women's Health Initiative, in women aged 50 to 59, the moderate PA group had significant weight loss compared with the sedentary group, whereas women in the 70 to 79 age group with higher PA showed attenuation of the expected age-related weight loss from sarcopenia and loss of lean body mass.[23]

Mental Health and Physical Activity

In addition, PA has an inverse relationship with adverse psychological symptoms, including depression and anxiety. The Pettee Gabriel and colleagues[12] review noted that a significant positive impact of PA on psychological symptoms was consistently observed across most studies. In SWAN, participants meeting guidelines for moderate intensity exercise had lower odds of clinically significant depressive symptoms, and the finding persisted over 10 years.[24] Karacan[25] reported positive benefits with reduced depressive mood, irritability, anxiety, and exhaustion after 3 and 6 months of an intervention that included an aerobic exercise program. In a randomized controlled intervention of Finnish women, psychological symptoms were collected twice daily using a mobile phone.[26] The prevalence of mood swings, but not irritability or depressive moods, was reduced preintervention -to postintervention.

Physical Activity and Physical Functioning

A key message to midlife women is the role of regular PA on PF. In the longitudinal SWAN analyses of PA trajectories, the participants that maintained high or moderate PA demonstrated significantly better PF than those who maintained low PA.[11] In a previous longitudinal SWAN analysis, higher baseline PA was independently associated with a 7% higher likelihood of high short form-36 (SF-36) physical role functioning and 10% greater likelihood of low SF-36 bodily pain scores.[27] The association between PA and physical role functioning was mediated by level of pain. Women may be motivated by pain to seek medical care, providing a teachable moment to talk about the association between PA and PF.

PHYSICAL FUNCTIONING

PF is assessed in a variety of ways, including self-reported and objective, performance-based measures, although the common goal is to measure the degree that one is able to complete tasks related to independent living or tasks that impact quality of life.[28] Self-reported measures of PF are an assessment of an individual's *perception* of limitations in functioning given the context of their own environment.[29] Objective measures of PF, such as grip strength or gait speed measures, are less vulnerable to the impact of individual-level factors. As such, self-reported and performance-based assessments of PF measure distinct, yet related domains.[30,31]

PF has long been studied in geriatric populations, with functional limitations being highly predictive of future poor outcomes, including disability, hospitalizations, nursing home admission, and mortality.[32,33] Although impairments in PF are most prevalent at older ages, the midlife period is an important life stage with respect to the *onset* of poor functioning, although risk factors for impairments can accumulate across the lifespan. Findings from an analysis conducted from 2000 to 2008 using data from 5 national US surveys, including NHANES, the National Health Interview Survey (NHIS), the Health and Retirement Study, the Medicare Current Beneficiary Survey, and the National Long Term Care Survey, suggest that the prevalence of limitations in activities of daily living (ADLs) is quite stable among older adults, and even slightly decreasing among those age 85+ years, but that the burden is increasing for midlife adults.[34] In NHIS, the number of 50- to 64-year-old individuals reporting difficulty with mobility tasks increased by approximately 10% from the 1997 to 1999 data collection cycle versus the 2005 to 2007 cycle.[35] Similarly, among 40 to 64 year olds in NHIS, the odds of reporting PF limitations or limitations in ADLs increased by 0.9% annually, and the increases were independent of increases in obesity.[36]

Those who have impairments at midlife have a high likelihood of developing further impairments or death within 10 years; however, regaining function and maintaining independence is also common.[37] SWAN has been instrumental in illustrating the prevalence of impairments during this life stage, and importantly describing the development of functional limitations during the menopause transition. At age 40 to 55,

81% of women in the SWAN cross-sectional study (N = 14,427) reported having no PF limitations; however, 10% reported some limitations, and an additional 9% reported substantial limitations.[38] These estimates were in line with those in the NHIS from a similar timeframe (midlife during the mid-1990s) that indicated that 15% of persons aged 45 to 64 reported having some functional limitations[39] and from a British cohort of adults aged 43 to 53 years in which 28% of participants had difficulty walking or stair climbing.[40] By the fourth SWAN visit when the cohort was between the ages of 45 and 57 years, 11% reported substantial limitations and approximately 30% reported moderate limitations.[41] At age 56 to 66 (SWAN visit 12), nearly 50% of women reported having at least some limitations.[42] The high prevalence of self-reported limitations during midlife was substantiated by findings from performance-based PF obtained from the Southeast Michigan cohort. Thirty-one percent of women from this cohort (includes 366 women from the Michigan SWAN site and 514 women the Michigan Bone Health and Metabolism Study, which followed the same protocol, mean age 47 years) walked at gait speeds below federal standards set for safely crossing pedestrian intersections (<1.22 m/s), and an additional 12% walked at speeds indicative of frailty in older adults (<1 m/s).[43]

In the United States, women have a longer life expectancy compared with men, but often live longer with disability.[44] Women have poorer levels of PF compared with men[45,46] and experience a more rapid decline in functioning.[47,48] Although the prevalence of PF limitations are positively correlated with age in both men and women, the emergence of declines in functioning often coincide with the timing of the menopausal transition.[49] Although poorer PF among perimenopausal as compared with premenopausal women can be attributed to health conditions and menopause-related symptoms,[50] the menopause-associated differences among late perimenopausal and postmenopausal women are largely independent of age and other health factors.[41,49] In SWAN, postmenopausal women and those with surgical menopause were 3 times more likely to report severe limitations in PF as compared with premenopausal women.[51] Postmenopausal and surgically menopausal women also have poorer performance-based PF and more rapid declines in functioning as compared with premenopausal or perimenopausal women.[51] Thus, reproductive aging and the associated hormonal and metabolic changes characteristic of the menopausal transition may play a role in this process, independent of chronologic aging.

Reproductive Aging and Physical Functioning

Work from SWAN demonstrated that greater reductions in estradiol and testosterone during this time were significantly associated with greater risk of PF limitations.[52] Furthermore, loss of muscle strength during menopause[48,53–55] has been associated with the physiologic declines in estradiol.[47,55] In some studies, muscle strength improved following exogenous hormone therapy.[47,56,57] In SWAN, women with poorer PF were more less likely to initiate use of hormone therapy, and the initiation of hormone therapy was associated with poorer subsequent PF.[58]

Body Composition Changes During Midlife and Physical Functioning

Although overall weight gain is primarily a product of chronologic aging, changes in body composition, or the relative proportion of fat mass to lean mass, is a function of both chronologic and reproductive aging.[59] Marked changes in body composition occur during the menopausal transition,[60] and greater fat mass and less skeletal muscle mass are associated with poorer performance-based PF measures, including gait speed and stair climb.[43] Furthermore, in longitudinal analyses, loss of lean mass across the midlife is predictive of slower gait speed and less leg strength.[61]

Inflammation Changes During Midlife and Physical Functioning

Women experience an exacerbated inflammatory response and alterations in homeostasis due to decreased levels of estrogen and the redistribution of adipose tissue that occurs during the menopausal transition.[62–64] In an SWAN analysis of black and white women, higher concentrations of C-reactive protein (CRP) and fibrinogen were associated with poorer self-reported PF.[65] In longitudinal analyses, higher concentrations of the proinflammatory biomarker CRP and hemostatic markers plasminogen activator inhibitor-1, tissue plasminogen activator-antigen, and Factor VIIc predicted poorer PF.[66]

One potential mechanism linking changes in body composition and inflammatory changes with PF may be the endocrine activity of adipose tissue through the secretion of adipokines, including leptin and adiponectin. Concentrations of the proinflammatory adipokines leptin and adiponectin are positively correlated with insulin resistance, lipid accumulation, and decreased oxidation of fatty acids in skeletal muscle.[67,68] In a longitudinal analysis of black and white SWAN women, higher baseline concentrations of leptin predicted poorer performance-based measures of PF mobility, including stair climb, sit-to-rise, 2-pound lift, and forward reach, but leptin was not associated with strength measures,[69] findings that persisted after adjustment for CRP. In the same analysis, baseline concentrations of adiponectin predicted quadriceps muscle strength but were not associated with any mobility-based measures of PF.

Midlife Mental and Physical Health and Physical Functioning

Approximately one-quarter of midlife women experience depressive symptoms.[70,71] In analyses of black and white women, higher scores (ie, more depressive symptoms) on the Center for Epidemiologic Studies-Depression scale were significantly associated with poorer performance-based PF, including sit-to-stand times and timed walk.[72] Furthermore, women who had incident depressive symptoms during follow-up experienced subsequent declines in performance-based PF, including 2-pound lift and stair climb times.

In terms of physical health conditions, a high prevalence of both peripheral nerve impairment and knee osteoarthritis has been reported among midlife women. Among black and white SWAN women from the Michigan site, the prevalence of peripheral nerve impairment was 14% to 19%.[73] In that same sample, the prevalence of moderate to severe radiographic knee osteoarthritis was 28%.[74] Women with peripheral nerve impairment had poorer PF performance, including stair climb and sit-to-stand.[75] Furthermore, age-related declines in stair climb time were twice as rapid for women with as compared with women without peripheral nerve impairment. Similarly, the presence of moderate to severe knee osteoarthritis was associated with 20% to 35% poorer performance in PF, including the timed walk and stair climb times.[76] Associations between mental and physical health measures and PF are likely bidirectional, as maintenance of PA and ability to continue functioning may be protective to long-term health outcomes.

Midlife Sociodemographic Factors and Physical Functioning

In addition to an understanding of psychological and physiologic predictors of poor PF, examination of sociodemographic and lifestyle correlates of functioning impairments is needed to help identify appropriate interventions to support healthy aging and prevent functioning impairments. One of the most notable sociodemographic measures associated with differences in PF is race/ethnicity. In SWAN, black women were more likely to report substantial PF limitations in cross-sectional analyses,[38] whereas Chinese and Japanese women had the greatest declines in PF over time.[42]

Modifiable lifestyle factors have been shown to be predictive of better midlife PF. In SWAN, better diet quality was associated with less PF limitations.[77] Greater intake of cholesterol, fat, or saturated fat was associated with 40% to 60% greater odds of having substantial PF limitations, and lower fruit, vegetable, and fiber intakes were inversely associated with self-reported PF. In SWAN, a healthy lifestyle score based on self-reported measures of smoking, PA, and diet was predictive of better PF, including faster timed walk and shorter chair stand times.[78] When considering each measure individually, the association between healthy lifestyle and PF was largely driven by PA.

Measures of PF are important as markers of healthy aging and are valuable to the understanding of future poor health outcomes. Poorer PF is associated with unfavorable cardiometabolic biomarkers[79,80] and worse vascular health indicators.[81] In older women, poor PF may be prognostic for cardiovascular disease.[82] In SWAN, women with poorer self-reported PF were more likely to experience incident metabolic syndrome in the next 10 years.[83]

SUMMARY

Functional limitations become more prevalent with age, but PF is a dynamic aspect of health, and recovery from limitations is possible.[37] PA interventions have been successful for preventing major mobility disability in older adults[84] and may be promising for maintaining function at younger ages. Arguably, interventions are needed to help women maintain functional status through midlife and into older ages. The rich longitudinal information in SWAN will continue to allow researchers to further investigate predictors at midlife that influence health well into old age. In addition, as the complete cohort reaches postmenopausal status, researchers can better define the role of reproductive aging on PA and PF.

ACKNOWLEDGMENTS

The authors would like to thank Allen M. Hallet, MS for computing the physical activity BRFSS (based on self-report) prevalence estimates and Eun Me Cha, MPH for computing the physical activity NHANES (based on accelerometry) prevalence estimates.

REFERENCES

1. Pettee Gabriel KK, Morrow JR Jr, Woolsey AL. Framework for physical activity as a complex and multidimensional behavior. J Phys Act Health 2012;9(Suppl 1): S11–8.
2. U.S. Department of Health and Human Services. 2008 Physical Activity Guidelines for Americans. Available at: www.health.gov/paguidelines. Accessed November 10, 2017.
3. CDC 2015 Behavioral Risk Factor Surveillance System. Available at: https://www.cdc.gov/brfss/annual_data/annual_data.html. Accessed November 10, 2017.
4. CDC National Health and Nutrition Examination Survey. Available at: http://www.cdc.gov/nchs/nhanes/nhanes_questionnaires.html. Accessed November 10, 2017.
5. Allender S, Hutchinson L, Foster C. Life-change events and participation in physical activity: a systematic review. Health Promot Int 2008;23(2):160–72.

6. Corder K, Ogilvie D, van Sluijs EM. Invited commentary: physical activity over the life course–whose behavior changes, when, and why? Am J Epidemiol 2009; 170(9):1078–81 [discussion: 1082–3].

7. Australian Longitudinal Study on Women's Health. Available at: http://ALSWH. org/. Accessed November 10, 2017.

8. Brown WJ, Heesch KC, Miller YD. Life events and changing physical activity patterns in women at different life stages. Ann Behav Med 2009;37(3):294–305.

9. Sowers MF, Crawford SL, Sternfeld B, et al. SWAN: a multicenter, multiethnic, community-based cohort study of women and the menopausal transition. In: Lobo R, Marcus R, Kelsey J, editors. Menopause: biology and pathobiology. San Diego (CA): Academic Press; 2000. p. 175–88.

10. Andruff H, Carraro N, Thompson A, et al. Latent class growth modelling: a tutorial. Tutor Quant Methods Psychol 2009;5(1):11–24.

11. Pettee Gabriel K, Sternfeld B, Colvin A, et al. Physical activity trajectories during midlife and subsequent risk of physical functioning decline in late mid-life: the Study of Women's Health Across the Nation (SWAN). Prev Med 2017;105: 287–94.

12. Pettee Gabriel K, Mason JM, Sternfeld B. Recent evidence exploring the association between physical activity and menopausal symptoms in midlife women: perceived risks and possible health benefits. Womens Midlife Health 2015;105: 1–28.

13. Gibson C, Matthews K, Thurston R. Daily physical activity and hot flashes in the Study of Women's Health Across the Nation (SWAN) flashes study. Fertil Steril 2014;101(4):1110–6.

14. Gjelsvik B, Rosvold EO, Straand J, et al. Symptom prevalence during menopause and factors associated with symptoms and menopausal age. Results from the Norwegian Hordaland Women's Cohort study. Maturitas 2011;70(4):383–90.

15. de Azevedo Guimaraes AC, Baptista F. Influence of habitual physical activity on the symptoms of climacterium/menopause and the quality of life of middle-aged women. Int J Womens Health 2011;3:319–28.

16. Newton KM, Reed SD, Guthrie KA, et al. Efficacy of yoga for vasomotor symptoms: a randomized controlled trial. Menopause 2014;21(4):339–46.

17. Sternfeld B, Guthrie KA, Ensrud KE, et al. Efficacy of exercise for menopausal symptoms: a randomized controlled trial. Menopause 2014;21(4):330–8.

18. Daley A, Stokes-Lampard H, Thomas A, et al. Exercise for vasomotor menopausal symptoms. Cochrane Database Syst Rev 2014;(11).

19. National Institutes of Health. National Institutes of Health State-of-the-Science Conference statement: management of menopause-related symptoms. Ann Intern Med 2005;142(12 Pt 1):1003–13.

20. Kline CE, Sui X, Hall MH, et al. Dose–response effects of exercise training on the subjective sleep quality of postmenopausal women: exploratory analyses of a randomised controlled trial. BMJ Open 2012;2(4):e001044.

21. Choi J, Guiterrez Y, Gilliss C, et al. Physical activity, weight, and waist circumference in midlife women. Health Care Women Int 2012;33(12):1086–95.

22. Lusk AC, Mekary RA, Feskanich D, et al. Bicycle riding, walking, and weight gain in premenopausal women. Arch Intern Med 2010;170(12):1050–6.

23. Sims ST, Larson JC, Lamonte MJ, et al. Physical activity and body mass: changes in younger versus older postmenopausal women. Med Sci Sports Exerc 2012; 44(1):89–97.

24. Dugan SA, Bromberger JT, Segawa E, et al. Association between physical activity and depressive symptoms: midlife women in SWAN. Med Sci Sports Exerc 2015; 47(2):335–42.

25. Karacan S. Effects of a long-term aerobic exercise on physical fitness and post-menopausal symptoms with menopausal rating scale. Sci Sports 2010;25(1): 39–46.

26. Moilanen JM, Mikkola TS, Raitanen JA, et al. Effect of aerobic training on meno-pausal symptoms–a randomized controlled trial. Menopause 2012;19(6):691–6.

27. Dugan SA, Everson-Rose SA, Karavolos K, et al. The impact of physical activity level on SF-36 role-physical and bodily pain indices in midlife women. J Phys Act Health 2009;6:33–42.

28. Painter P, Stewart AL, Caery S. Physical functioning: definitions, measurement and expectations. Adv Ren Replace Ther 1999;6(2):110–23.

29. Tomey KM, Sowers MR. Assessment of physical functioning: a conceptual model encompassing environmental factors and individual compensation strategies. Phys Ther 2009;89(7):705–14.

30. Wittink H, Rogers W, Sukiennik A, et al. Physical functioning: self-report and per-formance measures are related but distinct. Spine (Phila Pa 1976) 2003;28(20): 2407–13.

31. Bean JF, Olveczky DD, Kiely DK, et al. Performance-based versus patient-reported physical function: what are the underlying predictors? Phys Ther 2011;91(12):1804–11.

32. Guralnik JM, Simonsick EM, Ferrucci L, et al. A short physical performance bat-tery assessing lower extremity function: association with self-reported disability and prediction of mortality and nursing home admission. J Gerontol 1994; 49(2):M85.

33. Pennix BW, Ferrucci L, Leveille SG, et al. Lower extremity performance in nondis-abled older persons as a predictor of subsequent hospitalization. J Gerontol A Biol Sci Med Sci 2000;55(11):M691–7.

34. Freedman VA, Spillman BC, Andreski PM, et al. Trends in late life activity limita-tions in the United States: an update from five national surveys. Demography 2013;50(2):661–71.

35. Martin LG, Freedman VA, Schoeni RF, et al. Trends in disability and related chronic conditions among people ages fifty to sixty four. Health Aff (Millwood) 2010;29:725–31.

36. Martin LG, Schoeni RF. Trends in disability and related chronic conditions among the forty-and-over population: 1997-2010. Disabil Health J 2014;7(1 Suppl):S4–14.

37. Brown RT, Diaz-Ramirez LG, Boscardin WJ, et al. Functional impairment and decline in middle age: a cohort study. Ann Intern Med 2017;167(11):761–8.

38. Sowers M, Pope S, Welch G, et al. The association of menopause and physical functioning in women at midlife. J Am Geriatr Soc 2001;49(11):1485–92.

39. Adams PF, Marano MA. Current estimates from the National Health Interview Sur-vey, 1994. Vital Health Stat 10 1995;(193 Pt 1):1–260.

40. Murray ET, Hardy R, Strand BH, et al. Gender and life course occupational social class differences in trajectories of functional and limitations in midlife: findings from the 1946 British birth cohort. J Gerontol A Biol Sci Med Sci 2011;66(12): 1350–9.

41. Tseng LA, El Khoudary SR, Young EA, et al. The association of menopause status with physical function: the Study of Women's Health Across the Nation. Meno-pause 2012;19(11):1186–92.

42. Ylitalo KR, Karvonen-Gutierrez CA, Fitzgerald N, et al. Relationship of race-ethnicity, body mass index, and economic strain with longitudinal self-report of physical functioning: the Study of Women's Health Across the Nation. Ann Epidemiol 2013;23(7):401–8.

43. Sowers M, Jannausch ML, Gross M, et al. Performance-based physical functioning in African-American and Caucasian women at midlife: considering body composition, quadriceps strength, and knee osteoarthritis. Am J Epidemiol 2006;163(10):950–8.

44. Freedman VA, Wolf DA, Spillman BC. Disability-free life expectancy over 30 years: a growing female disadvantage in the US population. Am J Public Health 2016;106(6):1079–85.

45. Danneskiold-Samsoe B, Bartels EM, Bülow PM, et al. Isokinetic and isometric muscle strength in a healthy population with special reference to age and gender. Acta Physiol (Oxf) 2009;197(Suppl 673):1–68.

46. Kuh D, Bassey EJ, Butterworth S, et al, Musculoskeletal Study Team. Grip strength, postural control, and functional leg power in a representative cohort of British men and women: associations with physical activity, health status, and socioeconomic conditions. J Gerontol A Biol Sci Med Sci 2005;60(2):224–31.

47. Phillips SK, Rook KM, Siddle NC, et al. Muscle weakness in women occurs at an earlier age than in men, but strength is preserved by hormone replacement therapy. Clin Sci (Lond) 1993;84(1):95–8.

48. Samson MM, Meeuwsen IB, Crowe A, et al. Relationships between physical performance measures, age, height, and body weight in healthy adults. Age Ageing 2000;29:235–42.

49. Avis NE, Colvin A, Bromberger JT, et al. Change in health-related quality of life over the menopausal transition in a multi-ethnic cohort of middle-aged women: study of Women's Health Across the Nation. Menopause 2009;16(5):860–9.

50. Avis NE, Ory M, Matthews KA, et al. Health-related quality of life in a multiethnic sample of middle aged women: study of Women's Health Across the Nation (SWAN). Med Care 2003;41:1262–76.

51. Sowers M, Tomey K, Jannausch M, et al. Physical functioning and menopause states. Obstet Gynecol 2007;110(6):1290–6.

52. El Khoudary SR, McClure CK, VoPham T, et al. Longitudinal assessment of the menopausal transition, endogenous estradiol, and perception of physical functioning: the Study of Women's Health Across the Nation. J Gerontol A Biol Sci Med Sci 2014;69(8):1011–7.

53. Carville SF, Rutherford OM, Newham DJ. Power output, isometric strength and steadiness in the leg muscles of pre- and postmenopausal women; the effects of hormone replacement therapy. Eur J Appl Physiol 2006;96(3):292–8.

54. Cooper R, Mishra G, Clennell S, et al. Menopausal status and physical performance in midlife: findings from a British birth cohort study. Menopause 2008; 15(6):1079–85.

55. Cauley JA, Gutai JP, Kuller LH, et al. The epidemiology of serum sex hormones in postmenopausal women. Am J Epidemiol 1989;129(6):1120–31.

56. Greeves JP, Cable NT, Reilly T, et al. Changes in muscle strength in women following the menopause: a longitudinal assessment of the efficacy of hormone replacement therapy. Clin Sci (Lond) 1999;97(1):79–84.

57. Skelton DA, Phillips SK, Bruce SA, et al. Hormone replacememt therapy increases isometric muscle strength of adductor pollicis in post-menopausal women. Clin Sci (Lond) 1999;96(4):357–64.

58. Hess R, Colvin A, Avis NE, et al. The impact of hormone therapy on health-related quality of life: longitudinal results from the Study of Women's Health Across the Nation. Menopause 2008;15(3):422–8.

59. Karvonen-Gutierrez C, Kim C. Association of mid-life changes in body size, body composition and obesity status with the menopausal transition. Healthcare (Basel) 2016;4(3) [pii:E42].

60. Sowers M, Zheng H, Tomey K, et al. Changes in body composition in women over six years at mid-life: ovarian and chronological aging. J Clin Endocrinol Metab 2007;92(3):895–901.

61. Sowers MR, Crutchfield M, Richards K, et al. Sarcopenia is related to physical functioning and leg strength in middle-aged women. J Gerontol A Biol Sci Med Sci 2005;60(4):486–90.

62. Gebara OC, Mittleman MA, Sutherland P, et al. Association between increased estrogen status and increased fibrinolytic potential in the Framingham Offspring Study. Circulation 1995;91(7):1952–8.

63. Pfeilschifter J, Köditz R, Pfohl M, et al. Changes in proinflammatory cytokine activity after menopause. Endocr Rev 2002;23(1):90–119.

64. Teede HJ, McGrath BP, Smolich JJ, et al. Postmenopausal hormone replacement therapy increases coagulation activity and fibrinolysis. Arterioscler Thromb Vasc Biol 2000;20(5):1404–9.

65. Tomey K, Sowers M, Zheng H, et al. Physical functioning related to C-reactive protein and fibrinogen levels in mid-life women. Exp Gerontol 2009;44(12):799–804.

66. McClure CK, El Khoudary SR, Karvonen-Gutierrez C. Prospective associations between inflammatory and hemostatic markers and physical functioning limitations in mid-life women: longitudinal results of the Study of Women's Health Across the Nation (SWAN). Exp Gerontol 2014;49:19–25.

67. Dyck DJ, Heigenhauser GJ, Bruce CR. The role of adipokines as regulators of skeletal muscle fatty acid metabolism and insulin sensitivity. Acta Physiol (Oxf) 2006;186(1):5–16.

68. Yang J. Enhanced skeletal muscle for effective glucose homeostasis. Prog Mol Biol Transl Sci 2014;121:133–63.

69. Karvonen-Gutierrez CA, Zheng H, Mancuso P, et al. Higher leptin and adiponectin concentrations predict poorer performance-based physical functioning in midlife women: the Michigan Study of Women's Health Across the Nation. J Gerontol A Biol Sci Med Sci 2016;71(4):508–14.

70. Woods NF, Mitchell ES. Pathways to depressed mood for midlife women: observations from the Seattle Midlife Women's Health Study. Res Nurs Health 1997;20:119–29.

71. Bromberger JT, Kravitz HM, Matthews K, et al. Predictors of first lifetime episodes of major depression in midlife women. Psychol Med 2009;39(1):55–64.

72. Tomey S, Sowers MR, Harlow S, et al. Physical functioning among mid-life women: associations with trajectory of depressive symptoms. Soc Sci Med 2010;71(7):1259–67.

73. Ylitalo KR, Herman WH, Harlow SD. Monofilament insensitivity and small and large nerve fiber symptoms in impaired fasting glucose. Prim Care Diabetes 2013;7(4):309–13.

74. Karvonen-Gutierrez C, Harlow SD, Mancuso P, et al. Association of leptin levels with radiographic knee osteoarthritis among a cohort of midlife women. Arthritis Care Res (Hoboken) 2013;65(6):936–44.

75. Ylitalo KR, Herman WH, Harlow SD. Performance-based physical functioning and peripheral neuropathy in a population-based cohort of mid-life women. Am J Epidemiol 2013;177(8):810–7.

76. Sowers M, Karvonen-Gutierrez CA, Jacobson JA, et al. Associations of anatomical measures from MRI with radiographically defined knee osteoarthritis score, pain, and physical functioning. J Bone Joint Surg Am 2011;93(3):241–51.

77. Tomey S, Sowers MR, Crandall C, et al. Dietary intake related to prevalent functional limitations in midlife women. Am J Epidemiol 2008;167(8):935–43.

78. Sternfeld B, Colvin A, Stewart A, et al. The impact of a healthy lifestyle on future physical functioning in midlife women. Med Sci Sports Exerc 2017;49(2):274–82.

79. Amiri P, Hosseinpanah F, Rambod M, et al. Metabolic syndrome predicts poor health-related quality of life in women but not in men: Tehran Lipid and Glucose Study. J Womens Health (Larchmt) 2010;19(6):1201–7.

80. Sowers M, Karvonen-Gutierrez CA, Palmieri-Smith R, et al. Knee osteoarthritis in obese women with cardiometabolic clustering. Arthritis Rheum 2009;61(10): 1328–36.

81. El Khoudary SR, Chen HY, Barinas-Mitchell E, et al. Simple physical performance measures and vascular health in late midlife women: the Study of Women's Health Across the Nation. Int J Cardiol 2015;182:115–20.

82. Newman AB, Simonsick EM, Naydeck BL, et al. Association of long-distance corridor walk performance with mortality, cardiovascular disease, mobility limitation, and disability. JAMA 2006;295(17):2018–26.

83. Ylitalo KR, Karvonen-Gutierrez C, McClure C, et al. Is self-reported physical functioning associated with incident cardiometabolic abnormalities or the metabolic syndrome? Diabetes Metab Res Rev 2016;32(4):413–20.

84. Pahor M, Guralnik JM, Ambrosius WT, et al. Effect of structured physical activity on prevention of major mobility disability in older adults: the LIFE Study randomized clinical trial. JAMA 2014;311(23):2387–96.

Genitourinary Changes with Aging

Caroline M. Mitchell, MD[a], L. Elaine Waetjen, MD[b],*

KEYWORDS

- Genitourinary syndrome of menopause • Vaginal dryness • Sexual dysfunction
- Urinary symptoms • Vulvar atrophy • Atrophic vaginitis

KEY POINTS

- Both chronologic aging and menopause affect the physical, physiologic, and microbiological characteristics of the genitourinary tract.
- The genitourinary syndrome of menopause is the currently recommended terminology to describe the constellation of genitourinary symptoms and signs associated with menopause.
- Genitourinary symptoms are frequently reported by midlife and older women, but these symptoms do not always correlate well with the signs of genitourinary aging.
- Genitourinary symptoms can have a significant impact on function, quality of life, and relationships, although many women do not seek treatment.

INTRODUCTION

The menopause transition is a critical time in aging of the female genitourinary tract. Circulating estradiol changes from cyclical, higher levels in premenopause to varying levels in perimenopause, to more constant, lower levels in postmenopause. With chronologic aging, factors such as weight gain, loss of muscle mass, immunosenescence, and medical morbidity can lead to functional decline. These co-occuring hormonal and physiologic changes combine with changes in older women's relationships and behaviors to increase the risk of bothersome genitourinary symptoms that significantly impact women's lives.

In this article, the authors detail what is known about the physical, physiologic, and microbiologic changes in the lower genitourinary tract associated with menopause and aging. They also review the 2014 North American Menopause Society's definition

Financial Disclosures: Dr C.M. Mitchell is a consultant for Symbiomix Therapeutics LLC. Dr L.E. Waetjen has no financial conflicts of interest or funding sources to disclose.
[a] Department of Obstetrics, Gynecology & Reproductive Biology, Vincent Center for Reproductive Biology, Massachusetts General Hospital, 55 Fruit Street, Boston, MA 02114, USA;
[b] Department of Obstetrics and Gynecology, University of California, Davis, 4860 Y Street, Suite 2500, Sacramento, CA 95817, USA
* Corresponding author.
E-mail address: lewaetjen@ucdavis.edu

of the Genitourinary Syndrome of Menopause (GSM) and present what is known about the epidemiology and impact of genitourinary aging: vulvovaginal, urinary and sexual symptoms.

GENITOURINARY CHANGES ASSOCIATED WITH AGING AND MENOPAUSE
The Vagina

The stratified squamous vaginal epithelium is estrogen responsive, layered over the immune-cell rich lamina propria,[1] and surrounded by layers of smooth muscle, collagen, and elastin.[2] As serum estrogen levels decrease, the vaginal epithelium and lamina propria thin, smooth muscle atrophies, blood flow to the vaginal area decreases, and collagen and tissue elasticity are lost.[3,4] In combination, these changes lead to a pale, thinner, more friable vaginal mucosa with less physiologic discharge.[5,6] Oral and topical estrogen therapy can reverse many of these changes, leading to increased blood flow and vaginal discharge.[7]

Vaginal tissue expression of estrogen receptors, particularly estrogen receptor-β, decreases significantly after menopause and is not restored by estrogen therapy.[8] Glycogen content in vaginal cells decreases,[9] limiting substrate for beneficial vaginal lactobacilli, leading to decreased colonization and elevated vaginal pH in some women.[10–12] The vaginal microbial community after menopause is more diverse, and often includes uropathogens such as *Escherichia coli* and common skin colonizers such as *Streptococcus*.[12,13] By molecular evaluation, 39% to 55% of postmenopausal women have a *Lactobacillus*-dominant (ie, >50% of sequences) vaginal microbial community.[10,12,13] Older studies using a Gram stain show a *Lactobacillus*-dominant community (ie, Nugent score 0–3) in 13% to 46%.[11,14]

In the postmenopausal genital mucosa, immune cell numbers are similar or slightly reduced compared with premenopause[1,15] and have the same cytolytic capacity.[16] Some studies show decreased cytokines and antiviral activity in cervicovaginal fluid after menopause.[17,18] In a cohort of Kenyan women with human immunodeficiency virus infection, serum cytokine and chemokine levels correlated more with age than menopause, although cervicovaginal lavage levels correlated with menopausal status.[19] In vitro studies using cervical explant tissue from premenopausal women versus postmenopausal women demonstrate increased cytokine production in response to challenge with human immunodeficiency virus, and greater viral replication in explants from postmenopausal women.[20] These data suggest that altered mucosal immune responses after menopause may increase susceptibility to genital infections.

The Vulva

The vulva is composed of the mons pubis, labia majora, labia minora, clitoris, vestibule, and hymen. The labia majora is mainly made up of fibroadipose tissue, and the labia minora is composed of dense connective tissue, erectile tissue, and elastic fibers.[21] Between the outer surfaces of the labia majora and inner labia minora, the cutaneous thickness and keratinization decrease and the estrogen receptor concentration increases. Compared with exposed skin, vulvar skin is more sensitive and shows higher permeability, occlusion, and hydration, as measured by transepidermal water loss, susceptibility to friction, and sensitivity to estrogen. Blood flow and innervation to the vulva is also higher than in other exposed skin surfaces.[22]

With aging and menopause, the vulva undergoes structural changes: a reduction of pubic hair and subcutaneous fat in the labia majora, decreased size of labia minora and vestibular bulbs,[23,24] retraction of the vaginal introitus and involution of hymenal carunculae with loss of elasticity,[25] and overall reduction in blood flow.[26] Although not as well-studied as the vagina, postmenopausal cell-mediated immunity in the vulva is less efficient,[27] and the ratio between proinflammatory cytokines and antiinflammatory mediators increases.[28] Contrary to expectations, barrier function, hydration, and susceptibility to friction do not objectively change across the lifespan[26] and sensation decreases.[29]

The vulvar microbiome, although again not as well-studied as the vagina, shows greater bacterial diversity of the labia majora versus minora. Microbial populations are primarily composed of commensals of the skin, gastrointestinal and vaginal bacteria, such as *Staphylococcus*, *E coli*, and *Lactobacillus* species.[30] Whether and how the microbiota of the vulva may be related to vulvar symptoms and conditions of aging and/or menopause is unclear.

Lower Urinary Tract

The relative contribution of aging versus menopause to changes in the lower urinary tract—bladder, urethra, and pelvic floor—is not well-studied. Aging is associated with bladder remodeling and decreased ratio of smooth muscle to collagen,[31] along with reduced bladder capacity, detrusor contraction strength, bladder sensation, urethral closure pressure, and urinary flow.[32–34] There is an increased prominence of the urethral meatus relative to the introitus[25] and a decrease in contractile coordination and strength in pelvic floor muscles.[35,36] Finally, aging-related changes in the central nervous system, in particular weaker signals in the bladder control network and/or changes in prefrontal cortical functioning, may be important in the lower urinary tract dysfunction seen in older women.[37]

The evidence suggesting an effect of menopause on the lower urinary tract is based largely on studies of exogenous estrogen treatment in postmenopausal women: changes reversed by estrogen treatment are presumed to be associated with lower estrogen levels. Estrogen receptors are found throughout the urinary tract, in the bladder, trigone, urethra, and the levator ani muscles,[8,38] and the balance of these receptors changes from before to after menopause.[8] In observational studies, estrogen administration after menopause increases urethral closure pressure[39] and urethral blood flow.[40] Estrogen use decreased the total collagen and increased collagen degradation products in the periurethral mucosa,[41] but was associated with increased high tensile strength collagen (type I) over the looser types (types III and V) in the deeper connective tissues of the pelvis.[42] Finally, exogenous estrogen promotes a *Lactobacillus*-dominant vaginal environment,[43] increases the presence of antimicrobial peptides in the bladder, and strengthens the intracellular barrier to bacterial invasion.[44]

Contrary to the previously accepted paradigm that urine is sterile, studies using culture-independent methods demonstrate a urinary microbiome with predominant species similar to the vagina and vulva: *Lactobacillus*, *Gardnerella*, *Streptococcus*, *Staphylococcus*, and *Corynebacteria*.[45] The postmenopausal urinary microbiome changes with estrogen treatment[46] and with symptoms and conditions that increase in prevalence with aging.[47]

GENITOURINARY SYNDROME OF MENOPAUSE

In 2014, the North American Menopause Society proposed replacing the negative and nonspecific term "vulvovaginal atrophy" with the neutral and specific term "genitourinary syndrome of menopause" (GSM). This name change is part of a movement to promote greater recognition and public discussion about the "collection of symptoms and signs associated with decreased estrogen levels that can involve the labia majora/minora, vestibule/introitus, clitoris, vagina, urethra, and bladder" (**Table 1**) that often go untreated but can significantly impact older women's quality of life.[25]

Although GSM is common, not all postmenopausal women develop GSM symptoms or signs, and not all genitourinary symptoms after menopause can be classified as GSM, that is, not all symptoms are associated with decreased estrogen levels and potentially treatable with topical or systemic estrogen. Indeed, GSM is a diagnosis of exclusion in perimenopausal and postmenopausal women. Although epidemiologic studies have not differentiated GSM from other etiologies of vulvovaginal, urinary, and sexual symptoms affecting midlife and older women, they do provide insight into the scope and impact of genitourinary aging.

VULVOVAGINAL SYMPTOMS: EPIDEMIOLOGY AND IMPACT

Up to 45% of postmenopausal women report some type of vulvovaginal symptom,[48,49] and of those with symptoms, dryness (55%–75%) and pain with intercourse (40%–44%) are the most common, followed by itching and irritation (18%–37%) and soreness/pain (18%–29%).[48,50–55] Several demographic factors have been associated with vulvovaginal symptoms. In one population-based study, report of vaginal dryness was associated with nonwhite race, diabetes, and lower body mass index.[52] A few studies show more bothersome vulvovaginal symptoms in women who are married or who are sexually active.[50,52,56]

There are few data to support a consistent biologic phenotype in women with vulvovaginal symptoms versus those without.[57] Physical signs of GSM correlate with report of symptoms in some studies[58,59] but not in many others.[6,12,57,60] Additionally, not all GSM symptoms even co-occur; reports of vaginal dryness and pain were significantly but only weakly correlated ($r = 0.4$).[61] In cross-sectional studies, by both culture and molecular detection methods, the composition of the vaginal microbiome was not associated with the presence of moderate to severe vulvovaginal symptoms,[13,52] although signs of vaginal "atrophy," pallor, loss of rugae, and friability, are associated with lower prevalence of vaginal *Lactobacillus*.[12] Although one study of 290 Mexican women showed no association between estrogen

Table 1 Genitourinary syndrome of menopause (GSM): symptoms and signs	
Symptoms	**Signs**
Genital dryness	Decreased moisture
Decreased lubrication with sexual activity	Decreased elasticity
Discomfort or pain with sexual activity	Labia minora resorption
Post-coital bleeding	Pallor/Erythema
Decreased arousal, orgasm, desire	Loss of vaginal rugae
Irritation/Burning/Itching of vulva or vagina	Tissue fragility/fissures/petechiae
Dysuria	Urethral eversion or prolapse
Urinary frequency/urgency	Loss of hymenal remnants
	Prominence of urethral meatus
	Introital retraction
	Recurrent urinary tract infections

Supportive findings: pH >5, increased parabasal cells on maturation index, and decreased superficial cells on wet mount or maturation index.

From Portman DJ, Gass ML, Vulvovaginal Atrophy Terminology Consensus Conference Panel. Genitourinary syndrome of menopause: new terminology for vulvovaginal atrophy from the International Society for the Study of Women's Sexual Health and the North American Menopause Society. Menopause 2014;21(10):1063–8; with permission.

receptor-α polymorphisms and severity of vaginal dryness,[62] a separate study of 177 Mexican women demonstrated an association with decreased lubrication during intercourse.[63] In a small group of 26 women, the quantity of vaginal fluid cytokines did not differ between women with and without vulvovaginal symptoms.[64,65]

Often, women believe these symptoms to be a normal part of menopause and do not seek treatment.[53] Of the 25% who do seek treatment, many report their physicians dismiss GSM symptoms as a normal part of aging.[53,66] However, vulvovaginal symptoms cause significant distress for women,[67,68] negatively impacting sexual function[69,70] and quality of life.[50] Depression, concomitant urinary incontinence (UI), a higher body mass index, and poorer general health increased the impact of vulvovaginal symptoms on daily functioning, self-concept, and/or body image.[67] The majority of women in relationships with vulvovaginal symptoms state that symptoms lead them to avoid intimacy (58%) or contribute to loss of libido (64%).[56] Approximately 30% of partners identify these symptoms as the main reason they stop engaging in sex.[56] Reduction in severity of GSM-related vulvovaginal symptoms is associated with improvement in the sexual function domain of the Menopause-Specific Quality of Life score.[70]

Other Vulvovaginal Conditions Associated with Aging

For the clinician, determining whether vulvovaginal complaints are GSM (and thus presumably responsive to estrogen treatment) or related to other genitourinary conditions with increased prevalence in older women can be challenging. Three vulvar dermatologic conditions have an increased prevalence in postmenopausal women: lichen sclerosus,[71,72] lichen planus,[73–75] and lichen simplex chronicus. All 3 entities can present with symptoms and signs similar to GSM (**Table 2**).

LOWER URINARY TRACT SYMPTOMS: EPIDEMIOLOGY AND IMPACT
Urinary Urgency and Frequency

Community-based estimates of urinary urgency and frequency prevalence range between 10% and 20% in postmenopausal women.[76,77] Structural changes associated with aging and menopause may lead to functional changes associated with urinary urgency and/or frequency: reduced bladder capacity, detrusor contraction strength, bladder sensation, urethral closure pressure, and urinary flow.[32,34] Alternatively, these symptoms can be related to behaviors or to urinary conditions unrelated to menopause, including idiopathic overactive bladder, detrusor overactivity associated with neurologic and medical conditions such as diabetes, and interstitial cystitis. There are no clear means of distinguishing GSM-related urinary urgency or frequency responsive to topical estrogen versus idiopathic symptoms. Urinary urgency and frequency symptoms, especially when associated with urge UI, are associated with depression, embarrassment, and shame and can limit social activities, ability to travel outside the home, occupational function, and relationships.[78]

Recurrent Urinary Tract Infection and Dysuria

About 8% to 11% of community-dwelling postmenopausal women report recurrent urinary tract infections (UTIs),[79] and about 7% to 13% report dysuria.[80] Postmenopausal women have greater susceptibility to recurrent UTI than premenopausal women. Aging-related higher postvoid residual urine volumes and reduced urinary

Table 2
Comparison of clinical and pathologic characteristics of genitourinary syndrome of menopause (GSM) and vulvar dermatoses with increased prevalence in postmenopausal women

	Menopause[48,50–55]	Lichen Sclerosus[115,116]	Lichen Planus[74,117]	Lichen Simplex Chronicus[117,118]
Skin color	Pale, Pink	Hypopigmented plaques or patches, "keyhole" distribution	Hyperpigmented, erythematous	Erythematous, white, gray
Skin appearance	Flat, dry, thin, petechiae	Thin, "cigarette paper," purpura, fissures	Eroded, friable, white reticulations	Thickened, lichenified plaques, excoriations, accentuated skin markings
Symptoms	Dryness (55%–75%) Dyspareunia (40%–44%) Itching/irritation (18%–37%) Soreness/pain (18%–29%)	Itching (89%) Soreness (69%) Pain/burning (9%) Dyspareunia (30%)	Pain (80%) Itching (65%) Irritation (48%) Dyspareunia (61%)	Itching Irritation
Etiology	Decreased serum estrogen	Autoimmune	Autoimmune	Chronic irritation, allergic contact dermatitis

flow are mechanical factors that increase the risk of recurrent UTI.[81] Vaginal colonization with the uropathogen *E coli* is inversely associated with vaginal *Lactobacillus* colonization; thus, the decrease in vaginal *Lactobacillus* after menopause may increase the risk for UTIs.[82] Topical vaginal estrogen has long been used to prevent the recurrence of UTIs in postmenopausal women, with a presumed mechanism of restoring vaginal *Lactobacillus* colonization.[79] Recurrent UTI and related dysuria symptoms have a significant impact on women's lives, including limiting activities, mental stress, depression, and the economic burden of multiple doctor visits and treatments.[83,84]

Other Urinary Symptoms Associated with Aging: Urinary Incontinence

UI is a frequently reported urinary symptom that increases in prevalence with aging, but is not included as a GSM symptom. In midlife, about 15% of community-dwelling women report moderate UI and 10% have severe UI; 25% of women wear protective undergarments.[85] In the Study of Women's Health Across the Nation, neither the development of clinically significant stress or urge UI (weekly or more) nor worsening of UI were associated with advancing menopausal stage, serum estradiol, or decrease in estradiol over time.[86–88] Rather, in postmenopausal women, both stress and urge UI worsens with exogenous estrogen use.[89,90] UI can affect women's lives negatively, leading to decreased quality of life[91,92] and significant morbidity, such as functional decline[93] and increased risk of falls and fractures in the elderly.[94] However, less than 40% of women report seeking treatment for their UI.[95]

SEXUAL FUNCTION AND DYSFUNCTION: EPIDEMIOLOGY AND IMPACT

In a survey of almost a thousand women over the age of 40, one-half reported sexual activity within the past month.[96] Among older women (mean age 72) with a partner, 35% reported sexual activity in the previous week.[97] Visual erotic stimuli lead to similar vaginal blood flow increases in premenopausal and postmenopausal women, suggesting that sexual responsiveness is preserved after menopause.[98,99] Some postmenopausal women discuss positive changes in sexual function after menopause owing to greater empowerment, less concern about pregnancy, and better communication of needs with partners.[100]

Although the frequency of sexual activity decreases in women with age and with worse general health[101,102] and sexual function scores worsen over the menopausal transition,[103] 60% to 75% of older women feel that sexuality is important to their well-being and overall quality of life.[101,104] In the Vaginal Health: Insights, Views and Attitudes survey, women reported that sexual GSM symptoms had the greatest negative life impact.[56] One of the most frequently reported GSM symptom is pain with intercourse, ranging in prevalence from 20% to 59%.[52–54,105,106] This symptom has also been associated with hypoactive sexual desire disorder,[107] avoiding sex,[3,108] and less sex.[61] Sexual pain may be the GSM symptom most likely to prompt women to seek treatment. Although a majority of women report vaginal dryness as their most bothersome GSM symptom (54%),[68] in two randomized clinical trials evaluating treatment for GSM symptoms, most women chose pain with intercourse as their most bothersome symptom (52%–60%).[70,109]

The physical signs of GSM are presumed to be the primary cause of most postmenopausal dyspareunia. Additionally, exogenous estrogen is associated with lower density of nerve fibers in the vaginal mucosa, suggesting that vaginal innervation may increase in response to lower estrogen levels, leading to increased pain sensation.[110]

Lower serum estradiol levels have been correlated with reports of vestibular pain with intercourse in postmenopausal women.[111] In an older study, women who remained sexually active had fewer physical signs of genitourinary aging, which supported the common notion that women must "use it or lose it"—that is, remain sexually active with intercourse or lose vaginal function.[112] However, in cross-sectional studies it is impossible to determine directionality of such a relationship; it is just as likely that GSM leads to decreased sexual activity. Longitudinal studies considering other factors associated with sexual dysfunction or distress, such as insomnia,[113] physical health, mood, and the presence of a partner,[114] are needed to better understand the relationship between the development of GSM symptoms and sexual functioning.

SUMMARY

The genitourinary changes associated with aging and menopause are highly variable in women and do not correlate well with genitourinary symptoms. However, the GSM, characterized by vulvovaginal and lower urinary tract symptoms, is prevalent and has a significant negative impact on women's lives. To fill important gaps in knowledge and identify modifiable factors to prevent development of GSM symptoms, research should focus on the underlying biology of genitourinary discomfort in postmenopausal women. A greater clinical awareness is also necessary; primary care doctors and gynecologists should regularly inquire about genitourinary symptoms as patients age and transition through menopause so that currently available, effective interventions can be provided to improve postmenopausal quality of life.

REFERENCES

1. Pudney J, Quayle AJ, Anderson DJ. Immunological microenvironments in the human vagina and cervix: mediators of cellular immunity are concentrated in the cervical transformation zone. Biol Reprod 2005;73(6):1253–63.
2. Yavagal S, de Farias TF, Medina CA, et al. Normal vulvovaginal, perineal, and pelvic anatomy with reconstructive considerations. Semin Plast Surg 2011; 25(2):121–9.
3. Calleja-Agius J, Brincat M. The effect of menopause on the skin and other connective tissues. Gynecol Endocrinol 2012;28(4):273–7.
4. Semmelink HJ, de Wilde PC, van Houwelingen JC, et al. Histomorphometric study of the lower urogenital tract in pre- and post-menopausal women. Cytometry 1990;11(6):700–7.
5. Bachmann G, Lobo RA, Gut R, et al. Efficacy of low-dose estradiol vaginal tablets in the treatment of atrophic vaginitis: a randomized controlled trial. Obstet Gynecol 2008;111(1):67–76.
6. Davila GW, Singh A, Karapanagiotou I, et al. Are women with urogenital atrophy symptomatic? Am J Obstet Gynecol 2003;188(2):382–8.
7. Semmens JP, Tsai CC, Semmens EC, et al. Effects of estrogen therapy on vaginal physiology during menopause. Obstet Gynecol 1985;66(1):15–8.
8. Gebhart JB, Rickard DJ, Barrett TJ, et al. Expression of estrogen receptor isoforms alpha and beta messenger RNA in vaginal tissue of premenopausal and postmenopausal women. Am J Obstet Gynecol 2001;185(6):1325–30 [discussion: 1330–1].
9. Mirmonsef P, Modur S, Burgad D, et al. Exploratory comparison of vaginal glycogen and Lactobacillus levels in premenopausal and postmenopausal women. Menopause 2015;22(7):702–9.

10. Brotman RM, Shardell MD, Gajer P, et al. Association between the vaginal micro-biota, menopause status, and signs of vulvovaginal atrophy. Menopause 2014; 21(5):450–8.

11. Hillier SL, Lau RJ. Vaginal microflora in postmenopausal women who have not received estrogen replacement therapy. Clin Infect Dis 1997;25(Suppl 2): S123–6.

12. Hummelen R, Macklaim JM, Bisanz JE, et al. Vaginal microbiome and epithelial gene array in post-menopausal women with moderate to severe dryness. PLoS One 2011;6(11):e26602.

13. Mitchell CM, Srinivasan S, Zhan X, et al. Vaginal microbiota and genitourinary menopausal symptoms: a cross-sectional analysis. Menopause 2017;24(10): 1160–6.

14. Burton JP, Reid G. Evaluation of the bacterial vaginal flora of 20 postmenopausal women by direct (Nugent score) and molecular (polymerase chain reaction and denaturing gradient gel electrophoresis) techniques. J Infect Dis 2002;186(12): 1770–80.

15. Meditz AL, Moreau KL, MaWhinney S, et al. CCR5 expression is elevated on en-docervical CD4+ T cells in healthy postmenopausal women. J Acquir Immune Defic Syndr 2012;59(3):221–8.

16. White HD, Yeaman GR, Givan AL, et al. Mucosal immunity in the human female reproductive tract: cytotoxic T lymphocyte function in the cervix and vagina of premenopausal and postmenopausal women. Am J Reprod Immunol 1997; 37(1):30–8.

17. Chappell CA, Isaacs CE, Xu W, et al. The effect of menopause on the innate anti-viral activity of cervicovaginal lavage. Am J Obstet Gynecol 2015;213(2): 204.e1-6.

18. Jais M, Younes N, Chapman S, et al. Reduced levels of genital tract immune bio-markers in postmenopausal women: implications for HIV acquisition. Am J Ob-stet Gynecol 2016;215(3):324.e1–10.

19. Sivro A, Lajoie J, Kimani J, et al. Age and menopause affect the expression of specific cytokines/chemokines in plasma and cervical lavage samples from fe-male sex workers in Nairobi, Kenya. Immun Ageing 2013;10(1):42.

20. Rollenhagen C, Asin SN. Enhanced HIV-1 replication in ex vivo ectocervical tis-sues from post-menopausal women correlates with increased inflammatory re-sponses. Mucosal Immunol 2011;4(6):671–81.

21. Deliveliotou AC, Creatsas G. Anatomy of the vulva. In: Farage M, Maibach HI, editors. The vulva: physiology and clinical management. 2nd edition. Boca Ra-ton (FL): CRC Press; 2017. p. 3–5.

22. Farage M, Maibach H. Tissue structure and physiology of the vulva. In: Farage M, Maibach HI, editors. The vulva: physiology and clinical management. 2nd edition. Boca Raton (FL): CRC Press; 2017. p. 6–13.

23. Basaran M, Kosif R, Bayar U, et al. Characteristics of external genitalia in pre- and postmenopausal women. Climacteric 2008;11(5):416–21.

24. Suh DD, Yang CC, Cao Y, et al. Magnetic resonance imaging anatomy of the fe-male genitalia in premenopausal and postmenopausal women. J Urol 2003; 170(1):138–44.

25. Portman DJ, Gass ML, Vulvovaginal Atrophy Terminology Consensus Confer-ence Panel. Genitourinary syndrome of menopause: new terminology for vulvo-vaginal atrophy from the International Society for the Study of Women's Sexual Health and the North American Menopause Society. Menopause 2014;21(10): 1063–8.

26. Farage M, Maibach H. Lifetime changes in the vulva and vagina. Arch Gynecol Obstet 2006;273(4):195–202.

27. Summers PR, Hunn J. Unique dermatologic aspects of the postmenopausal vulva. Clin Obstet Gynecol 2007;50(3):745–51.

28. Farage M, Wehmeyer K, Fadayel G, et al. Biomolecular markers and physical measures in the urogenital area. In: Farage M, Maibach HI, editors. The vulva: physiology and clinical management. 2nd edition. Boca Raton (FL): CRC Press; 2017. p. 69–80.

29. Connell K, Guess MK, Bleustein CB, et al. Effects of age, menopause, and co-morbidities on neurological function of the female genitalia. Int J Impot Res 2005;17(1):63–70.

30. Brown CJ, Wong M, Davis CC, et al. Preliminary characterization of the normal microbiota of the human vulva using cultivation-independent methods. J Mod Microbiol 2007;56(Pt 2):271–6.

31. Lepor H, Sunaryadi I, Hartanto V, et al. Quantitative morphometry of the adult human bladder. J Urol 1992;148(2 Pt 1):414–7.

32. Pfisterer MH, Griffiths DJ, Rosenberg L, et al. Parameters of bladder function in pre-, peri-, and postmenopausal continent women without detrusor overactivity. Neurourol Urodyn 2007;26(3):356–61.

33. Pfisterer MH, Griffiths DJ, Schaefer W, et al. The effect of age on lower urinary tract function: a study in women. J Am Geriatr Soc 2006;54(3):405–12.

34. Madersbacher S, Pycha A, Schatzl G, et al. The aging lower urinary tract: a comparative urodynamic study of men and women. Urology 1998;51(2):206–12.

35. Huang WC, Yang JM. Menopause is associated with impaired responsiveness of involuntary pelvic floor muscle contractions to sudden intra-abdominal pressure rise in women with pelvic floor symptoms: a retrospective study. Neurourol Urodyn 2018;37(3):1128–36.

36. Alperin M, Cook M, Tuttle LJ, et al. Impact of vaginal parity and aging on the architectural design of pelvic floor muscles. Am J Obstet Gynecol 2016; 215(3):312.e1-9.

37. Griffiths DJ, Tadic SD, Schaefer W, et al. Cerebral control of the lower urinary tract: how age-related changes might predispose to urge incontinence. Neuro-image 2009;47(3):981–6.

38. Copas P, Bukovsky A, Asbury B, et al. Estrogen, progesterone, and androgen receptor expression in levator ani muscle and fascia. J Womens Health Gend Based Med 2001;10(8):785–95.

39. Fantl JA, Cardozo L, McClish DK. Estrogen therapy in the management of urinary incontinence in postmenopausal women: a meta-analysis. First report of the Hormones and Urogenital Therapy Committee. Obstet Gynecol 1994; 83(1):12–8.

40. Tsai E, Yang C, Chen H, et al. Bladder neck circulation by Doppler ultrasonography in postmenopausal women with urinary stress incontinence. Obstet Gynecol 2001;98(1):52–6.

41. Jackson S, James M, Abrams P. The effect of oestradiol on vaginal collagen metabolism in postmenopausal women with genuine stress incontinence. BJOG 2002;109(3):339–44.

42. Moalli PA, Talarico LC, Sung VW, et al. Impact of menopause on collagen subtypes in the arcus tendineous fasciae pelvis. Am J Obstet Gynecol 2004;190(3): 620–7.

43. Shen J, Song N, Williams CJ, et al. Effects of low dose estrogen therapy on the vaginal microbiomes of women with atrophic vaginitis. Sci Rep 2016;6:24380.

44. Luthje P, Hirschberg AL, Brauner A. Estrogenic action on innate defense mechanisms in the urinary tract. Maturitas 2014;77(1):32–6,

45. Brubaker L, Wolfe AJ. The female urinary microbiota, urinary health and common urinary disorders. Ann Transl Med 2017;5(2):34.

46. Thomas-White KJ, Taege S, Johansen D, et al. Bladder and vaginal microbiomes have a corresponding shift following estrogen treatment in postmenopausal women. [Abstract 940.4]. FASEB J 2017;31(1).

47. Pearce MM, Zilliox MJ, Rosenfeld AB, et al. The female urinary microbiome in urgency urinary incontinence. Am J Obstet Gynecol 2015;213(3):347.e1-11.

48. Nappi RE, Kokot-Kierepa M. Vaginal health: insights, views & attitudes (VIVA) - results from an international survey. Climacteric 2012;15(1):36–44.

49. Santoro N, Komi J. Prevalence and impact of vaginal symptoms among postmenopausal women. J Sex Med 2009;6(8):2133–42.

50. DiBonaventura M, Luo X, Moffatt M, et al. The association between vulvovaginal atrophy symptoms and quality of life among postmenopausal women in the United States and Western Europe. J Womens Health (Larchmt) 2015;24(9):713–22.

51. Domoney C, Currie H, Panay N, et al. The CLOSER survey: impact of postmenopausal vaginal discomfort on women and male partners in the UK. Menopause Int 2013;19(2):69–76.

52. Huang AJ, Moore EE, Boyko EJ, et al. Vaginal symptoms in postmenopausal women: self-reported severity, natural history, and risk factors. Menopause 2010;17(1):121–6.

53. Kingsberg SA, Krychman M, Graham S, et al. The Women's EMPOWER Survey: identifying women's perceptions on vulvar and vaginal atrophy and its treatment. J Sex Med 2017;14(3):413–24.

54. Kingsberg SA, Wysocki S, Magnus L, et al. Vulvar and vaginal atrophy in postmenopausal women: findings from the REVIVE (REal Women's VIews of Treatment Options for Menopausal Vaginal ChangEs) survey. J Sex Med 2013;10(7):1790–9.

55. Palma F, Xholli A, Cagnacci A, as the Writing Group of the AGATA Study. Management of vaginal atrophy: a real mess. Results from the AGATA study. Gynecol Endocrinol 2017;33(9):702–7.

56. Simon JA, Kokot-Kierepa M, Goldstein J, et al. Vaginal health in the United States: results from the vaginal health: insights, views & attitudes survey. Menopause 2013;20(10):1043–8.

57. Greendale GA, Zibecchi L, Petersen L, et al. Development and validation of a physical examination scale to assess vaginal atrophy and inflammation. Climacteric 1999;2(3):197–204.

58. Le Donne M, Caruso C, Mancuso A, et al. The effect of vaginally administered genistein in comparison with hyaluronic acid on atrophic epithelium in postmenopause. Arch Gynecol Obstet 2011;283(6):1319–23.

59. Simon JA, Archer DF, Kagan R, et al. Visual improvements in vaginal mucosa correlate with symptoms of VVA: data from a double-blind, placebo-controlled trial. Menopause 2017;24(9):1003–10.

60. Gass MI , Cochrane BB, Larson JC, et al. Patterns and predictors of sexual activity among women in the hormone therapy trials of the women's health initiative. Menopause 2011;18(11):1160–71.

61. Thomas HM, Bryce CL, Ness RB, et al. Dyspareunia is associated with decreased frequency of intercourse in the menopausal transition. Menopause 2011;18(2):152–7.

62. Aguilar-Zavala H, Perez-Luque EL, Luna-Martinez F, et al. Symptoms at post-menopause: genetic and psychosocial factors. Menopause 2012;19(10): 1140–5.

63. Malacara JM, Perez-Luque EL, Martinez-Garza S, et al. The relationship of estrogen receptor-alpha polymorphism with symptoms and other characteristics in post-menopausal women. Maturitas 2004;49(2):163–9.

64. Kollmann Z, Bersinger N, von Wolff M, et al. Vaginal cytokines do not correlate with postmenopausal vulvovaginal symptoms. Gynecol Endocrinol 2015;31(4): 317–21.

65. Stute P, Kollmann Z, Bersinger N, et al. Vaginal cytokines do not differ between postmenopausal women with and without symptoms of vulvovaginal irritation. Menopause 2014;21(8):840–5.

66. Utian WH, Maamari R. Attitudes and approaches to vaginal atrophy in postmenopausal women: a focus group qualitative study. Climacteric 2014;17(1):29–36.

67. Hunter MM, Nakagawa S, Van Den Eeden SK, et al. Predictors of impact of vaginal symptoms in postmenopausal women. Menopause 2016;23(1):40–6.

68. Palma F, Xholli A, Cagnacci A. as the writing group of the As. The most bothersome symptom of vaginal atrophy: evidence from the observational AGATA study. Maturitas 2018;108:18–23.

69. Nappi RE, Nijland EA. Women's perception of sexuality around the menopause: outcomes of a European telephone survey. Eur J Obstet Gynecol Reprod Biol 2008;137(1):10–6.

70. Pinkerton JV, Bushmakin AG, Komm BS, et al. Relationship between changes in vulvar-vaginal atrophy and changes in sexual functioning. Maturitas 2017;100: 57–63.

71. Fruchter R, Melnick L, Pomeranz MK. Lichenoid vulvar disease: a review. Int J Womens Dermatol 2017;3(1):58–64.

72. Goldstein AT, Marinoff SC, Christopher K, et al. Prevalence of vulvar lichen sclerosus in a general gynecology practice. J Reprod Med 2005;50(7):477–80.

73. Ball SB, Wojnarowska F. Vulvar dermatoses: lichen sclerosus, lichen planus, and vulval dermatitis/lichen simplex chronicus. Semin Cutan Med Surg 1998;17(3): 182–8.

74. Cooper SM, Wojnarowska F. Influence of treatment of erosive lichen planus of the vulva on its prognosis. Arch Dermatol 2006;142(3):289–94.

75. Eisen D. The vulvovaginal-gingival syndrome of lichen planus. The clinical characteristics of 22 patients. Arch Dermatol 1994;130(11):1379–82.

76. Coyne KS, Sexton CC, Vats V, et al. National community prevalence of overactive bladder in the United States stratified by sex and age. Urology 2011;77(5): 1081–7.

77. Irwin DE, Milsom I, Hunskaar S, et al. Population-based survey of urinary incontinence, overactive bladder, and other lower urinary tract symptoms in five countries: results of the EPIC study. Eur Urol 2006;50(6):1306–14 [discussion: 1314–5].

78. Kinsey D, Pretorius S, Glover L, et al. The psychological impact of overactive bladder: a systematic review. J Health Psychol 2016;21(1):69–81.

79. Perrotta C, Aznar M, Mejia R, et al. Oestrogens for preventing recurrent urinary tract infection in postmenopausal women. Cochrane Database Syst Rev 2008;(2):CD005131.

80. Erekson EA, Li FY, Martin DK, et al. Vulvovaginal symptoms prevalence in postmenopausal women and relationship to other menopausal symptoms and pelvic floor disorders. Menopause 2016;23(4):368–75.

81. Raz R, Gennesin Y, Wasser J, et al. Recurrent urinary tract infections in post-menopausal women. Clin Infect Dis 2000;30(1):152–6.

82. Gupta K, Stapleton AE, Hooton TM, et al. Inverse association of H2O2-producing lactobacilli and vaginal Escherichia coli colonization in women with recurrent urinary tract infections. J Infect Dis 1998;178(2):446–50.

83. Wagenlehner F, Wullt B, Ballarini S, et al. Social and economic burden of recurrent urinary tract infections and quality of life: a patient web-based study (GESPRIT). Expert Rev Pharmacoecon Outcomes Res 2018;18(1):107–17.

84. Renard J, Ballarini S, Mascarenhas T, et al. Recurrent lower urinary tract infections have a detrimental effect on patient quality of life: a prospective, observational study. Infect Dis Ther 2015;1:125–35.

85. Sampselle CM, Harlow SD, Skurnick J, et al. Urinary incontinence predictors and life impact in ethnically diverse perimenopausal women. Obstet Gynecol 2002;100(6):1230–8.

86. Waetjen LE, Feng WY, Ye J, et al. Factors associated with worsening and improving urinary incontinence across the menopausal transition. Obstet Gynecol 2008;111(3):667–77.

87. Waetjen LE, Ye J, Feng WY, et al. Association between menopausal transition stages and developing urinary incontinence. Obstet Gynecol 2009;114(5): 989–98.

88. Waetjen LE, Johnson WO, Xing G, et al. Serum estradiol levels are not associated with urinary incontinence in midlife women transitioning through menopause. Menopause 2011;18(12):1283–90.

89. Hendrix SL, Cochrane BB, Nygaard IE, et al. Effects of estrogen with and without progestin on urinary incontinence. JAMA 2005;293(8):935–48.

90. Grodstein F, Lifford K, Resnick NM, et al. Postmenopausal hormone therapy and risk of developing urinary incontinence. Obstet Gynecol 2004;103(2):254–60.

91. Botlero R, Bell RJ, Urquhart DM, et al. Urinary incontinence is associated with lower psychological general well-being in community-dwelling women. Menopause 2010;17(2):332–7.

92. Margareta N, Ann L, Othon L. The impact of female urinary incontinence and urgency on quality of life and partner relationship. Neurourol Urodyn 2009;28(8): 976–81.

93. Omli R, Hunskaar S, Mykletun A, et al. Urinary incontinence and risk of functional decline in older women: data from the Norwegian HUNT-study. BMC Geriatr 2013;13:47.

94. Brown JS, Vittinghoff E, Wyman JF, et al. Urinary incontinence: does it increase risk for falls and fractures? Study of Osteoporotic Fractures Research Group [see comments]. J Am Geriatr Soc 2000;48(7):721–5.

95. Waetjen LE, Xing G, Johnson WO, et al, Study of Women's Health Across the Nation (SWAN). Factors associated with reasons incontinent midlife women report for not seeking urinary incontinence treatment over 9 years across the menopausal transition. Menopause 2018;25(1):29–37.

96. Trompeter SE, Bettencourt R, Barrett-Connor E. Sexual activity and satisfaction in healthy community-dwelling older women. Am J Med 2012;125(1):37–43.e31.

97. Wang V, Depp CA, Ceglowski J, et al. Sexual health and function in later life: a population-based study of 606 older adults with a partner. Am J Geriatr Psychiatry 2015;23(3):227–33.

98. Laan E, van Lunsen RH. Hormones and sexuality in postmenopausal women: a psychophysiological study. J Psychosom Obstet Gynaecol 1997;18(2):126–33.

99. Suh DD, Yang CC, Cao Y, et al. MRI of female genital and pelvic organs during sexual arousal. J Psychosom Obstet Gynaecol 2004;25(2):153–62.

100. Thomas HN, Hamm M, Hess R, et al. Changes in sexual function among midlife women: "I'm older... and I'm wiser". Menopause 2018;25(3):286–92.

101. Lindau ST, Schumm LP, Laumann EO, et al. A study of sexuality and health among older adults in the United States. N Engl J Med 2007;357(8):762–74.

102. Lee DM, Nazroo J, O'Connor DB, et al. Sexual health and well-being among older men and women in England: findings from the English Longitudinal Study of Ageing. Arch Sex Behav 2016;45(1):133–44.

103. Avis NE, Colvin A, Karlamangla AS, et al. Change in sexual functioning over the menopausal transition: results from the Study of Women's Health Across the Nation. Menopause 2017;24(4):379–90.

104. Cain VS, Johannes CB, Avis NE, et al. Sexual functioning and practices in a multi-ethnic study of midlife women: baseline results from SWAN. J Sex Res 2003;40(3):266–76.

105. Minkin MJ, Reiter S, Maamari R. Prevalence of postmenopausal symptoms in North America and Europe. Menopause 2015;22(11):1231–8.

106. Flynn KE, Carter J, Lin L, et al. Assessment of vulvar discomfort with sexual activity among women in the United States. Am J Obstet Gynecol 2017;216(4): 391.e1–8.

107. Worsley R, Bell RJ, Gartoulla P, et al. Prevalence and predictors of low sexual desire, sexually related personal distress, and hypoactive sexual desire dysfunction in a community-based sample of midlife women. J Sex Med 2017;14(5):675–86.

108. Stenberg A, Heimer G, Ulmsten U, et al. Prevalence of genitourinary and other climacteric symptoms in 61-year-old women. Maturitas 1996;24(1–2):31–6.

109. Mitchell CM. Effects of Vagifem vs. Replens vs. placebo on most bothersome vaginal symptoms. Philadelphia: North American Menopause Society; 2017.

110. Griebling TL, Liao Z, Smith PG. Systemic and topical hormone therapies reduce vaginal innervation density in postmenopausal women. Menopause 2012;19(6): 630–5.

111. Kao A, Binik YM, Amsel R, et al. Biopsychosocial predictors of postmenopausal dyspareunia: the role of steroid hormones, vulvovaginal atrophy, cognitive-emotional factors, and dyadic adjustment. J Sex Med 2012;9(8):2066–76.

112. Leiblum S, Bachmann G, Kemmann E, et al. Vaginal atrophy in the postmenopausal woman. The importance of sexual activity and hormones. JAMA 1983; 249(16):2195–8.

113. Kling JM, Manson JE, Naughton MJ, et al. Association of sleep disturbance and sexual function in postmenopausal women. Menopause 2017;24(6):604–12.

114. Thomas HN, Thurston RC. A biopsychosocial approach to women's sexual function and dysfunction at midlife: a narrative review. Maturitas 2016;87:49–60.

115. Burrows LJ, Creasey A, Goldstein AT. The treatment of vulvar lichen sclerosus and female sexual dysfunction. J Sex Med 2011;8(1):219–22.

116. Cooper SM, Gao XH, Powell JJ, et al. Does treatment of vulvar lichen sclerosus influence its prognosis? Arch Dermatol 2004;140(6):702–6.

117. Moyal-Barracco M, Wendling J. Vulvar dermatosis. Best Pract Res Clin Obstet Gynaecol 2014;28(7):946–58.

118. Kellogg Spadt S, Kusturiss E. Vulvar dermatoses: a primer for the sexual medicine clinician. Sex Med Rev 2015;3(3):126–36.

Cognitive Changes with Reproductive Aging, Perimenopause, and Menopause

Kelly N. Morgan, PsyD[a],*, Carol A. Derby, PhD[b,c,1],
Carey E. Gleason, PhD, MS[d]

KEYWORDS

- Estrogens • Cognition • Menopause • Study of women across the nation
- Hormone therapy • Women's Health Initiative
- Kronos early estrogen prevention study
- Early versus late intervention trial with estradiol

KEY POINTS

- Estrogens influence neuroprotective and neurotrophic mechanisms underlying various cognitive processes in addition to regulating sexual and reproductive characteristics.
- Longitudinal studies of cognition in the menopausal transition suggest transient, reduced practice effects or encoding over repeated assessment in perimenopause as opposed to declines in performance.
- Although the WHI/WHIMS trials reflected cognitive harm after exogenous hormone treatment, confounders in the study design have since been identified.

Continued

Disclosure Statement: No disclosures.

Funding: KEEPS Continuation Grant number: NIH-NIA 1RF1AG057547; GRECC article number: 002 to 2018 (C. Gleason). The Study of Women's Health Across the Nation (SWAN) has grant support from the National Institutes of Health (NIH), DHHS, through the National Institute on Aging (NIA), the National Institute of Nursing Research (NINR) and the NIH Office of Research on Women's Health (ORWH) (Grants U01NR004061; U01AG012505, U01AG012535, U01AG012531, U01AG012539, U01AG012546, U01AG012553, U01AG012554, U01AG012495) (C. Derby).

The content of this article is solely the responsibility of the authors and does not necessarily represent the official views of the NIA, NINR, ORWH, or the NIH.

[a] Division of Neuropsychology, The Institute of Living/Hartford Hospital, 200 Retreat Avenue, Research Building 6th Floor, Hartford, CT 06106, USA; [b] Saul R. Korey Department of Neurology, Albert Einstein College of Medicine, 1410 Pelham Parkway South, Bronx, NY 10461, USA; [c] Department of Epidemiology and Population Health, Albert Einstein College of Medicine, 1300 Morris Park Ave, Bronx, NY 10461, USA; [d] Division of Geriatrics, Department of Medicine, University of Wisconsin School of Medicine and Public Health, Madison Geriatric Research Education and Clinical Center (GRECC) (11G), Wm S. Middleton Memorial Veterans Hospital, 2500 Overlook Terrace, Madison, WI 53706, USA

[1] Present address: 1225 Morris Park Avenue, Van Etten Room 3C5D, Bronx, NY 10461.

* Corresponding author.

E-mail address: Kelly.Morgan2@hhchealth.org

Obstet Gynecol Clin N Am 45 (2018) 751–763
https://doi.org/10.1016/j.ogc.2018.07.011
0889-8545/18/© 2018 Elsevier Inc. All rights reserved.

obgyn.theclinics.com

Continued

- Large clinical trials, such as KEEPS-Cog and ELITE, have shown neither deleterious nor beneficial cognitive outcomes with hormone therapy when women are metabolically healthy and treatment commences at or shortly after the menopausal transition.
- A number of questions regarding hormone therapy remain, particularly the optimal duration of hormone therapy administration and pharmacogenomic interactions related to treatment.

INTRODUCTION

Cognitive decline and dementia are a growing public health problem, with the worldwide prevalence of dementia expected to triple by 2050.[1] Evidence suggests that midlife may be a critical period in the natural course of dementia.[2] For women, understanding the effects of reproductive aging on cognition in midlife and beyond remains a topic of great interest, particularly given that estrogens are involved in a number of cellular pathways that underlie brain function.[3] Of particular interest is whether the perimenopause is a therapeutic window in which hormone therapy may prevent cognitive decline. To contextualize this emerging evidence, this article summarizes mechanisms that may link hormones to cognitive function, briefly discusses evidence from observational studies of the longitudinal changes in cognition occurring over the menopause transition, and concludes with discussions of the emergent evidence from clinical trials of estrogen therapy administered around menopause and remaining gaps in our understanding of the cognitive effects of menopausal hormone therapy.

MECHANISMS LINKING ESTROGEN WITH NEURAL AND COGNITIVE PROCESSES

Estrogen receptors (ERs) are plentiful in areas of the brain controlling memory and executive cognitive function.[4] ER isoforms are differentially expressed within the brain,[5,6] respond to estradiol in unique ways,[7,8] and initiate numerous intracellular and extracellular actions in both neural and peripheral substrates.[9] For instance, the ER isoform, ER-β, is expressed primarily in the cerebral cortex and hippocampus, whereas ER-α signaling occurs largely in magnocellular cholinergic neurons of the basal forebrain.[5,10] In aging, memory function is affected by shifts in the ratio between ER-α and ER-β and subsequent modifications in estrogen-regulated gene transcription.[11,12]

The means through which estrogens elicit brain effects are varied, and include alterations in neurotransmission as well as neurotrophic and neuroprotective actions. Estradiol has been shown to enhance cell growth and differentiation through the regulation of genomic processing and growth factor subtypes.[13,14] Particularly relevant to memory formation, estradiol promotes cell growth and survival through trophic mechanisms of basal forebrain and hippocampal neurons, regions involved in memory and executive cognitive function. Estrogens have been found to elevate dendritic spine density and synaptogenesis in the cornu ammonis 1 field of the hippocampus[15,16] and prefrontal cortex.[17,18] Estradiol is also associated with an increase in neurogenesis of the dentate gyrus.[19] Although both progesterone and estradiol have been shown to increase excitatory synapses and dendritic spine density,[20] only estrogens enhance cornu ammonis 1 long-term potentiation, a critical factor in episodic memory formation.[21]

Further, estradiol has been shown to attenuate neurodegenerative processes associated with Alzheimer's disease (AD), the most common type of dementia.[22] In particular, estradiol has been shown to attenuate tau hyperphosphorylation[23] and deposition of amyloid β,[24] and has also been shown to ameliorate the inflammatory sequelae of amyloid β.[25]

Estrogen and Brain Metabolism

Estradiol may also effect cognitive processes by maintaining glycolytic metabolism,[26] an important indicator of healthy aging. Estrogenic signaling promotes glycolytic over ketogenic metabolism by acting as a critical regulator of the glycolytic pathway. Moreover, estrogens maintain healthy mitochondrial bioenergetics[27] through the regulation of Ca^{2+} homeostasis, protection against free radical proliferation, trafficking of cholesterol, and clearance of amyloid β.[27] Cellular accumulation of amyloid β is often hastened by reduced mitochondrial bioenergetics followed by subsequent hypometabolism.[27] Importantly, reinstating estrogenic systems does not necessarily reverse glycolytic dysfunction. Multiple studies now point to the presence of a critical period for the introduction of exogenous estrogens and a healthy cell bias. Specifically, exogenous estrogen may support glycolytic metabolism in healthy neuronal cells or exacerbate pathologic burden in the setting of neurodegeneration.[3,28,29]

In addition to the effects of exogenous estrogen, menopause-associated shifts in endogenous estrogens may cause glycolytic dysregulation. For example, a drastic decrease in estrogen acutely disables the cell's recruitment and use of glucose for aerobic glycolysis, thus, shifting metabolism to a ketogenic phenotype. The ketogenic metabolic process is far less efficient and requires recruitment of ketone bodies from peripheral organs while concurrently initiating the fatty acid oxidation pathway. The fatty acid oxidation pathway breaks down local myelin sheath and is increasingly activated with the depletion of ketone body reserves.[29] The shift to ketogenesis triggers increased accumulation of mitochondrial amyloid β and oxidative stress,[30] as well as progressive hypometabolism and white matter changes in areas implicated in the pathogenesis of AD.[31,32] Further, the impact of estrogen on insulin-regulating mechanisms, such as glucose transporter isoforms,[33] insulin-like growth factor-1, and insulin-degrading enzyme, is likely critical in maintaining insulin and glucose homeostasis and promoting healthy metabolism in neural substrates, particularly in regions that are vulnerable to the pathology of AD, such as the hippocampus.[34]

Estrogenic Neuroprotection

Estradiol exhibits neuroprotection in models of oxidative stress, excitatory neurotoxicity, ischemia, and apoptosis.[35–37] As noted, estradiol is critical to Ca^{2+} homeostasis and initiates downstream signaling that promotes neuroprotection through long-term and acute reactions.

Estradiol has also been shown to reduce oxidative stress, where disruption of the electron transporter chain can trigger impaired synthesis of adenosine triphosphate and an increase in reactive oxygen species. The culmination of such dysregulation could, thus, cause cell damage as well as neurodegenerative processes.[38,39] Relevant to AD and related dementias, estradiol seems to decrease the amyloid burden by increasing antioxidants, such as glutaredoxin, peroxiredoxin-V, and manganese superoxide dismutase.[26,40]

In summary, estrogens are influential in various neural cellular systems, suggesting mechanisms through which the menopausal decline in estrogen could interfere with cognitive functioning. To examine this hypothesized effect, the following section reviews findings from longitudinal observational studies of cognition across the menopause transition.

LONGITUDINAL DATA REGARDING THE EFFECT OF MENOPAUSAL HORMONE CHANGES ON COGNITIVE FUNCTION

Although memory complaints are common during menopause,[41] longitudinal data regarding the impact of menopausal hormone changes on cognitive function are limited. Most longitudinal studies of cognitive aging have focused on individuals over the age of 65; few have examined both hormone trajectories and cognitive performance across the menopausal transition and thus there are few data regarding the relative contributions of chronologic and reproductive aging to cognitive function. Only 2 longitudinal cohort studies have reported longitudinal cognitive data for women transitioning through menopause, the Kinmen Women-Health Investigation (KIWI)[42] and the Study of Women's Health Across the Nation (SWAN).[43] As reviewed by Greendale and colleagues (2011),[44] both studies observed decrements in cognitive function specifically in perimenopause. The effects were subtle, evidenced by reduced "learning effects" over repeated cognitive assessments rather than by a decline in cognitive performance. The KIWI was limited to only 18 months of follow-up of initially premenopausal women.[42] In SWAN, premenopausal and postmenopausal women showed improvements over 4 annual assessments, whereas women who were late perimenopausal did not.[43]

Whether trajectories of menopausal hormones predict later cognitive decline remains an unanswered question. This question is currently under investigation in the ongoing SWAN study, which is the only large cohort to have characterized hormone changes and cognition over the entire menopause transition. The multisite study began in 1996, enrolling 3302 women at 7 clinical centers across the United States.[45] Women were initially 42 to 52 years of age and were premenopausal or early perimenopausal. To date, more than 20 years of follow-up have documented hormone trajectories across the menopausal transition and have identified heterogeneity in the rates and patterns of change across women.[46] Cognitive assessments began at the fourth annual SWAN visit and are ongoing. These data will provide new information regarding both the short- and long-term cognitive effects of the endogenous hormone changes occurring during the menopause.

In the following sections, the authors examine efforts to mitigate the cognitive and physiologic changes in menopause, reviewing data from intervention trials and attempts to address gaps in our understanding of the cognitive effects of menopausal hormone therapy.

HORMONE THERAPY TRIALS AND EMERGING SUPPORT FOR THE CRITICAL WINDOW HYPOTHESIS

Although early observational and basic science studies revealed promising cognitive and neuroprotective outcomes from hormone therapy, large clinical trials such as the Women's Health Initiative (WHI) and Women's Health Initiative Memory Study (WHIMS), exposed significant risks, including cognitive risks, associated with treatment.[47,48] Over time, findings revealed that age at initiation of hormone therapy may be a primary contributing factor to discrepancies between studies reflecting treatment benefits in cognition from those that suggested harm. That is, a critical window of treatment initiation is a key determinant in positive versus deleterious outcomes.

Women's Health Initiative Hormone and Cognition Therapy Trials

Given the positive effects seen in both basic science and observational epidemiologic studies, the WHI/WHIMS findings of an increased risk of cognitive impairment and dementia were stunning. In the massive WHI trial, 161,809 women aged 50 to 79 years participated in various clinical trials between 1993 and 1998. In the hormone treatment trial, more than 27,000 women were administered a combination of oral estrogen (conjugated equine estrogen [CEE]) and progesterone (medroxyprogesterone acetate [MPA]), CEE alone (if hysterectomized), or placebo over a period of 5.2 years, at which time the study was discontinued owing to adverse outcomes, particularly increased incidence of invasive breast cancer in CEE + MPA group, and an increased risk of stroke and blood clots in the CEE + MPA and CEE-alone trials.[47]

The WHIMS included 4532 postmenopausal women in the WHI hormone therapy trial who were 65 years of age at study baseline and free of clinical dementia. WHIMS women completed cognitive assessments at annual in-clinic assessments and via semiannual mailed questionnaires. Findings from this substudy revealed that CEE + MPA treatment offered minimal protection against cognitive decrements and actually increased the likelihood of dementia.[48] A similar but statistically insignificant finding was evident in the CEE-alone group. Critically, all participants were several years beyond the menopausal transition at WHIMS baseline.[49]

The cognitive effects noted in the seminal WHI and WHIMS studies were supported by imaging findings. In the WHIMS-MRI study, former hormone therapy users exhibited decreased hippocampal, frontal, and total brain volumes, although there was no evidence to suggest between-group differences in ischemic burden.[50] Importantly, at study baseline, lower global cognition[51] and increased white matter lesion burden[52] were found to be significant moderators of structural change, suggesting that individuals with poorer neurologic health at treatment outset were likely to experience deleterious outcomes.[53]

The WHI ancillary Study of Cognitive Aging assessed long-term cognitive effects after hormone therapy. The study included a sample of 2305 postmenopausal WHIMS participants who completed a comprehensive cognitive battery after the cessation of study treatment with hormone therapy or placebo. Those who received CEE alone showed neither beneficial nor deleterious cognitive effects[54] and those who received CEE + MPA demonstrated decreased verbal learning and memory over a 4- to 5-year span.[55] Neither group experienced significant effects on affective symptoms.[54,55]

Emerging Support for the Critical Window Hypothesis

In contrast, multiple previous studies revealed benefits of hormone therapy use when treatment commenced proximal to the menopause transition. For example, 727 women who initiated hormone therapy around menopause (n = 81) performed better than untreated women on verbal fluency and memory tasks.[56] Treated women exhibited improved verbal memory years later versus untreated women, who generally demonstrated declines in performance at follow-up.[56] These results were consistent with those of women receiving hormone therapy shortly after oophorectomy.[57] Moreover, Bagger and colleagues (2005)[58] indicated that women receiving hormone therapy in a randomized trial over 2 to 3 years around the menopause transition showed a decreased incidence of impaired cognition by 64% in follow-up testing occurring between 5 and 15 years later.

Similarly, 428 women who received hormone therapy before age 56 outperformed those who were treated after age 56 on verbal fluency, psychomotor speed, and global cognition measures (ie, the Mini-Mental Status Examination)[59] in a cross-sectional study. By contrast, the group of women in this study who received hormone therapy after 56 years of age exhibited worse global cognition than the group that never received treatment.[59] Consistent with these findings, a study of women with a mean of age of 48.8 years at treatment outset and duration of 5.2 years outperformed women who never received treatment on mental flexibility and global cognition tasks, as well as those women whose treatment duration was 14.30 years on average.[60] An observational study (the Cache County cohort) revealed a similar pattern of findings, where former voluntary hormone therapy users who initiated treatment shortly after menopause demonstrated lower risk of developing AD than current users who were older.[61]

Supporting this hypothesized timing-dependent pattern, a secondary analysis of the WHIMS data (the Women's Health Initiative Memory Study-Young [WHIMS-Y]) surveyed data from 1326 participants ages 50 to 55 years from the WHI CEE-alone trials, in which treatment commenced shortly after menopause. Results from Espeland and colleagues (2013)[62] indicated that women who received hormone therapy exhibited no declines or improvements in cognition in the years after treatment discontinuation. In contrast, women aged 65 to 79 years and receiving treatment showed persisting declines in working memory, executive functioning, and global cognition regardless of hysterectomy status or drug formulation.

In total, these studies supported the idea that hormone therapy treatment can promote both detrimental or beneficial effects on cognitive health,[9] depending on the timing of administration. Specifically, administration of exogenous hormones must occur in a narrow window of time around the menopausal transition to be useful in treating symptoms of estrogen depletion.[28,63–65] The importance of timing is secondary to the health of underlying cells and substrates (ie, the healthy cell bias and intact mitochondrial bioenergetics) and, as noted, women in the WHIMS trials were 65 years of age and older. Imaging data reinforce this timing hypothesis.[66,67]

In addition to the evidence increasing the importance of timing of estrogen administration, a number of other factors seem to contribute to disparate results in hormone therapy research, including the heterogeneous effects of varied routes of administration, hormone formulations, and treatment schedules (ie, continuous vs pulsed administration). These factors have been shown to influence treatment outcomes regardless of treatment timing.[68,69] The WHIMS trial, for instance, used a combination of synthetic progestin (MPA) and estrogen. Nilsen and Brinton (2003)[70] argued that MPA might oppose the neuroprotective effects of estradiol in vitro in hippocampal neurons, specifically highlighting findings of adverse effects of CEE + MPA on verbal memory performance. Women having been treated with MPA formulations exhibited declines in verbal memory performance even when therapy was started soon after the menopause (mean age, 52 years).[69]

Additional variables likely contributing to disparate outcomes in hormone therapy research include, but are not limited to, factors in reproductive history, such as age at menarche, advanced age of last pregnancy, increased duration of reproductive period, and historical oral contraceptive use, each being positively correlated with cognition in advancing age (Early versus Late Intervention Trial with Estradiol [ELITE] and WISH trials).[71]

Observation of the healthy user bias and critical window hypothesis have driven efforts to inform who might benefit from hormone therapy and for whom treatment would be contraindicated, thus spurring further concentration on bioenergetic functioning. For example, in 2015, Espeland and colleagues[72] reevaluated the WHIMS data and noted outcomes varied depending on the presence or absence of diabetes. Women who had type II diabetes randomized to the CEE group were at greater risk of developing cognitive impairment and probable dementia versus age-matched peers without diabetes and those with diabetes who were randomized to placebo. Women with diabetes in the CEE-alone group were at further increased risk for cognitive impairment and probable dementia. These findings were not associated with prior cognitive functioning, history of cardiovascular disease, obesity status, prediabetes, or hypertension, and results were sustained 10 years after termination. Espeland

and colleagues (2015)[72] argued that individuals metabolically reliant on ketogenesis would experience exacerbated metabolic dysregulation with the reintroduction of estrogens. That is, exogenous administration would likely suppress existing ketogenic processes before glycolytic metabolism could be restored and, therefore, escalate bioenergetic dysregulation. Women treated with CEE + MPA presumably did not experience compounded cognitive deficits, because the MPA opposed estrogen's actions on ketogenic metabolism.

ADDRESSING GAPS IN UNDERSTANDING AFTER THE WOMEN'S HEALTH INITIATIVE TRIALS

Several recent studies have aimed to explain discrepant findings around the cognitive risks and benefits of hormone therapy. The following such studies were designed not only to address conflicting outcomes, but to resolve remaining controversies in the literature. The Kronos Early Estrogen Prevention Study-Cognitive and Affective Study (KEEPS-Cog), an ancillary study of the large, randomized controlled KEEPS trial (primarily focused on cardiovascular outcomes of hormone therapy), was designed to investigate alterations in cognition and mood after hormone treatment in early menopause.[73] The KEEPS-Cog study revealed findings that were consistent with those of the WHIMS-Y trial.[74] A total of 662 early menopausal women treated with transdermal estradiol + micronized progesterone, low-dose CEE + micronized progesterone, or placebo exhibited neither significant increases nor decreases in performance on measures of attention or memory compared with placebo. However, participants who received oral CEE showed fewer depression and anxiety symptoms over the course of 4 years. All women were within 3 years of their final menstrual period and were neither hysterectomized nor oophorectomized. Further, KEEPS-Cog researchers used a transdermal estradiol formulation as well as a lower CEE dose than that of the WHIMS. Finally, estrogen was opposed with a micronized progestin in a pulsed fashion to better approximate cyclic exposure and naturally occurring progesterone, whereas the WHIMS trial used a continuous MPA administration.[74] These key differences in study design and enrollment likely contributed to the discrepant findings between the KEEPS-Cog and the WHIMS. The KEEPS participants will be reevaluated approximately a decade after randomization in the KEEPS-Continuation Study, which will investigate long-term cognitive and mood outcomes of menopausal HT, as well as neuroimaging correlates of brain health and AD-related biomarkers.

Last, the ELITE trial, another large randomized control trial, included both women who were within 6 years of menopause and those who were 10 or more years outside of menopause, with the intent to further examine the window of opportunity hypothesis.[75] In this trial, women with recent or remote (>10 years after FMP) menopausal transition status received oral estradiol for up to 5 years. Like KEEPS-Cog and the WHIMS-Y studies, ELITE findings revealed no cognitive harm or benefit for younger women. In contrast with the WHIMS, the ELITE data suggested no harm or benefit on cognition for the women randomized to hormone therapy 10 years after menopause.

SUMMARY: IMPLICATIONS FOR CLINICAL PRACTICE

Overall, cognitive complaints are common among middle-aged women and analyses suggest that women experience subtle cognitive changes during the menopausal transition that are not explained by confounding variables, such as vasomotor symptoms, mood, sleep disturbance, etc.[76] Current data suggest that these changes may be transient and whether they predict continued cognitive decline at older ages is currently being explored. Whether the patterns and rates of change in hormones over the menopause transition predict changes in cognitive function remains a critical question.

The conclusion that menopausal hormone therapy will not induce cognitive harm is supported by the accumulation of recent and large controlled trials, specifically when treatment is initiated at or near the menopausal transition and women are characterized as metabolically healthy. However, further characterization is needed to discern those who will benefit from those who will not, and those women for whom treatment is contraindicated entirely. Ideally, a woman seeking to manage symptoms occurring during the menopausal transition would have specific and personalized guidance, such that she need not carry undue concerns, or be unaware of real risks.

Supporting the need for personalizing medical consultation, a recent KEEPS publication specifically examined the pharmacogenomic interactions of hormone therapy (ie, transdermal 17β-estradiol [50 μg/d], oral CEE [0.45 mg/d], each combined with progesterone [200 mg/d], or placebo and 764 candidate single nucleotide polymorphisms). Outcomes included carotid artery intima-medial thickness and coronary artery calcification in 403 women 4 years after randomization in the KEEPS. Miller and colleagues (2016)[77] described a pharmacogenomic interaction in the carotid artery intima-medial thickness innate immunity pathway such that genetic variants seemed to interact with hormone therapy status to affect cardiovascular phenotypes. Other suggested genetic variations that may interact with hormone therapy include noninnate immunity pathway factors such as single nucleotide polymorphisms involved in the coagulation cascade, changes in beta-adrenergic receptors after the menopause, and triglyceride, fasting blood glucose, and diastolic blood pressure status. Certainly, the interaction of hormones and conventional cardiovascular risk factors such as hypercholesterolemia, hypertension, and type II diabetes would be important to consider, because these factors can exacerbate calcium accumulation in coronary arteries. In total, further research is necessary to elucidate how ER polymorphisms contribute to cardiovascular disease and the implications of pharmacogenomic interaction with hormone therapy.[77]

Aside from pharmacogenomic interactions, many more general questions remain unanswered regarding hormone therapy use at menopause. For example, what time period of use is optimal for cognitive health while minimizing risks of cancers and cardiovascular morbidities? Findings to date support the use of brief, low-dose hormone therapy treatment[78–81]; however, the precise definition of brief remains uncertain.

The KEEPS represented one of the first attempts to partially approximate the premenopausal status with menopausal hormone therapy. The trial used 4 years of a native estrogen, 17β-estradiol, comparing this form of hormone therapy with the commonly prescribed oral CEE (0.45 mg/d) and placebo. The KEEPS used a pulsed-dose of a natural hormonal progesterone analogue (micronized progestin) in contrast with a continuous, synthetic progesterone (MPA). To our knowledge, no studies have attempted to fully mimic the premenopausal hormone cycles with menopausal hormone therapy, effectively delaying the transition or attenuating the abruptness of change. Data from such a trial would clarify why women's risk for cardiovascular disease shifts upward with menopause[82] and why women evidence differential risk for AD dementia compared with men.[83,84]

Altogether, data are still needed to guide the health care of women entering the menopausal transition. Specifically, data are needed to assist women in making personalized and informed decisions regarding management of their menopausal symptoms and the prevention of future adverse health outcomes.

REFERENCES

1. World Health Organization. Available at: http://www.who.int/mediacentre/factsheets/fs362/en/. Accessed December 15, 2017.
2. Karlamangla AS, Lachman ME, Han W, et al. Evidence for cognitive aging in midlife women: Study of Women's Health Across the Nation. PLoS One 2017; 12:e0169008.
3. Brinton RD. Estrogen regulation of glucose metabolism and mitochondrial function: therapeutic implications for prevention of Alzheimer's disease. Adv Drug Deliv Rev 2008;60:1504–11.
4. McEwen BS. Invited review: estrogens effects on the brain: multiple sites and molecular mechanisms. J Appl Physiol (1985) 2001;91:2785–801.
5. Shughrue PJ, Lane MV, Merchenthaler I. Comparative distribution of estrogen receptor-alpha and -beta mRNA in the rat central nervous system. J Comp Neurol 1997;388:507–25.
6. Toran-Allerand CD, Guan X, MacLusky NJ, et al. ER-X: a novel, plasma membrane-associated, putative estrogen receptor that is regulated during development and after ischemic brain injury. J Neurosci 2002;22:8391–401.
7. Lauber AH, Mobbs CV, Muramatsu M, et al. Estrogen receptor messenger RNA expression in rat hypothalamus as a function of genetic sex and estrogen dose. Endocrinology 1991;129:3180–6.
8. Patisaul HB, Whitten PL, Young L. Regulation of estrogen receptor beta mRNA in the brain: opposite effects of 17beta-estradiol and the phytoestrogen, coumestrol. Brain Res Mol Brain Res 1999;67:165–71.
9. Hara Y, Waters EM, McEwen BS, et al. Estrogen effects on cognitive and synaptic health over the lifecourse. Physiol Rev 2015;95:785–807.
10. Shughrue PJ, Scrimo PJ, Merchenthaler I. Estrogen binding and estrogen receptor characterization (ERα and ERβ) in the cholinergic neurons of the rat basal forebrain. Neuroscience 2000;96:41–9.
11. Foster TC. Role of estrogen receptor alpha and beta expression and signaling on cognitive function during aging. Hippocampus 2012;22:656–69.
12. Han X, Aenlle KK, Bean LA, et al. Role of estrogen receptor α and β in preserving hippocampal function during aging. J Neurosci 2013;33:2671–83.
13. Lee SJ, McEwen BS. Neurotrophic and neuroprotective actions of estrogens and their therapeutic implications. Annu Rev Pharmacol Toxicol 2001;41:569–91.
14. Toran-Allerand CD. The estrogen/neurotrophin connection during neural development: is co-localization of estrogen receptors with the neurotrophins and their receptors biologically relevant? Dev Neurosci 1996;18:36–48.
15. Hao J, Janssen WGM, Tang Y, et al. Estrogen increases the number of spinophilin-immunoreactive spines in the hippocampus of young and aged female rhesus monkeys. J Comp Neurol 2003;465:540–50.
16. Sakamoto H, Mezaki Y, Shikimi H, et al. Dendritic growth and spine formation in response to estrogen in the developing Purkinje cell. Endocrinology 2003;144:4466–77.
17. Maki PM. Estrogen effects on the hippocampus and frontal lobes. Int J Fertil Womens Med 2005;50:67–71.
18. Tang Y, Janssen WGM, Hao J, et al. Estrogen replacement increases spinophilin-immunoreactive spine number in the prefrontal cortex of female rhesus monkeys. Cereb Cortex 2004;14:215–23.
19. Barha CK, Galea LAM. Influence of different estrogens on neuroplasticity and cognition in the hippocampus. Biochim Biophys Acta 2010;1800:1056–67.

20. Woolley CS, McEwen BS. Roles of estradiol and progesterone in regulation of hippocampal dendritic spine density during the estrous cycle in the rat. J Comp Neurol 1993;336:293–306.

21. Foy MR, Henderson VW, Berger TW, et al. Estrogen and neural plasticity. Curr Dir Psychol Sci 2000;9:148–52.

22. McKhann GM, Knopman DS, Chertkow H, et al. The diagnosis of dementia due to Alzheimer's disease: recommendations from the National Institute on Aging and the Alzheimer's Association workgroup. Alzheimers Dement 2011;7:263–9.

23. Alvarez-de-la-Rosa M, Silva I, Nilsen J, et al. Estradiol prevents neural tau hyperphosphorylation characteristic of Alzheimer's disease. Ann N Y Acad Sci 2005; 1052:210–24.

24. Yue X, Lu M, Lancaster T, et al. Brain estrogen deficiency accelerates Abeta plaque formation in an Alzheimer's disease animal model. Proc Natl Acad Sci U S A 2005;102:19198–203.

25. Thomas T, Bryant M, Clark L, et al. Estrogen and raloxifene activities on amyloid-beta-induced inflammatory reaction. Microvasc Res 2001;61:28–39.

26. Nilsen J, Irwin RW, Gallaher TK, et al. Estradiol in vivo regulation of brain mitochondrial proteome. J Neurosci 2007;27:14069–77.

27. Yao J, Brinton RD. Estrogen regulation of mitochondrial bioenergetics: implications for prevention of Alzheimer's disease. Adv Pharmacol 2012;64:327–71.

28. Maki PM. Critical window hypothesis of hormone therapy and cognition: a scientific update on clinical studies. Menopause 2013;20:695–709.

29. Morris AA. Cerebral ketone body metabolism. J Inherit Metab Dis 2005;28: 109–21.

30. Young KJ, Bennett JP. The mitochondrial secret(ase) of Alzheimer's disease. J Alzheimers Dis 2010;20(Suppl 2):S381–400.

31. Kuczynski B, Targan E, Madison C, et al. White matter integrity and cortical metabolic associations in aging and dementia. Alzheimers Dement 2010;6: 54–62.

32. Zhang Y, Schuff N, Jahng GH, et al. Diffusion tensor imaging of cingulum fibers in mild cognitive impairment and Alzheimer disease. Neurology 2007;68:13–9.

33. Rettberg JR, Yao J, Brinton RD. Estrogen: a master regulator of bioenergetic systems in the brain and body. Front Neuroendocrinol 2014;35:8–30.

34. Schiöth HB, Craft S, Brooks SJ, et al. Brain insulin signaling and Alzheimer's disease: current evidence and future directions. Mol Neurobiol 2012;46:4–10.

35. Dubal DB, Zhu H, Yu J, et al. Estrogen receptor alpha, not beta, is a critical link in estradiol-mediated protection against brain injury. Proc Natl Acad Sci U S A 2001; 98:1952–7.

36. Goodman Y, Bruce AJ, Cheng B, et al. Estrogens attenuate and corticosterone exacerbates excitotoxicity, oxidative injury, and amyloid beta-peptide toxicity in hippocampal neurons. J Neurochem 1996;66:1836–44.

37. Pike CJ. Estrogen modulates neuronal Bcl-xL expression and beta-amyloid-induced apoptosis: relevance to Alzheimer's disease. J Neurochem 1999;72: 1552–63.

38. Lin MT, Beal MF. Mitochondrial dysfunction and oxidative stress in neurodegenerative diseases. Nature 2006;443:787–95.

39. Yao J, Petanceska SS, Montine TJ, et al. Aging, gender and APOE isotype modulate metabolism of Alzheimer's Abeta peptides and F-isoprostanes in the absence of detectable amyloid deposits. J Neurochem 2004;90:1011–8.

40. Nilsen J, Brinton RD. Mitochondria as therapeutic targets of estrogen action in the central nervous system. Curr Drug Targets CNS Neurol Disord 2004;3:297–313.

41. Sullivan Mitchell E, Fugate Woods N. Midlife women's attributions about perceived memory changes: observations from the Seattle Midlife Women's Health Study. J Womens Health Gend Based Med 2001;10:351–62.

42. Fuh JL, Wang SJ, Lee SJ, et al. A longitudinal study of cognition change during early menopausal transition in a rural community. Maturitas 2006; 53:447–53.

43. Greendale GA, Huang MH, Wight RG, et al. Effects of the menopause transition and hormone use on cognitive performance in midlife women. Neurology 2009; 72:1850–7.

44. Greendale GA, Derby CA, Maki PM. Perimenopause and cognition. Obstet Gynecol Clin North Am 2011;38:519–35.

45. Sowers MF, Crawford SL, Sternfeld B, et al. SWAN: a multicenter, multiethnic, community-based cohort study of women and the menopausal transition. In: Lobo RA, Kelsey J, Marcus R, editors. Menopause biology and pathobiology. San Diego (CA): Academic Press; 2000. p. 175–88.

46. Tepper P, Randolph JF Jr, McConnell DS, et al. Trajectory clustering of estradiol and follicle-stimulating hormone during the menopausal transition among women in the Study of Women's Health across the Nation (SWAN). J Clin Endocrinol Metab 2012;97:2872–80.

47. Rossouw JE, Anderson GL, Prentice RL, et al. Risks and benefits of estrogen plus progestin in healthy postmenopausal women: principal results From the Women's Health Initiative randomized controlled trial. JAMA 2002;288:321–33.

48. Shumaker SA, Legault C, Rapp SR, et al. Estrogen plus progestin and the incidence of dementia and mild cognitive impairment in postmenopausal women: the Women's Health Initiative Memory Study: a randomized controlled trial. JAMA 2003;289:2651–62.

49. Coker LH, Espeland MA, Rapp SR, et al. Postmenopausal hormone therapy and cognitive outcomes: the Women's Health Initiative Memory Study (WHIMS). J Steroid Biochem Mol Biol 2010;118:304–10.

50. Coker LH, Hogan PE, Bryan NR, et al. Postmenopausal hormone therapy and subclinical cerebrovascular disease: the WHIMS-MRI Study. Neurology 2009; 72:125–34.

51. Espeland MA, Rapp SR, Shumaker SA, et al. Conjugated equine estrogens and global cognitive function in postmenopausal women: Women's Health Initiative Memory Study. JAMA 2004;291:2959–68.

52. Resnick SM, Espeland MA, Jaramillo SA, et al. Postmenopausal hormone therapy and regional brain volumes: the WHIMS-MRI Study. Neurology 2009;72:135–42.

53. McCarrey AC, Resnick SM. Postmenopausal hormone therapy and cognition. Horm Behav 2015;74:167–72.

54. Resnick SM, Espeland MA, An Y, et al. Effects of conjugated equine estrogens on cognition and affect in postmenopausal women with prior hysterectomy. J Clin Endocrinol Metab 2009;94:4152–61.

55. Resnick SM, Maki PM, Rapp SR, et al. Effects of combination estrogen plus progestin hormone treatment on cognition and affect. J Clin Endocrinol Metab 2006; 91:1802–10.

56. Jacobs DM, Tang MX, Stern Y, et al. Cognitive function in nondemented older women who took estrogen after menopause. Neurology 1998;50:368–73.

57. Verghese J, Kuslansky G, Katz MJ, et al. Cognitive performance in surgically menopausal women on estrogen. Neurology 2000;55:872–4.

58. Bagger YZ, Tanko LB, Alexandersen P, et al. Early postmenopausal hormone therapy may prevent cognitive impairment later in life. Menopause 2005;12:12–7.

59. MacLennan AH, Henderson VW, Paine BJ, et al. Hormone therapy, timing of initiation, and cognition in women aged older than 60 years: the REMEMBER pilot study. Menopause 2006;13:28–36.

60. Matthews K, Cauley J, Yaffe K, et al. Estrogen replacement therapy and cognitive decline in older community women. J Am Geriatr Soc 1999;47:518–23.

61. Zandi PP, Carlson MC, Plassman BL, et al. Hormone replacement therapy and incidence of Alzheimer disease in older women - the Cache County Study. JAMA 2002;288:2123–9.

62. Espeland MA, Shumaker SA, Leng I, et al. Long term effects on cognitive function of postmenopausal hormone therapy prescribed to women aged 50-55 years. JAMA Intern Med 2013;235:649–57.

63. Gibbs RB, Gabor R. Estrogen and cognition: applying preclinical findings to clinical perspectives. J Neurosci Res 2003;74:637–43.

64. Sherwin BB. Estrogen therapy: is time of initiation critical for neuroprotection? Nat Rev Endocrinol 2009;5:620–7.

65. Zhang Q, Han D, Wang R, et al. C terminus of Hsc70-interacting protein (CHIP)-mediated degradation of hippocampal estrogen receptor-alpha and the critical period hypothesis of estrogen neuroprotection. Proc Natl Acad Sci U S A 2011; 108:E617–24.

66. Kantarci K, Lowe VJ, Lesnick TG, et al. Early postmenopausal transdermal 17β-estradiol therapy and amyloid-β deposition. J Alzheimers Dis 2016;53:547–56.

67. Kantarci K, Zuk SM, Gunter JL, et al. Effects of hormone therapy on brain structure. Neurology 2016;87:887–96.

68. Kang JH, Grodstein F. Postmenopausal hormone therapy, timing of initiation, APOE and cognitive decline. Neurobiol Aging 2012;33:1129–37.

69. Maki PM, Gast MJ, Vieweg AJ, et al. Hormone therapy in menopausal women with cognitive complaints: a randomized, double-blind trial. Neurology 2007;69: 1322–30.

70. Nilsen J, Brinton RD. Divergent impact of progesterone and medroxyprogesterone acetate (Provera) on nuclear mitogen-activated protein kinase signaling. Proc Natl Acad Sci U S A 2003;100:10506–11.

71. Karim R, Dang H, Henderson VW, et al. Effect of reproductive history and exogenous hormone use on cognitive function in mid- and late life. J Am Geriatr Soc 2016;64:2448–56.

72. Espeland MA, Brinton RD, Hugenschmidt C, et al. Impact of type 2 diabetes and postmenopausal hormone therapy on incidence of cognitive impairment in older women. Diabetes Care 2015;38:2316–24.

73. Wharton W, Gleason CE, Miller VM, et al. Rationale and design of the Kronos Early Estrogen Prevention Study (KEEPS) and the KEEPS cognitive and affective sub study (KEEPS Cog). Brain Res 2013;1514:12–7.

74. Gleason CE, Dowling NM, Wharton W, et al. Effects of hormone therapy on cognition and mood in recently postmenopausal women: findings from the randomized, controlled KEEPS-cognitive and affective study. PLoS Med 2015;12:1–26.

75. Henderson VW. Gonadal hormones and cognitive aging: a midlife perspective. Womens Health (Lond) 2011;7:81–93.

76. Greendale GA, Wight RG, Huang MH, et al. Menopause-associated symptoms and cognitive performance: results from the Study of Women's Health Across the Nation. Am J Epidemiol 2010;171:1214–24.

77. Miller VM, Jenkins GD, Biernacka JM, et al. Pharmacogenomics of estrogens on changes in carotid artery intima-medial thickness and coronary arterial calcification: Kronos Early Estrogen Prevention Study. Physiol Genomics 2016;48:33–41.

78. Gordon JL, Rubinow DR, Elsenlohr-Moul TA, et al. Efficacy of transdermal estradiol and micronized progesterone in the prevention of depressive symptoms in the menopause transition: a randomized clinical trial. JAMA Psychiatry 2018. https://doi.org/10.1001/jamapsychiatry.2017.3998.

79. Hale GE, Shufelt CL. Hormone therapy in menopause: an update on cardiovascular disease considerations. Trends Cardiovasc Med 2015;25:540–9.

80. Johnson SR, Ettinger B, Macer JL, et al. Uterine and vaginal effects of unopposed ultralow-dose transdermal estradiol. Obstet Gynecol 2005;105:779–87.

81. Samsioe G, Hruska J. Optimal tolerability of ultra-low-dose continuous combined 17beta-estradiol and norethisterone acetate: laboratory and safety results. Climacteric 2010;13:34–44.

82. Morselli E, Santos RS, Criollo A, et al. The effects of oestrogens and their receptors on cardiometabolic health. Nat Rev Endocrinol 2017;13:352–64.

83. Altmann A, Tian L, Henderson VW, et al. Sex modifies the APOE-related risk of developing Alzheimer disease. Ann Neurol 2014;75:563–73.

84. Ungar L, Altmann A, Greicius MD. Apolipoprotein E, gender, and Alzheimer's disease: an overlooked, but potent and promising interaction. Brain Imaging Behav 2014;8:262–73.

UNITED STATES POSTAL SERVICE ®

Statement of Ownership, Management, and Circulation
(All Periodicals Publications Except Requester Publications)

1. Publication Title	2. Publication Number	3. Filing Date
OBSTETRICS AND GYNECOLOGY CLINICS OF NORTH AMERICA	000 – 276	9/18/2018

4. Issue Frequency	5. Number of Issues Published Annually	6. Annual Subscription Price
MAR, JUN, SEP, DEC	4	$313.00

7. Complete Mailing Address of Known Office of Publication *(Not printer) (Street, city, county, state, and ZIP+4®)*

ELSEVIER INC.
230 Park Avenue, Suite 800
New York, NY 10169

Contact Person
STEPHEN R. BUSHING

Telephone *(Include area code)*
215-239-3688

8. Complete Mailing Address of Headquarters or General Business Office of Publisher *(Not printer)*

ELSEVIER INC.
230 Park Avenue, Suite 800
New York, NY 10169

9. Full Names and Complete Mailing Addresses of Publisher, Editor, and Managing Editor *(Do not leave blank)*

Publisher *(Name and complete mailing address)*

TAYLOR E BALL, ELSEVIER INC.
1600 JOHN F KENNEDY BLVD. SUITE 1800
PHILADELPHIA, PA 19103-2899

Editor *(Name and complete mailing address)*

KERRY HOLLAND, ELSEVIER INC.
1600 JOHN F KENNEDY BLVD. SUITE 1800
PHILADELPHIA, PA 19103-2899

Managing Editor *(Name and complete mailing address)*

PATRICK MANLEY, ELSEVIER INC.
1600 JOHN F KENNEDY BLVD. SUITE 1800
PHILADELPHIA, PA 19103-2899

10. Owner *(Do not leave blank. If the publication is owned by a corporation, give the name and address of the corporation immediately followed by the names and addresses of all stockholders owning or holding 1 percent or more of the total amount of stock. If not owned by a corporation, give the names and addresses of the individual owners. If owned by a partnership or other unincorporated firm, give its name and address as well as those of each individual owner. If the publication is published by a nonprofit organization, give its name and address.)*

Full Name	Complete Mailing Address
WHOLLY OWNED SUBSIDIARY OF REED/ELSEVIER, US HOLDINGS	1600 JOHN F KENNEDY BLVD. SUITE 1800 PHILADELPHIA, PA 19103-2899

11. Known Bondholders, Mortgagees, and Other Security Holders Owning or Holding 1 Percent or More of Total Amount of Bonds, Mortgages, or Other Securities. If none, check box ▶ ☐ None

Full Name	Complete Mailing Address
N/A	

12. Tax Status *(For completion by nonprofit organizations authorized to mail at nonprofit rates) (Check one)*
The purpose, function, and nonprofit status of this organization and the exempt status for federal income tax purposes:

☒ Has Not Changed During Preceding 12 Months
☐ Has Changed During Preceding 12 Months *(Publisher must submit explanation of change with this statement)*

PS Form **3526**, July 2014 *(Page 1 of 4 (see instructions page 4))* PSN: 7530-01-000-9931   PRIVACY NOTICE: See our privacy policy on www.usps.com.

---

13. Publication Title		14. Issue Date for Circulation Data Below
OBSTETRICS AND GYNECOLOGY CLINICS OF NORTH AMERICA		JUNE 2018

15. Extent and Nature of Circulation			Average No. Copies Each Issue During Preceding 12 Months	No. Copies of Single Issue Published Nearest to Filing Date
a. Total Number of Copies *(Net press run)*			219	295
b. Paid Circulation *(By Mail and Outside the Mail)*	(1)	Mailed Outside-County Paid Subscriptions Stated on PS Form 3541 *(Include paid distribution above nominal rate, advertiser's proof copies, and exchange copies)*	59	71
	(2)	Mailed In-County Paid Subscriptions Stated on PS Form 3541 *(Include paid distribution above nominal rate, advertiser's proof copies, and exchange copies)*	0	0
	(3)	Paid Distribution Outside the Mails Including Sales Through Dealers and Carriers, Street Vendors, Counter Sales, and Other Paid Distribution Outside USPS®	98	122
	(4)	Paid Distribution by Other Classes of Mail Through the USPS *(e.g., First-Class Mail®)*	0	0
c. Total Paid Distribution *(Sum of 15b (1), (2), (3), and (4))*		▶	157	193
d. Free or Nominal Rate Distribution *(By Mail and Outside the Mail)*	(1)	Free or Nominal Rate Outside-County Copies included on PS Form 3541	51	86
	(2)	Free or Nominal Rate In-County Copies Included on PS Form 3541	0	0
	(3)	Free or Nominal Rate Copies Mailed at Other Classes Through the USPS *(e.g., First-Class Mail)*	0	0
	(4)	Free or Nominal Rate Distribution Outside the Mail *(Carriers or other means)*	0	0
e. Total Free or Nominal Rate Distribution *(Sum of 15d (1), (2), (3) and (4))*		▶	51	86
f. Total Distribution *(Sum of 15c and 15e)*		▶	208	279
g. Copies not Distributed *(See Instructions to Publishers #4 (page #3))*		▶	11	16
h. Total *(Sum of 15f and g)*		▶	219	295
i. Percent Paid *(15c divided by 15f times 100)*		▶	75.48%	69.18%

If you are claiming electronic copies, go to line 16 on page 3. If you are not claiming electronic copies, skip to line 17 on page 3.

16. Electronic Copy Circulation		Average No. Copies Each Issue During Preceding 12 Months	No. Copies of Single Issue Published Nearest to Filing Date
a. Paid Electronic Copies	▶	0	0
b. Total Paid Print Copies (Line 15c) + Paid Electronic Copies (Line 16a)	▶	157	193
c. Total Print Distribution (Line 15f) + Paid Electronic Copies (Line 16a)	▶	208	279
d. Percent Paid (Both Print & Electronic Copies) (16b divided by 16c × 100)	▶	75.48%	69.18%

☒ I certify that 50% of all my distributed copies (electronic and print) are paid above a nominal price.

17. Publication of Statement of Ownership

☒ If the publication is a general publication, publication of this statement is required. Will be printed
in the **DECEMBER 2018** issue of this publication.   ☐ Publication not required.

18. Signature and Title of Editor, Publisher, Business Manager, or Owner		Date
STEPHEN R. BUSHING - INVENTORY DISTRIBUTION CONTROL MANAGER	*[signature]* Stephen R. Bushing	9/18/2018

I certify that all information furnished on this form is true and complete. I understand that anyone who furnishes false or misleading information on this form or who omits material or information requested on the form may be subject to criminal sanctions (including fines and imprisonment) and/or civil sanctions (including civil penalties).

PS Form **3526**, July 2014 *(Page 3 of 4)*   PRIVACY NOTICE: See our privacy policy on www.usps.com

Moving?

Make sure your subscription moves with you!

To notify us of your new address, find your **Clinics Account Number** (located on your mailing label above your name), and contact customer service at:

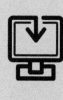

Email: journalscustomerservice-usa@elsevier.com

800-654-2452 (subscribers in the U.S. & Canada)
314-447-8871 (subscribers outside of the U.S. & Canada)

Fax number: 314-447-8029

Elsevier Health Sciences Division
Subscription Customer Service
3251 Riverport Lane
Maryland Heights, MO 63043

*To ensure uninterrupted delivery of your subscription, please notify us at least 4 weeks in advance of move.

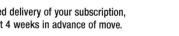

Printed and bound by CPI Group (UK) Ltd, Croydon, CR0 4YY

03/10/2024

01040391-0020